Philosophical Essays on Dreaming

Philosophical Essays on Dreaming

EDITED BY

CHARLES E. M. DUNLOP

Essay Index

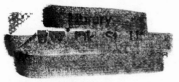

Cornell University Press   ITHACA AND LONDON

First published 1977 by Cornell University Press.
Published in the United Kingdom by Cornell University Press Ltd.,
2–4 Brook Street, London W1Y 1AA.

International Standard Book Number (cloth) 0-8014-1015-0
International Standard Book Number (paper) 0-8014-9862-7
Library of Congress Catalog Card Number 77-4582
Printed in the United States of America by Vail-Ballou Press, Inc.
*Librarians: Library of Congress cataloging information
appears on the last page of the book.*

To Jaakko Hintikka

At this moment it does indeed seem to me that it is with eyes awake that I am looking at this paper; that this head which I move is not asleep, that it is deliberately and of set purpose that I extend my hand and perceive it; what happens in sleep does not appear so clear nor so distinct as does all this. But in thinking over this I remind myself that on many occasions I have in sleep been deceived by similar illusions, and in dwelling carefully on this reflection I see so manifestly that there are no certain indications by which we may clearly distinguish wakefulness from sleep that I am lost in astonishment. And my astonishment is such that it is almost capable of persuading me that I do dream.

Descartes, *Meditation I*

An hour earlier, when the two officials of the People's Commissariat of the Interior were hammering on Rubashov's door, in order to arrest him, Rubashov was just dreaming that he was being arrested.

Koestler, *Darkness at Noon*

Preface

Although the topic of dreaming has intrigued philosophers for centuries, it has only recently begun to receive undivided philosophical attention. Such a resurgence of interest is welcome, not only because of the intrinsic appeal of the subject, but also because of important connections between dreaming and issues in epistemology, philosophy of language, and philosophy of science. One aim of the present anthology is to make those connections explicit. Of further significance is the fact that dreaming has undergone extensive experimental investigation, yielding what Frederick Snyder has called "the most thorough test yet given to any psycho-physical relationship." [1] Some of the results are discussed by philosophers in this book.

To date, contemporary analytic philosophy has produced only one monograph on dreaming, and hardly more than fifty articles. This situation has its bright side, however. Many of the articles which have appeared are of some philosophical importance, and it has seemed worthwhile to collect them in a single volume. At present, the set of essays in this collection and Norman Malcolm's monograph *Dreaming* constitute the most significant contemporary philosophical writings on dreaming. [2]

1. "The Physiology of Dreaming," in Milton Kramer, ed., *Dream Psychology and the New Biology of Dreaming* (Springfield, Ill., and Fort Lauderdale, 1969), p. 18.
2. With one exception: Hilary Putnam's "Dreaming and 'Depth Grammar' "; earlier copyright agreements made its inclusion in this volume impossible. Put-

I am grateful to a number of people for their helpful criticism and generous support of this project. Useful suggestions at the early stages came from Romane Clark, L. Nathan Oaklander, and David H. Sanford. I am much indebted to Michael Jubien, Ralf Meerbote, William E. Morris, and two anonymous referees from Cornell University Press for their prompt, detailed, and constructive comments on later drafts of my Introduction. My thanks are due also to the University of Michigan Research and Special Projects Fund for financial support, and to Ronda Bloomfield and Diana O'Hanisain for their expert and cheerful typing of a manuscript filled with notational idiosyncrasies.

Acknowledgment is made to Routledge & Kegan Paul Ltd. and to Humanities Press Inc. for permission to quote from Norman Malcolm's *Dreaming* in the Introduction to this volume.

Finally, I owe a great deal to my wife, Lynn, for helping me keep my professional endeavors in a proper perspective, and to my good friends Bill and Mary Jane Lockwood, for offering sustenance, humor, and insight during some very difficult times.

CHARLES E. M. DUNLOP

Flint, Michigan

nam's paper appears in Ronald Butler, ed., *Analytical Philosophy,* First Series (Oxford, 1966), and has recently been reprinted in Hilary Putnam, *Mind, Language and Reality* (Cambridge, 1975).

Contents

Philosophical Essays on Dreaming

CHARLES E. M. DUNLOP

Introduction

I. Dreams, Deception, and Skepticism

A. Dreaming and Perceiving

Since philosophical discussions of dreaming have long been associated with problems of skepticism, it comes as little surprise that the recent revival of interest in dreaming should have begun by following a similar course. In fact, the essays by O. K. Bouwsma and Margaret Macdonald share both a common purpose and a common methodology. They are aimed at overthrowing Cartesian dream skepticism, and they agree that the key to this epistemological problem lies in the examination of ordinary, everyday discourse. This way of doing philosophy is criticized by R. M. Yost and Donald Kalish, who view their own critique of Macdonald as having "some bearing on the work of authors who philosophize as she does." And perhaps it does, but the remaining essays in this volume demonstrate that the relevant methodological issues are still far from settled.

With occasional exceptions, the first three papers proceed with a limited amount of attention to the question of what dreaming is. While this may turn out to be an important shortcoming, it is at least readily understandable from one point of view. Despite the fact that Descartes was committed to a particular analysis of dreaming (involving the presentation of "ideas" during sleep), his skeptical argument makes no reference to, and does not logically presuppose, that account. Hence, it may appear that discussions of dream skepticism can develop independently of some particular theory about the nature of dreaming. The point can be illustrated as follows:

(1) (a) Dreaming, like waking perception, involves the presentation of "ideas."

(b) The "ideas" which occur during sleep are qualitatively similar to those occurring in waking perception.

(c) Therefore, I cannot tell whether my presently occurring "ideas" constitute a dream, or a waking perception.

(2) (a) On past occasions I have dreamt that I was in front of the fireplace, when in fact I was in bed asleep.

(b) On some such occasions I was deceived.

(c) Therefore, although I am at this moment convinced that I am awake and perceiving the fireplace, I must admit that I *may* instead be asleep and dreaming.

Descartes' argument is certainly compatible with (1), but his actual presentation is closer to (2). And since (2), unlike (1), could be accepted by a philosopher who does not recognize "ideas," "sense-data," and the like, it might seem that the problem of dream skepticism need not be bothered by questions concerning the nature of dreaming. But this conclusion is premature. Argument (2), while not committed to "ideas," does presuppose that dreaming involves, or accompanies, some kinds of mental activity during sleep. And Norman Malcolm's challenge to this thesis provides a new attack on skepticism.[1]

Before coming to that, however, it will be useful to measure some of the earlier attempts to meet Descartes' challenge. According to O. K. Bouwsma, Descartes' dream argument begins with the "fact" that he is sitting in front of the fire, etc., passes on to a recollection that on previous occasions he has dreamt the very same thing, and concludes that the alleged fact may not be a fact at all, but only a dream. Bouwsma writes:

Clearly Descartes has abandoned the original distinction, the fact that I am here, etc., and the fact that I dreamed that I am here, etc., upon the basis of which he elaborated his argument. In order to find out whether he is awake or not, he must depend upon facts of the sort he began with. He continues however to use language which is significant

---

1. In fairness, it should be added that Margaret Macdonald anticipates Malcolm's work in certain respects, but she fails to make any systematic use of the point under discussion.

only in terms of the distinctions which he has abandoned. The questions "Am I awake?" "Am I asleep?" are questions about bodies. Since he has ruled out bodies as within the range of the application of these terms, his language is now meaningless.

It is perhaps not clear what theory of meaning Bouwsma's remarks presuppose, but his criticism that Descartes forsakes the initial distinction between waking and dreaming deserves comment. Descartes' premise, which presupposes that we can make the distinction, and his conclusion, which denies that we can, are certainly at odds with one another. It is possible, however, that there is no defect in Descartes' reasoning; instead, he may be using a *reductio ad absurdum* argument against the view that qualitative features of "ideas" are sufficient by themselves to warrant the distinction between waking and dreaming.[2] If so, skepticism in the First Meditation is preserved.

Apart from the verdict on this point, however, Bouwsma's paper remains of further interest. His discussion of the personal pronoun's significance in sentences of the form "X is (am, are, etc.) asleep," and his connection of this point with a discussion of meaningfulness, strikingly anticipate some of Norman Malcolm's remarks on the same topic. And his insightful comparison of dreams, nonveridical perceptions, and mirror images bears close reading in conjunction with Macdonald's essay.

An important question connected with Descartes' dream argument is whether there is enough similarity between dreams and waking life to support the claim that dreams may deceive us in the manner of waking illusions. Macdonald's primary aim in "Sleeping and Waking" is to argue that there is not. Through a consideration of "the logic of discourse about waking realities and illusions," she urges "that none of the criteria appropriate to waking life apply to dreams." Illusions and hallucinations, she maintains, normally occur in a context of "real" things, whereas the objects of dreams do not. "[T]he dreamer cannot wake to exclaim, 'Thank goodness, there isn't a real corpse on the floor.' For the dream corpse never was on the floor to which he wakes and the murder may have been

2. For an elaboration of this view, see Harry G. Frankfurt, *Demons, Dreamers, and Madmen* (Indianapolis and New York, 1970), Chapter 5.

dreamed to occur ten years ago and not five minutes before he wakes on Friday, 18th April, 1952."

Now, it is not difficult to see the distinction which Macdonald apparently has in mind. For while I often dream that an object exists without dreaming that it exists at any particular time or place, I do not visually misperceive or hallucinate an object without assigning it some spatio-temporal location. But, as the passage just quoted suggests, Macdonald maintains further that there is no continuity whatever between dreams and waking life: "When a dreamer wakes his dream vanishes and its contents cannot, therefore, be checked for they no longer exist in any context for comparison. They may be remembered but not corrected."

These remarks are clearly aimed at undermining skepticism. But an unwelcome result seems to be that Macdonald is committed to a much stronger thesis than she probably intended to hold; namely, that we *never* dream that anything happens in the physical world. The reason is that if I *did* sometimes have such dreams, then I should be able to discover, at least occasionally, that my dream description was or was not an accurate description of the world. If my dreams issued in any beliefs about the world, then certain discoveries would show them to be true or false. But, already committed to a radical disparity between the objects of perception and the objects of dreams, Macdonald writes: "[D]reams are neither corrigible nor incorrigible; the notion of corrigibility cannot significantly be applied to dreams." The price required for this conclusion, however, seems unduly high.

Macdonald's view on the incorrigibility of dreams leads her to maintain that "while dreaming, a dreamer cannot significantly be said to know or truly or mistakenly believe any proposition about the contents of his dreams." (This conclusion may also have been reached by way of a more general thesis that dreams do not involve any occurrent mental activity; Macdonald's position here is not entirely clear.) [3] And she adds:

3. Yost and Kalish provide some further evidence that Macdonald subscribed to the generalized version. In that form, as they point out, it is an unsupported premise. But her more limited claim concerning knowledge and belief follows from the view that dreams are neither corrigible nor incorrigible.

"From the fact that I saw the Hebrides in a dream it does not follow that I *saw* any more than that which I saw was the Hebrides. Nor does it follow that I seemed to see or thought I saw." These, along with similar remarks scattered throughout her paper, contain the seeds of a crucial point which, generalized, comes to this:

(1) In my dream I ϕ-ed [believed, thought, saw, seemed to see, etc.] that P

does *not* entail

(2) (While asleep) I ϕ-ed that P.

It is always possible for (1) to be true and (2) false, *even* when "ϕ" is replaced by "dream." This point can be made clearest by noticing that (1) is equivalent [4] to

(1') I dreamt that I ϕ-ed that P.

If "dream" is now substituted for "ϕ", sentence (1') will read as follows:

(1'') I dreamt that I dreamt that P.

But (1'') is compatible with the negation of an instance of (2) again substituting "dream" for "ϕ"):

(2' neg) (While asleep) I did not dream that P.

Therefore, since (1'') is a substitution-instance of (1), and since (1'') is consistent with (2' neg) (the negation of a substitution-instance of (2)), it follows that (1) does not entail (2). It might be noted, incidentally, that in the present example "dreams" behaves like "believes," since

(3) A believes that he believes that P

does not entail

(4) A believes that P. [5]

The failure of the entailment from (1) to (2) (a point made also by Malcolm) can scarcely be overstressed. For while it does not rule out ϕ-ing during sleep, it does rule out a quick argument in favor of ϕ-ing during sleep. R. M. Yost and Donald Kalish, for example, think that (2) can be *derived* from (1). In fact, however, expressions such as "in my dream" and "I dreamt" normally operate in part as disclaimers, indicating that what follows is not to be construed as the report of actual oc-

4. Cf. Malcolm's "Dreaming and Skepticism," Sec. II (final paragraph).
5. See Jaakko Hintikka, *Knowledge and Belief* (Ithaca, 1962), pp. 123–125.

currences.[6] Thus, in the sentence "I dreamt that I believed that my great-grandmother was still alive," the expression "I dreamt" signals that "I believed that my great-grandmother was still alive" is not to be taken literally.

Yost and Kalish find Macdonald holding, not just that (1) fails to entail (2), but that (e.g.) "I dreamt that I believed that my great-grandmother was still alive" entails "While dreaming, it is logically impossible that I believed that my great-grandmother was still alive." For they attribute to Macdonald the following view, which they label "A-1a":

(A-1a) Any sentence of the form
    X dreamt that he . . . O
where "O" refers to part of the contents of the dream and the blank is to be filled by a transitive verb, implies the corresponding sentence of the form
    while dreaming, it is logically impossible that X . . . O.

This is a stronger thesis yet, but Yost and Kalish do provide textual evidence for their interpretation. In any case, equipped with (A-1a), Yost and Kalish criticize Macdonald's entire argument as "inelegant," claiming that it introduces superfluous assumptions when it could be made to rest on (A-1a) alone. They further argue that (A-1a) is false, and that Macdonald's essay fails to refute skepticism. The charge of inelegance especially merits a brief discussion.

Yost and Kalish attempt to sustain their charge by considering three Cartesian premises which Macdonald opposes, and arguing that her refutation of each could be made to depend exclusively on (A-1a). But the arguments that they produce in each case seem defective. Consider, for example, one claim which Macdonald does want to refute—the claim that (as Yost and Kalish put it)

while dreaming, Descartes mistakenly believed the statement 'This is a hand' to be true. [Editor's emphasis]

They go on to write:

We have here an instance of (A-1a); the blank has been filled by 'believes to be true' and 'O' has been replaced by the sentence 'This is a real hand'. Given this instance of (A-1a) and the fact that *Descartes did*

---

6. For a fuller treatment of this point see the last few paragraphs of Macdonald's essay. Cf. Norman Malcolm, *Dreaming* (London, 1962), pp. 88, 94–98.

dream that he believed the sentence 'This is a real hand' to be true, it follows that, while dreaming, it is logically impossible that Descartes believed the sentence 'This is a real hand' to be true. . . . Thus, we maintain not only that (A-1a) is a necessary premise in Macdonald's argument . . . but also that it is sufficient. [Editor's emphasis]

Of significance here is a conflation of two expressions:
  (a) believing, while dreaming, that I see a hand
and
  (b) dreaming that I believe that I see a hand.[7]
Expression (b) says that the belief was dreamt, while (a) maintains that the belief actually occurred. Yost and Kalish attribute (b) to Descartes. But Descartes was concerned with a state of affairs like (a); he did not even consider situation (b). Nor does Macdonald attribute situation (b) to Descartes. Thus, (A-1a), even if it is an accurate reflection of *one* of Macdonald's points, is simply inapplicable to the Cartesian premise under discussion here. The charge of inelegance, therefore, must be reconsidered.

Macdonald's treatment of skepticism is based upon the numerous differences she finds between dreams and waking illusions. "For if what is said of one state is nonsensical when applied to the other, then this provides at least one certain mark by which to distinguish between them." In their final paragraphs, Yost and Kalish dispute the adequacy of this solution (Cf. Section X of Malcolm's essay). But we can begin to see that little more progress can be made in the absence of a clearer account of what dreaming is and is not. After all, the skeptical problem is generated by an alleged possibility of continual confusion between dreams and waking life. Since the possibility in question is partly a conceptual one, it can hardly be evaluated properly before dreaming is located on the conceptual map. Macdonald has provided a beginning, but does not offer a comprehensive analysis. And the alternative approach proposed by Yost and Kalish seems both oversimplified and incorrect: "To say that one dreams is to say that one sees, hears, touches, etc. while asleep." If this account were literally accu-

---

7. The conflation, however, is not the result of an oversight. For Yost and Kalish write: "[w]e should maintain, with Descartes, that if anyone dreams that he believes, doubts, expects, desires, etc., then he really does."

rate, then to say that one dreams of petting one's dog would be to say that one pets his dog during sleep. At the very least, then, the formulation is careless. Perhaps a better version would be: To say that one dreams is to say that one has visual, auditory, tactile, etc. experiences during sleep. It may still be doubted, however, whether just *any* experience during sleep should count as a dream; in any case, this proposal requires an extended defense. Norman Malcolm's work helps to fill a vacuum left by the discussion so far, providing a new approach to dreaming. And Malcolm's arguments, if they are accepted, will complete the destruction of the Cartesian view of dreaming, and with it Cartesian dream skepticism.

B. *Norman Malcolm's View*

Malcolm's study of dreaming first appeared in an article, "Dreaming and Skepticism" (reproduced in this anthology), and was later elaborated in his monograph, *Dreaming.*[8] As the list on page 21 demonstrates, there is considerable overlap between the two works, but the reader cannot expect to obtain a complete picture of Malcolm's position without careful scrutiny of both.

Both D and DS represent a direct attack on what might be called "received opinion," or the "traditional approach" to dreaming, for Malcolm claims that dreams are *not* identical with images, thoughts, or emotions occurring in sleep. Despite Malcolm's contention that his view stems from a close adherence to our common conceptual framework, the concept of dreaming which emerges has struck many readers as paradoxical, if not downright false. Nonetheless, the care with which his argument proceeds demands that it be given serious attention. In fact, the significance of Malcolm's work can be measured in part by the critical literature that it has engendered; virtually every philosophical article on dreaming published since 1959 addresses some aspect of Malcolm's writings.

The following account of Malcolm's position draws from both D and DS, in order to facilitate understanding of some of

8. Hereafter, the abbreviations "DS" and "D" will serve for "Dreaming and Skepticism" and *Dreaming* (respectively); reference will be made to sections in DS and to pages in D.

Chapter Headings in D.	Corresponding Sections in DS.
1. Introduction	Introduction
2. Asserting That One Is Asleep	II
3. Judging That One Is Asleep	II
4. A Comparison of 'I Am Asleep' and 'I Am in Pain'	
5. Two Objections	
6. The Criteria of Sleep	I
7. Phenomena Resembling Sleep	
8. Sound Asleep	I, X
9. Judgments in Sleep	III, VII
10. Applications to Other Mental Phenomena	II, III
11. Dreaming as an Exception	IV
12. The Concept of Dreaming	IV, V, VIII
13. Temporal Location and Duration of Dreams	VIII
14. A Queer Phenomenon [Dream-telling]	VIII
15. Continuity between Dreams and Waking Life	IV (footnote 9)
16. Dreams and Skepticism	II, III, VI, VII, X
17. The Principle of Coherence	XI
18. Do I Know I Am Awake?	VII

the points in the critical essays. But it is necessarily incomplete, and should be construed as an attempt to illuminate, not epitomize.

As Malcolm himself observes (D, 1-4), philosophers from Aristotle to Russell have regarded dreams as conscious mental states present during sleep. Many psychologists appear to have shared this view also. These facts alone would make a refutation of the position highly significant. But there is a matter of additional interest since, as we have already seen, the traditional approach to dreaming appears to provide an important foothold for skepticism. If Malcolm's thesis is correct, therefore, it looks as if a famous skeptical argument has been destroyed.

Malcolm's basic strategy is to point out an incompatibility between occurrent mental activity and a (sound) sleeping state. His argument is initially directed against the possibility of making assertions and judgments during sleep, but he later maintains that the same argument, *mutatis mutandis,* can be used to rule out other types of mental activity as well. To take the case of assertions first, Malcolm argues (DS, II) that anyone who asserted that he was asleep would thereby falsify his claim; like the assertion (i) that I am unconscious, the assertion (ii) that I am asleep is self-defeating (D, 5–7). The very fact that these assertions are made shows them to be false.

Now, someone might object that the assertions under discussion, even if self-defeating, are so for different reasons. The first one could be absurd because unconscious people cannot have the awareness that assertions require; the second could be absurd, not because sleepers are unconscious (as Malcolm sometimes tends to assume; Cf. D, 12, 36; DS, IX) but because sleepers lack the voluntary abilities requisite for making assertions. If so, might it still not be the case that sleepers make judgments? Malcolm's answer is that the supposition that they do would be logically impossible to verify, because any behavior showing that a judgment was made would *ipso facto* show that the person was not (sound) asleep (Cf. D, 29–31, 36; DS, II). This is clearly a point just about verification, but it is quickly associated with a doctrine about meaning. For Malcolm adds that the notion of a sleeper's making judgments "is senseless in the sense that nothing can count in favour of either its truth or falsity" (D, 37).

The same argument can be employed to exclude, in the sense of impossibility of verification, the occurrence of *any* mental phenomena (images, beliefs, etc.) during sleep. The sleeper cannot be questioned about their occurrence while he is asleep, for any response on his part would falsify the hypothesis that he *is* asleep. And physiological evidence, for reasons which will be mentioned later, is of no help. Finally, the sleeper cannot be consulted after awakening, since we have no independent means of establishing the veracity of his testimony. In the absence of an independent check, the testimony must be discounted (D, 11).

Malcolm's view so far seems to involve two distinct theses: [9] (1) that hypotheses concerning the presence of mental activity

9. This observation is made by Pears.

during sleep are, in a certain way, self-contradictory; [10] (2) that such hypotheses are logically impossible to *verify* (D, 10–11; 36). The difference is crucial inasmuch as a theory of meaning is concerned, but as an attack on skepticism perhaps either version will suffice. For "if one cannot have thoughts while sound asleep, one cannot be *deceived* while sound asleep" (DS, III).[11] As far as *this* point is concerned, it appears to matter little whether the "cannot" signifies meaninglessness ("impossibility of verification") or logical impossibility. To see this more clearly, it is necessary only to take note of two passages where Malcolm confronts dream skepticism.

In the notion of the dream of sound sleep there is no foothold for philosophical skepticism. It is an error to say that a person *cannot tell* whether he is awake or sound asleep and dreaming. For this implies (a) that he might *think* he was awake and yet be sound asleep—which is impossible. And it implies (b) that he might think he was sound asleep and yet be awake. Now (b), unlike (a), is not impossible: but the thought that the man has—namely, that he is sound asleep—is self-contradictory (in the special sense that I explained),[12] and a little reflection could teach him that it is. Whether or not a particular person would see this point of logic, in any case no general ground for skepticism is provided. [DS, VII]

According to the view expressed here, skepticism involves a kind of logical contradiction. In *Dreaming,* however, Malcolm's challenge to skepticism rests squarely on the notion of senselessness (impossibility of verification):

My contribution (if it is one) to this renowned skeptical problem has been to try to show that the sentence 'I am not awake' is strictly senseless and does not express a possibility that one can think. This is to say

10. "The kind of self-contradiction is this: if someone claims that he is sound asleep then it follows that he is not what he claims. It is an assertion that would necessarily be false each time it was made. . . . [T]here is the same kind of self-contradiction in wondering or conjecturing whether one is sound asleep, or in being in doubt about it." (DS, II; cf. D, 7).

11. Notice that this claim is correct only if "thoughts" is replaced by "beliefs." Notice also, however, that Malcolm provides no argument against the view that we may hold beliefs while asleep. In fact, one can properly be said to hold beliefs (and to be deceived in virtue of them) even at times when one's mind is a blank. Perhaps one could even *acquire* beliefs in such circumstances, though this is admittedly not the sort of premise envisaged by most proponents of dream skepticism.

12. See Footnote 10.

that when the sentence 'I am not awake' is used to make a statement, there is not another possible statement which is its proper negation. There are not two things for me to decide between, one that I am awake the other that I am not awake. There is nothing to decide, no choice to make, nothing to find out. I cannot pass from not knowing whether I am awake or dreaming to knowing I am awake. To say 'I don't know whether I am awake or dreaming' would be to imply that 'I am dreaming' makes sense and expresses a possibility. Therefore the sentence 'I don't know whether I am awake or dreaming' cannot be a proper description of my condition, being itself a piece of nonsense. [D, 118]

But the question remains whether either of these approaches successfully undercuts skepticism. The following counter-argument to Malcolm suggests itself: Granting that the sentence "I don't know whether I am awake or dreaming" does not express a real possibility, it is still to be decided whether I am really uttering this sentence or only dreaming that I am uttering it. It will not help to argue that "Since I am considering this question, I must be awake", for again I may ask "Am I really considering it, or only dreaming that I am?" And so on, *ad infinitum.* Malcolm himself mentions, and appears to accept, a similar argument (D, 117–118).[13] He then adds that his intention is not "to propose a piece of reasoning by which someone can arrive at the knowledge that he is awake" (D, 118), even though his aim *is* evidently to expose the errors on which dream skepticism rests (D, 120). The upshot is that Malcolm's challenge to dream skepticism is somewhat obscure.[14]

Malcolm's rejection of traditional opinions about the nature of dreaming calls for revision of some closely allied notions as well. In this respect, his account of how dream reports function is especially noteworthy. The view to which Descartes was committed, and to which current investigators often subscribe,

13. Notice, however, that even if this argument is accepted, it does not entail that if I am dreaming then I am deceived. Contrary to what many philosophers have supposed, "*a* dreamt that *p*" does not entail "*a* was deceived," just because some dreams are like fictions which we do not take seriously. Furthermore, if Malcolm is correct in maintaining that "dreams" is never replaceable by "believes," the Cartesian problem about dream *deception* vanishes. Deception is impossible in the absence of false belief.

14. Another argument against skepticism, only implicit in *Dreaming,* is discussed in Charles E. M. Dunlop, "Performatives and Dream Skepticism," *Philosophical Studies,* 25 (1974), 295–297.

maintains that dream reports describe experiences which took place during sleep—and that such reports, being only contingently connected with the dream, may or may not accurately reflect dream content. But according to Malcolm, there are no states of consciousness in sleep; hence it follows that dream reports are not descriptions of experiences at all (at least not in the conventional sense of "description"). Yet these reports play a fundamental role in our concept of dreaming: "What we must say, although it seems paradoxical, is that the concept of dreaming is derived, not from dreaming, but from descriptions of dreams, i.e. from the familiar phenomenon that we call 'telling a dream' " (D, 55). If this seems paradoxical, it becomes all the more so if we bear in mind Malcolm's theory that the "familiar phenomenon" does not occur subsequent to experiences in sleep. It is hardly surprising, therefore, that he regards dream-telling as a "queer phenomenon" (D, 86). A fact to be accepted, but not explained, is that one often awakens in the morning and tells stories "under the influence of an impression—as if one was faithfully recalling events that one witnessed" (D, 86). When a person does this we say "He dreamt" (Cf. DS, VIII).

At this point one may wish to protest that Malcolm's theory leaves too many matters unresolved. Where, for example, do our waking impressions come from? And why do people awaken in the morning and tell such odd stories? But Malcolm's reply is that such questions are wrong-headed; his intention has been to say what dreaming is *not*, rather than to say what dreaming is. The reason for this may be discovered in Malcolm's reliance on *criteria* for answering questions about dreaming. While criteria may be used to rule with certainty on the presence or absence of something, they do not at the same time yield definitions (D, 60). Specifically, the "criterial" approach, although it may exclude items with which dreams have traditionally identified (images, judgments, etc.), tends to reject as unintelligible the question "What is dreaming?" (D, 59). For dream-telling, as the criterion of dreaming, affords no answer to the question, and "there can only be as much precision in the concept of dreaming as is provided by the common criterion of dreaming" (D, 75). "In a lecture Wittgenstein once said that it is an important thing in philosophy to know when to *stop*. If we cease to ask *why* it is that sometimes when people wake up they relate stories in the past tense under the influence of an impression, then we will see dream-telling as it is—a remarkable human phenomenon, a part of the natural history of man, something *given*, the foundation for the concept of dreaming" (D, 87).

Malcolm's account of how dream reports function suggests a close parallel between dream-telling and story-telling. Indeed, the expression "I dreamt" often operates in a manner analogous to "Let's suppose" (D, 85–86). But whereas "Let's suppose" suggests that the described events did not occur, telling a dream does not entail that the dream did not occur. On the contrary, a person's dream report is our criterion of his having dreamt. One must nonetheless be wary of calling dreams "occurrences." Unlike rainstorms, they do not take place in "physical time" (D, 75), although Malcolm does not elaborate on his assumption that there is a sense of "event" which is conceptually independent of date and duration.

To this last point he would probably reply that no elaboration is needed; talk about dreams as occurrences is misleading because it is too easily associated with the false, traditional account of dreaming. Instead, we should focus on the language-game of dream-telling. But those who find room in ordinary discourse for the expression "Dreams occur during sleep" may find this response unsatisfactory. In a similar vein, they may question Malcolm's treatment of "remembering dreams." Ordinarily, if at time *t* I remember that *x* occurred, it follows that at some time prior to *t* I was aware that *x* occurred. Having argued, however, that awareness is incompatible with sleep, Malcolm is prevented from listing prior awareness as a necessary condition of remembering a dream. He suggests, therefore, that "there is no warrant for thinking that 'remembering a dream' carries exactly the same implications as 'remembering a physical occurrence' " (D, 58).[15] But even granting that there are different uses of "remember," it can be argued that Malcolm is understating the matter. If *all* other uses of "remem-

15. Cf. Malcolm's "A Definition of Factual Memory," reprinted in his *Knowledge and Certainty* (Englewood Cliffs, 1963), esp. pp. 239–240.

ber" carry at least the implication of prior awareness, there is little basis for maintaining that this condition is dispensable in the case of "remembering" dreams. Here, as with "Dreams are occurrences," Malcolm desires to render his theory consonant with common usage. But for this he appears to pay a price, because the senses of "occurs" and "remembers" to which his theory of dreaming is committed are rather uncommon.

It has been mentioned that the relationship between dream reports and dreams is "criterial," but just what does this mean? Unfortunately, Malcolm does not address the question directly, although he does provide some scattered clues. The following points may be made:

(1) If C is a criterion of X, then C gives conditions whose presence settles with certainty questions about the presence or absence of X (D, 60–61).

(2) If C and C' are both criteria of X, there may be cases where C and C' yield contradictory statements about the presence or absence of X. In such cases one criterion may overrule the other (D, 22–26).

(3) If C is a criterion of X, then C does not provide a *definition* of X (D, 60).

(4) If C is a criterion of X, then C is not (numerically) identical with X (D, 59–60).

(5) If C is a criterion of X, then C and X are not logically independent of each other (D, 60).

(6) If C is a criterion of X, then C must be employed in order to teach someone the concept "X" (D, 81).

(7) If C is a criterion of X, then C determines the content of the concept "X" (D, 75);

(8) If C is a criterion of X, then, in instances where C is present, we have a paradigm case of X (D, 27–28; 80–81).

(9) If C is a criterion of X, then the introduction of a new criterion (C') of X is permissible only if C' entails no "radical conceptual changes" vis-à-vis X (D, 81).

Many of these propositions have already been employed, more or less explicitly, in the discussion. But the last three deserve special consideration here, because they give rise to consequences which have provoked a good deal of critical attention (Cf. Sections III and IV below). In the first place, (7) and (8) leave us with a multiplicity of concepts of sleeping and dreaming. "With adults and older children there are the two criteria of behavior and testimony; with animals and human infants there is only the one criterion of behaviour. The concept of sleep is not exactly the same in the two cases" (D, 23). And a man in the throes of a nightmare is in a state "so unlike the paradigms of normal sleep that it is at least problematic whether it should be said that he was 'asleep' when those struggles were going on" (D, 62–63). "To say that a man who is walking is 'asleep' is a new use of the expression" (D, 27). "[I]t is better, I think, to say that in psychoanalysis there is a different concept of dreaming than to say that in psychoanalysis one finds out what one really dreamt" (D, 57n).

The second consequence to be mentioned concerns (9), which implies that current experimental studies of dreaming are seriously misguided. The reason is that the investigators often make claims about dreaming which are so at variance with our common concept that they amount to a radical conceptual change (D, 81; cf. DS, VIII). "Without an adequate realization of what they are doing," says Malcolm, "[the investigators] are proposing a new concept in which the notions of location and duration in physical time and the subjective/objective distinction will all have a place. We ought to consider the consequences of these stipulations and ask ourselves whether it is appropriate to call this creation a concept of *dreaming*" (D, 80). This result, if generalized, has repercussions which extend far beyond dreaming. It suggests that any scientific inquiry must head off collision with common concepts, or be charged with making pronouncements that are wholly irrelevant to those things (if any) in the world to which our common concepts apply.

So far as the present topic is concerned, however, the alleged incompatibility between common concept and scientific inquiry exists only if the former is what Malcolm takes it to be. And it is surely difficult to understand how the common concept, when brought to our attention, could seem so unfamiliar. Partly for this reason, though for others as well, most recent writings on dreaming have defended "received opinion." To these we may now turn.

II. Dreaming and Consciousness

As might be expected, Malcolm's provocative thesis has generated a number of replies. A summary of even those reproduced in this anthology would be neither desirable nor feasible; however, it may be fruitful to survey (here, and in Sections III and IV) their contributions to several major topics. Still, it will be seen that the topical divisions are somewhat artificial, since the subjects are ultimately interconnected.

A. *Judgments in Sleep*

As was pointed out in the previous section, Malcolm begins his argument in *Dreaming* by suggesting that the sentence "I am asleep" can never be truly *asserted;* he then goes on to consider whether it could be used correctly to express a *judgment.* He concludes, of course, that it could not, "for to know that a person uses those words correctly we should sometimes have to observe him judging that he is asleep *while* he is asleep. And that is the absurdity" (D, 35). To appreciate the force of this argument it is important to bear in mind Malcolm's contention that all mental activity during sleep may be ruled out in a similar fashion.

It may appear, however, that this approach does not adequately preserve the distinction between judging and asserting. Consider, for example, what would normally be involved in observing a *waking* person judge that he was depressed: we would have to hear him assert that he was depressed. In such a case we would be deciding whether he judged, on the grounds of whether he asserted. But although our evidence for someone's making a judgment is often that he makes an assertion, it does not follow that judgments are impossible in contexts where (for one reason or another) assertions are precluded. A. J. Ayer considers this point with respect to dreaming:

> To say that it is impossible to judge what one cannot assert is in this instance to beg the question. For if we define 'assertion' in such a way that in order to make an assertion it is necessary to be awake, we thereby make room for the possibility of judging what one cannot assert; it may be held to be possible just in those cases where the person who makes the judgment is asleep. It may also be held that there could not be such cases; but this must then be established on other grounds.

Now, it is true that Malcolm appears to conflate judging and asserting, but this is not just an oversight. For he subscribes to the view (D, 9–10) that there is a correlation between a person's *understanding* a particular sentence and his *using* it in circumstances which make it true. Presumably, then, the absence of this "correlation" would at least strongly suggest that the person did not understand the sentence in question, and therefore could not use it to make judgments.

Unfortunately, this argument of Malcolm's cannot be used to eliminate the possibility of judgments in sleep, since, as Malcolm himself admits, the "correlations" do not amount to necessary conditions—or, for that matter, to criteria. Nonetheless, he later maintains (D, 36) "that in order for the sentence to have a *correct* use one would sometimes have to say it when the thing one said was *true*." The principle implicit here—that someone understands a sentence only if he sometimes uses it to say something true—is highly restrictive, for it entails that a person's claim to make judgments in sleep could be tested (if at all) only when he was asleep. But this result seems to rule out the rather obvious suggestion that the person be consulted when he awakens. If upon awakening someone reported having made a judgment in sleep, why should his testimony not be accepted? Malcolm's reply is that "if we have no way of establishing how to use the sentence [to make a judgment] *other* than by appeal to his testimony, then we cannot appeal to his testimony" (D, 11). It may not be obvious, however, why independent corroboration of the subject's waking testimony should be required. There seem to be numerous cases where corroboration is not available, but this does not generally cast doubt upon the speaker's claim. E.g., I tied my shoes yesterday when nobody was watching, and five minutes ago I envisioned a unicorn but told no one about it. Malcolm considers this point: "But note that we have said that he did not, in fact, give any sign of it. He *could* have done so. Whereas it is false that a man who is sound asleep could, while he is sound asleep, give any signs or indications that a certain thought was occurring to him or that he was experiencing some sensation. For any sign of this would also be a sign that he was at least partly awake" (DS, VII). This reply is insufficient, however. If the person in fact gave no sign, what further advantage is secured by the mere possibility of his having done so? Malcolm's view [16] can be better understood by examining a passage where he replies to a critic: "I am assuming it to be an *a priori* truth that whenever a thought occurs to a person or he experiences a feeling he could, at the time, give expression to the thought or feeling. I mean that this is always logically possible, not that it is always physically or psychologically possible." [17] A reply is suggested in John V. Canfield's paper ("Judgments in Sleep"), where we are invited to consider the following judgment: 'I am sitting perfectly still.' A person cannot express that judgment while he is making it. And since, according to Malcolm, we could verify someone's claim to have made that judgment *only* through his subsequent testimony, we are debarred from using his testimony. If this is true, it would seem impossible to verify that someone understands the judgment 'I am sitting perfectly still.' But, as Canfield notes: "Everyone who understands English sentences understands the sentence 'I am sitting perfectly still. . . .' One method of verification would be simply to ask the person to describe the circumstances under which he would apply the sentence to himself."

Perhaps Malcolm is not left without a reply, however. He might contend that occurrent mental activity is not incompatible with such things as sitting perfectly still. "But having some conscious experience, no matter what, is not what is meant by being asleep" (D, 12). Strictly speaking, Malcolm is perfectly correct here; the trouble is that if "having a dream" were substituted for "being asleep" in the quotation, many people would hold him to be wrong. And *that* is where an important issue lies.

B. *Sleep and Experience*

Throughout his writings on dreaming, Malcolm tends to connect wakefulness with consciousness, and sleep (in the "primary

16. It should be noted that while the passage just quoted from DS, along with the next passage to be quoted, represent Malcolm's earlier view, he does not think himself committed to it in D. See his 1966 footnote to DS.

17. "Dreaming and Skepticism: A Rejoinder," *Australasian Journal of Philosophy,* 35 (1957), 207–208.

or basic" sense) with unconsciousness. If this view were correct, it would (as Malcolm observes) rule out not only judgments in sleep, but images, thoughts, and sensations as well. But it might be objected that the connections drawn here by Malcolm are too restrictive. Even granting that sleepers are not conscious of everything that waking people are, it does not follow that they have no awareness at all; David F. Pears suggests that the awareness associated with a dream might be similar to "some trance-like state, like that of a person who has been drugged, or even of someone who is totally absorbed in a work of art." [18] Malcolm even agrees that asthma victims may dream of suffocating while having real feelings of suffocation, but he adds that those sufferers are not fully asleep (D, 99). Nonetheless, this sort of case would seem to provide some basis for extrapolating to the conclusion that dreamers who *are* fully asleep may enjoy some level of consciousness. And since behavioral criteria of dreaming appear admissible in some borderline cases, they might be invoked in the central or paradigm cases as well.

Of course, it is just this sort of extrapolation that Malcolm wishes to prevent. His strategy is to claim that no behavioral criterion exists for the dreams of subjects who are sound asleep, and therefore that awareness in these cases cannot be established. Furthermore, if a behavioral criterion were introduced, the concept of dreaming would be altered. But this second point needs careful scrutiny (cf. Section III below). As Pears remarks in a slightly different context: "[Malcolm] says that his criterion is the one that we use, and that it fixes the primary concept of dreaming (D, 74, 79, 80, 81, 82). But . . . he never justifies his assertion that it fixes the primary concept, and not just part of the concept of dreaming."

The need to justify Malcolm's testimonial criterion of dreaming becomes all the more pressing if one refuses to grant the entailment from "asleep" to "unconscious." For, given that re-

18. Such cases of awareness may or may not be susceptible to verbal description by the subject himself; their not being so, however, does not automatically preclude their being genuine cases of awareness. For an interesting discussion of some senses of "awareness," see D. C. Dennett, *Content and Consciousness* (London and New York, 1969), Ch. 6, esp. pp. 114–126.

fusal, one might argue that some of the behavioral manifestations (including neurophysiological evidence) of mental activity during waking life can be brought to bear on questions about the nature of dreaming. Such reflections form a major part of Daniel C. Dennett's important paper, "Are Dreams Experiences?" where it is suggested that "the received view is more vulnerable to empirical disconfirmation than its status as the received view would lead us to expect." Furthermore, Dennett regards Malcolm's antitraditional conclusions as vulnerable to the same sort of empirical disconfirmation. In assessing this position, it is important to keep in mind that "empirical" is operating in the absence of any precise distinction between "theory" and "observation"; [19] hence, Dennett concludes that "it is an *open* and *theoretical* question whether dreams fall inside or outside the boundary of experience."

If, as Dennett maintains, the question is open and theoretical, then it *might* turn out in some way that dreams are not properly to be regarded as experiences.[20] But what reasons are there for thinking that this could happen? Dennett begins by envisaging a scientific elaboration of the received view, according to which dreams involve a "presentation" during sleep. An alleged difficulty with this version of the received view is its inability to provide a natural explanation of those dreams which present a sequence of events climaxed by an episode that turns out to have been occasioned by some environmental stimulus. Citing "precognition" as the explanation available to received theory,[21] Dennett introduces an alternative possibility: "per-

19. Indeed, a current view is that all scientific data are to some extent "theory-laden." See, for example, P. K. Feyerabend, "Explanation, Reduction, and Empiricism," in H. Feigl and G. Maxwell, eds., *Minnesota Studies in the Philosophy of Science*, vol. III (Minneapolis, 1962), pp. 28–97; Thomas S. Kuhn, *The Structure of Scientific Revolutions* (Chicago and London, 1962), esp. Ch. 10; or Mary Hesse, *The Structure of Scientific Inference* (Berkeley and Los Angeles, 1974), Ch. 1. Unfortunately, Dennett's paper does not address in any detail the role played by theoretical considerations in empirical theories of dreaming.

20. Notice that Malcolm apparently has no objection to saying that dreams are experiences, *if* this is taken to mean simply that people do dream (D, 58). But given his view that sleepers are unconscious, he cannot allow dreams to be experiences in the sense in which conscious mental phenomena are experiences.

21. It seems obvious that the received view has more plausible accounts than this at its disposal. But an even more fundamental question concerns the *kind*

haps there is a 'library' of undreamt dreams with various indexed endings, and the bang or bump or buzz [i.e., the environmental stimulus] has the effect of retrieving an appropriate dream and inserting it, cassette-like, in the memory mechanism." This suggestion has the merit of explaining "precognitive" dreams, but carries the consequence that dreams are not experiences, for they would lack a presentation process altogether. In his generalization of the cassette theory, however, Dennett confronts the question of when those dreams are composed, and admits that

a . . . likely finding of the cassette-theorist would be that the composition process occurs during sleep, and more particularly, during periods of rapid eye movements, with characteristic EEG patterns. One might even be able to "translate" the composition process; that is, predict dream recollections from data about the composition process. This theory looks suspiciously like the elaboration of the received theory, except for lacking the presentation process. Cassette narratives, we are told, are composed in narrative order, and long narratives take longer to compose, and the decay time for cassettes in storage is usually quite short; normally, the dream one "recalls" on waking was composed just minutes earlier, a fact attested to by the occasional cases of content-relativity [22] in one of the byproducts of cassette composition: rapid eye movements. On this theory dream memories are produced just the way the received theory says they are, except for one crucial thing: the process of dream-memory production is entirely unconscious, involves no awareness or experiencing at all.

But if *this* version is accepted, it is no longer clear that the cassette theory offers any advantage over received opinion in accounting for "precognitive" dreams. After all, if "the dream one 'recalls' on waking was composed just minutes earlier," then we still have the question of how dream content managed to merge with the waking stimulus. And at least some of the answers available to cassette theorists could serve received opinion

---

of evidence that is relevant in adjudicating between the received view and the alternative about to be introduced.

22. As Dennett elsewhere elaborates: "A person whose REMs are predominantly horizontal is awakened and reports a dream in which he watched two people throwing tomatoes at each other. A predominantly vertical pattern in REMs is correlated with a dream report of picking basketballs off the floor and throwing them up at the basket."

equally well. One possibility is that an environmental stimulus can come to represent many different things as it is worked into dream content. There seems in any case to have been little systematic investigation of the processes involved; hence, it is premature to suggest that the cassette theory offers a significant explanatory advantage here.

Nevertheless, the very talk of "advantage" points to a particular methodological path—one which offers an alternative to Malcolm's view that questions concerning dreaming are to be answered or dismissed on purely conceptual grounds. As Dennett remarks: "Once we grant that subjective, introspective or retrospective evidence does not have the authority to settle questions about the nature of dreams—for instance, whether dreams are experiences—we have to turn to the other data, the behavior and physiology of dreamers, and to the relative strengths of the theories of these, if we are to settle the question, a question which the subject is not in a privileged position to answer." Given this position, it appears conceivable that the cassette theory of dreaming could even someday gain widespread popular acceptance. Under such a view, dreams would not count as experiences and (if one presently accepts received opinion) the concept of dreaming might be said to have changed. This imagined development may seem as shocking to some readers as Malcolm's view seemed to staunch defenders of received opinion. But conceptual alteration (as well as abandonment) is no novelty in the history of ideas.

III. Criteria, Meaning, and Conceptual Change

The importance of criteria in Malcolm's view of dreaming can scarcely be overstressed. Earlier, an attempt was made to canvas his various remarks on the subject, and it was mentioned that Malcolm regards dream-telling as the sole criterion of dreaming. This latter point is of special interest, for it marks off an asymmetry between Malcolm's account of sleeping, and his account of dreaming. Whereas sleep is said to admit of two criteria [23]—behavior, used to determine that someone *is* asleep,

23. Robert Caldwell's paper argues, however, that Malcolm fails to establish either testimony or behavior as a criterion of sleep. Pears discusses the question of a behavioral criterion of dreaming.

and testimony, used to determine that someone *was* asleep (D, 22–23; DS, I)—the case of dreaming presents only the criterion of testimony. Hence, it is possible to determine whether someone dreamt, but not that someone is dreaming.

In the context of Malcolm's rejection of "received opinion," this approach is readily understandable. For if behavior were admitted as a criterion of dreaming, then sense could be made of the thesis that dreams occur in "physical time," and an avenue would open up for the "verification" of memory-claims and for physiological studies concerned with dreaming. Still, the question of whether there *is* a behavioral criterion of dreaming lingers on. Nightmares would seem to provide at least one case where an affirmative answer is correct, since we do of course have a behavioral test for them. And if nightmares are dreams, and if dreams occur in sleep, it follows that at least sometimes we have a behavioral means of determining that someone is dreaming. Malcolm's reply would be that he is concerned primarily with the dream of sound sleep, and that nightmares do not afford an instance of *that* (cf. D, 62–63). But this is based on the apparent assumption that if something is not fairly close to being paradigm case of *X,* then it is at best problematically a case of *X* (cf. D, 30). And such an assumption seems false. Furthermore, if, as Malcolm admits, a man undergoing a nightmare is difficult to arouse (D, 62), it would be natural to conclude that he *is* sound asleep (Cf. D, 22; DS, I).[24]

Whether or not a behavioral criterion of dreaming exists, an important cluster of issues concerning criteria remains. Criteria, for Malcolm, are not only supposed to provide a way of settling questions with certainty, but are also thought to yield a method of teaching. Thus, it appears that Malcolm would regard conditions C_1 . . . C_n as criteria for X if they picked out a *paradigm case* of X—i.e., a case which would normally be used to teach someone the meaning of "X" (cf. D, 80–81).

[I]t is obvious that no one would teach the word 'asleep' ostensively by using examples of people who are shouting or walking. These cases would be at a considerable distance from the paradigms. [D, 27–28]

24. Notice that from Malcolm's rejection of behavior as a criterion of dreaming it does not follow that behavior is irrelevant to dreaming. On at least some occasions it may provide evidence that a sleeper will later relate a dream. See D, 62.

If after waking from sleep a child tells us that he saw and did and thought various things, none of which could be true, and if his relation of these incidents has spontaneity and no appearance of invention, then we may say to him 'It was a dream'. [D, 55]

These quotations suggest two theses: (1) the content of at least many of our concepts is a direct function of those conditions which pick out paradigm cases to which the concepts may be applied; (2) these concepts must be learned from paradigm cases in which they are exemplified. Some fundamental issues are involved here which cut across the philosophy of language and the philosophy of mind; they may be indicated briefly.

The appeal to the paradigm case as a prerequisite of teaching has a slightly old-fashioned ring to it today, although of course it did not fifteen years ago. In any event, it seems quite possible to teach someone the meaning of "asleep" by pointing to examples of people who are in fact only (successfully) *pretending* to be asleep (cf. Robert L. Caldwell, p. 169). Furthermore, it is by no means clear that a child could learn the meaning of "dream" only through a language-game such as that described by Malcolm, for our ordinary concept of dreaming does not appear to be very much like what Malcolm takes it to be. Charles S. Chihara and Jerry A. Fodor suggest that

our notion of a dream is that of a mental event having various properties that are required in order to explain the characteristic features of the dream-behavior syndrome. For example, dreams occur during sleep, have duration, sometimes cause people who are sleeping to murmur or to toss, can be described in visual, auditory, or tactile terms, are sometimes remembered and sometimes not, are sometimes reported and sometimes not, sometimes prove frightening, sometimes are interrupted before they are finished, etc. But if these are the sorts of facts that characterize our concept of dream, then there seems to be nothing which would, in principle, prevent a child who never dreamed from arriving at this notion.

There is a deeper issue yet, however. Malcolm seems committed to the thesis that we learn the use of various sentences in paradigmatic situations, *and,* consequently, that there is no important, systematic connection between past-tense and present-tense, or between first-person and certain third-person sentences: "A connection in sense between 'I am asleep' and 'He is asleep' is exactly what cannot be established, since the fulfillment of the criterion of *truth,* relative to the third person sentence, can play no part in the fulfillment of the criterion of *understanding,* relative to the first person sentence" (D, 17).[25] A principle which can be distilled from the quotation is this: From the fact that a person understands a third-person sentence, *S,* and that he knows how to use a large number of first-person and third-person sentence pairs, it cannot be concluded that he even probably understands the (related) first-person use of *S.* But this principle is by no means beyond dispute, as Hilary Putnam has pointed out:

In the first place, the use of many sentences is *projected* from the use of simpler sentences. For example, no one learns the use of the sentence 'If she had been wearing a red dress, it would have been easier to pick her out' from paradigmatic cases: one inductively projects the use of this sentence from the use of simpler but related sentences, e.g., 'She is wearing a red dress', 'It was easy to pick her out', 'If you has asked, I would have given it to you', 'If you hadn't jerked your hand the glass wouldn't have broken', etc., these last two sentences being of the form 'If A had been the case B would have happened.' Notice that even these simpler sentences would mainly be projections: one would not learn the use of 'She is wearing a red dress' and 'She is not wearing a red dress' separately. One would project the use of the latter sentence from one's familiarity with other sentence–negated-sentence pairs. And similarly with past-present, active-passive, etc.: one learns to project one form given the other.[26]

Although Putnam does not explicitly mention "projecting" from third-person sentences to first-person sentences, it seems quite clear that he would argue analogously in the case of "He is asleep" and "I am asleep." The concept of projection quite obviously stands in need of elaboration. Still, it should be apparent that the dispute between paradigm case advocates and "projectionists" raise profound questions in learning theory, the theory of meaning, and the philosophy of mind, many of which are just beginning to be explored.

A second point to be discussed was Malcolm's view that conceptual content is a strict function of the "criteria" for the concept's application. To put it another way, each concept is held

25. Malcolm later modified his view on this subject. See his *Problems of Mind* (New York, 1971), 87–91.
26. "Dreaming and 'Depth Grammar,' " in R. J. Butler, ed., *Analytical Philosophy,* 1st ser. (Oxford, 1966), p. 229.

to apply ("unproblematically") only to paradigm-like situations; movement away from the paradigm case necessitates the introduction of a *different* (though perhaps related) concept.[27] Hence, the concept of sleep is different in the following cases: normal, undisturbed sleep (D, 29–31); sleep-walking (D, 27); nightmares, when the sleeper is calling out or tossing about (D, 28); small children and animals (D, 23). Furthermore, the concept of dreaming, as it is used by experimentalists, is not the same as the everyday concept of dreaming; the scientists are in fact proposing a "new concept" (D, 80).

It will be possible only to suggest where the dispute lies. To begin, it can be argued that Malcolm's view here does not at all accord with out intuitions. As Chihara and Fodor suggest, it is profitable to "compare Malcolm's . . . concepts of sleep with a case where it really does seem natural to say that a special concept of sleep has been employed, viz., where we say of a hibernating bear that it sleeps through the winter."

Why does Malcolm think that the adoption of a new criterion of dreaming would introduce a new concept of dreaming? There seem to be two main reasons. First, it allegedly would follow that "people would have to be *informed* on waking up that they had dreamt or not—instead of their informing us, as it now is" (D, 80). Second, in order to teach a person "the new concept of dreaming, we should have to explain the physiological experiment that provides the new criterion" (D, 81). Nonetheless, each of these points must face a possible rebuttal. (1) Even if the scientists are introducing a new (behavioral) criterion of dreaming (a point denied by E. M. Curley in "Dreaming and Conceptual Revision") Malcolm fails to explain why it could not supplement, rather than replace, the testimonial criterion. If it could (compare Malcolm's two criteria of sleep), then, although people might sometimes be informed that they had dreamt, it would not follow that they *must* be informed. And even if dream reports were entirely abandoned in favor of the physiological criterion, it is argued by Chihara that Malcolm's conclu-

27. It is not clear how much movement away from the paradigm Malcolm would allow before claiming that a new concept has been introduced. But lhe passages to be mentioned suggest that each paradigm applies only to a rather narrow range of cases.

sion would *still* not hold: "We do not use a person's memory claim that he had been to the movies yesterday as the criterion for determining that he had been to the movies, but does it follow from this that a person who had gone to the movies would have to be informed of this fact the next day?" Malcolm would say, of course, that while the concept of memory *requires* the possibility of independent, public verification, the concept of dreaming does not even *permit* this. But since this is precisely the point at issue, it cannot be employed as a rejoinder. (2) Chihara also asks:

But why could not the child first learn what dreams are as we now do and later learn how scientists test dream reports? Is the case we are considering so different from the case of a child acquiring the concept of distance? It is difficult to explain to a child complicated methods of measuring distances using precise optical instruments, and even more difficult to explain the methods by which scientists measure immense astronomical distances. Would Malcolm also say that the use of the term 'distance', where neither rod nor string is employed in measuring, 'would spring from confusion and result in confusion'?

One more example may be cited. Putnam reports that the criteria for identifying acids have changed over the past several centuries, due mostly to our increasingly sophisticated theoretical apparatus. Has this introduced a new concept of acid? In some ways perhaps, but in at least one sense, clearly not. What was a paradigm case of acid in the eighteenth century is still so in the twentieth century. Putnam writes: "It is true that we can today speak of a few acids that could not have been *identified as such* by eighteenth century criteria. If the eighteenth century chemist had insisted that there *could not be,* say, an acid too weak to turn litmus paper red (or to give any taste at all) as he understood the term, then perhaps we should say that a change of meaning had occurred. But who supposes that an eighteenth century chemist could have so insisted?" [28] Putnam goes on to suggest several ways of telling when a change of meaning has occurred. Still, this is only a beginning; questions concerning criteria, concepts, and conceptual change are far from settled,

28. "Dreaming and 'Depth Grammar,'" p. 220.

and in fact are currently receiving a great deal of philosophical attention.[29]

IV. Memory and the "Independent Verification" Requirement

It seems natural to think that if a person reported having had imagery during his previous night's sleep, we would be entitled to take him at his word. If we did so, however, according to Malcolm, we would not be receiving the report as a memory claim at all—at least not as anything like a paradigm case. For memory claims must be susceptible to public checks. In the case envisaged, it would be impossible to know whether the report was correct (or incorrect) (cf. D, 57).

This argument is discussed by Frederick Siegler, who accepts the idea that "if there were never any possibility of an appeal beyond one's own memory there could be no such thing as remembering." But Siegler goes on to argue that "this does not exclude the existence of a class of memory reports that *cannot in principle* be publicly checked, or *cannot in practice* be publicly checked." The question is still open, perhaps, of how the dream case is to be described. Is it a case of "remembering" (where public checks are often available) applied to dreams, or is it a case of "remembering a dream" (where checks are never available)? If Siegler is correct, however, its being the latter does not preclude its being subsumed under the former.

Vere C. Chappell is another critic of Malcolm's claim that memory reports concerning dreams do not permit the usual questions about "correct" and "incorrect." Chappell concedes

29. A few recent examples are: Arthur I. Fine, "Consistency, Derivability, and Scientific Change," *Journal of Philosophy*, 54 (1967), 231–240; Saul Kripke, "Identity and Necessity," in Milton Munitz, ed., *Identity and Individuation* (New York, 1971), pp. 135–166; Saul Kripke, "Naming and Necessity," in Donald Davidson and Gilbert Harman, eds., *Semantics of Natural Language* (Dordrecht, 1972), pp. 253–355, 763–769; Kathryn Pyne Parsons, "On Criteria of Meaning Change," *British Journal for the Philosophy of Science*, 22 (1971), 131–144; Hilary Putnam, "Meaning and Reference," *Journal of Philosophy*, 70 (1973), 699–711; Hilary Putnam, "The Meaning of 'Meaning,'" reprinted in Hilary Putnam, *Mind, Language and Reality* (Cambridge, 1975), pp. 215–271. See also the collection of papers in Glenn Pearce and Patrick Maynard, eds., *Conceptual Change* (Dordrecht, 1973).

"that Malcolm and Wittgenstein are right in holding that if no objective test of . . . a memory [of public phenomena] were possible, the memory could not, logically, be correct or incorrect." But he argues that "it does not follow that the memory of a necessarily private phenomenon—a particular sensation or a dream, say—must meet the same condition of objective testability to qualify as correct or incorrect." But then what sort of test must it meet? Chappell suggests a kind of coherence test: reviewing the dream events, along with putative memories of hitherto forgotten elements of the dream. "The one memory corroborates the other because the two do accord with each other."

Malcolm objects to this procedure on the grounds that dreams are often unpredictable and incoherent. As he puts it, you cannot really argue against a child "if he says that in his dream the train left from the filling station. In a dream a train does not have to run on tracks, and there is no 'usually' about it." [30] Now, if what Chappell is advocating were a strict coherence procedure, this reply would be conclusive. But Chappell's suggestion *seems* to be just that we often (successfully) apply certain mnemonic techniques in order to "bring back" memory details, and, further, that we often "immediately recognize" the recovered details as being correct. We do in fact accomplish this with respect to public phenomena, so why should we not also accomplish it in the case of remembering dreams? Malcolm would reply that the two cases are quite different, inasmuch as the memory claims of the former kind can be checked. But his argument about memory seems to rest on Wittgenstein's *Philosophical Investigations,* paragraphs 56 and 265. And Chappell notes that both of those paragraphs deal with a special *case* of memory: memory images. So, even if Wittgenstein is right, Malcolm cannot use the argument unless he shows either (a) that the argument can be generalized to *other* cases of remembering, or (b) that remembering dreams necessarily involves the use of memory images.

As we have just seen, Malcolm's rejection of "received opinion" about dream recollection is based largely on the claim that

30. This reply and others by Malcolm are printed in footnotes to Chappell's paper. The one quoted appears in note 8.

the putative memories are not open to independent verification. Essentially the same requirement leads him to reject the idea that physiological data could ever provide a way of determining whether (and when) mental activity occurs during sleep.

> If it were established, for example, that whenever a person makes a judgment the electrical output of a certain region of his brain rises or falls in some characteristic way, the occurrence of this electrical phenomenon in a sleeping person would not provide any probability that the sleeper was making a judgment. The imagined correlation would, of necessity, have been established only for the case of people who were awake, since the criteria for saying some person made a judgment could not be fulfilled when he was asleep. The attempt to extend the inductive reasoning to the case of sleeping persons would yield a conclusion that was logically incapable of confirmation. It would be impossible to know whether this conclusion was true or false. [D, 43]

This claim is taken up by Charles Landesman:

> An advocate of the view that dreams may consist of judgments will argue that the inaccessibility of judgments made while asleep is a contingent matter in respect to the species 'judgment' just as the inaccessibility of an instance of talking to oneself is a contingent matter in respect to the species 'talking to oneself,' and that the validity of Malcolm's argument hinges upon the arbitrary decision to include the contingent inaccessibility with the description of the event itself so as to make its inaccessibility a logical matter. It would be begging the question to reply that the inaccessibility of judgments made while asleep is not contingent, for this reply would represent a *decision* to determine contingency or the lack of it by reference to the subspecies rather than the species of event. What is possible or impossible relative to some x is a function not merely of the x-in-itself but also of our choice of description. Describing someone as a bachelor excludes the possibility of his being married, but describing him as a man does not.

The argument here is rather compact, but may be interpreted as follows. If we can have (e.g.) physiological evidence for someone's making a judgment, and there seems to be no reason why Malcolm should deny that we might (at least in *some* cases), then we should have a means of detecting judgments in sleep. To deny this, as Malcolm does, is to deny arbitrarily that "judgment in sleep" is just another case of "judgment." Malcolm would reply that the first premise in the argument is false—i.e., that we do not have physiological evidence for judgments *simpliciter,* but only for waking judgments. This response, Landesman suggests, merely illustrates the charge of "arbitrariness."

Now, Landesman's remarks about choices of description are important, but it cannot be fairly maintained that Malcolm's view on the inaccessibility of judgments in sleep is purely arbitrary. For he does set forth some independent arguments, some of which were mentioned in II-A above. Whether those arguments are satisfactory, of course, is another matter altogether.

Malcolm's apparent adherence to the principle that the conclusion of certain inductive inferences must be independently verifiable has seemed to some critics to preclude the possibility of any science which makes use of a theoretical term. Drawing on several examples from the history of science, Chihara and Fodor conclude "that there exist patterns of justificatory argument which are not happily identified either with appeals to symptoms or with appeals to criteria, and which do not in any obvious way rest upon such appeals." What would the correct procedure look like? In reviewing the experimental work of William C. Dement and Nathaniel A. Kleitman, E. M. Curley writes:

What they were operating with was, not a criterion, but a theory, which says that dreaming occurs in conjunction with a particular physiological process. This theory had already been made more or less probable by previous experiments. If the theory is correct, then the duration of the physiological process should be a reliable indicator of the duration of the dream. One way of testing the theory is to check the results of using that way of measuring the duration of the dream against those we get by asking the dreamer. If there is a good agreement between these two supposed indices of dream duration, then we infer that they are indeed both measures of the same thing.

With this sort of reflection, the debate between Malcolm and some of his critics again comes into sharp focus. Throughout D and DS it is maintained that statements about mental activity during sleep cannot be *verified;* the reply being offered here is that such statements can at least be *confirmed.* On Malcolm's account, the absence of possible verification points in the direction of meaninglessness; on the alternative view, the presence of significant experimentally determined psychophysical correlations may yield genuine insights into the nature of dreaming. These differences reflect a fundamental disagreement in approach to what Chihara and Fodor have called the "hoary problem" of other minds. A methodological verdict, however, should perhaps await some discussion of the recent experimental literature.

V. The Relevance of Contemporary Dream Research
A. Dreaming and REM Sleep

The vast amount of experimental literature on the topic of sleep and dreaming owes its origin largely to a result published by Eugene Aserinsky and Nathaniel Kleitman in 1953.[31] In monitoring the sleep of twenty normal adults, Aserinsky and Kleitman discovered the occurrence of periodic, synchronous rapid eye movements; these rapid eye movement periods each lasted about twenty minutes, and recurred several times during seven hours of sleep. The experimenters conjectured that such eye movements were associated with dreaming. Indeed, subjects awakened during those periods generally reported a dream, whereas subjects awakened at other times during sleep generally did not. Aserinsky and Kleitman concluded that "this method furnishes the means of determining the incidence and duration of periods of dreaming." [32]

Another, now-classic study by Dement and Kleitman [33] corroborated the earlier result, and introduced new findings and suggestions as well. In this experiment, dream reports were elicited eighty percent of the time from subjects who were awakened during periods of rapid eye movement (abbreviated REM), while subjects awakened during periods of no rapid eye movement (NREM) reported dreams only seven percent of the time. Dement and Kleitman concluded that dreaming occurs

31. "Regularly Occurring Periods of Eye Motility, and Concomitant Phenomena, during Sleep," *Science,* 118 (1953), 273–274.
32. Ibid., p. 274.
33. William C. Dement and Nathaniel A. Kleitman, "The Relation of Eye Movements during Sleep to Dream Activity: An Objective Method for the Study of Dreaming," *Journal of Experimental Psychology,* 53 (1957), 339–346. Reprinted in Wilse B. Webb, ed., *Sleep: An Experimental Approach* (New York and Toronto, 1968), pp. 78–89. Hereafter cited as "Dement and Kleitman," with page references to Webb.

during REM periods, and suggested that "The few instances of dream recall during NREM periods are best accounted for by assuming that the memory of the preceding dream persisted for an unusually long time." [34] Furthermore, Dement and Kleitman introduced what has come to be known as the "scanning hypothesis"—the idea that REMs reflect the dreamer's surveillance of a visual field. Their argument for this was based on alleged correlations between eye movement direction and dream content; however, as we shall see, the scanning hypothesis is extremely controversial.

The occurrence of REM periods during sleep has been observed again and again, and is beyond dispute. Subsequent electroencephalographic (EEG) studies of sleep have also revealed four distinct stages of sleep, and it has often been assumed, perhaps incorrectly,[35] that Stages I–IV represent progressively "deeper" levels of sleep. In any case, REM periods are clearly associated with EEG Stage I,[36] and have also been correlated with increase and variation in respiratory rate, reduction in blood pressure, acceleration and variation of heart rate,[37] frequent penile erections,[38] loss of muscle tone,[39] and greatly increased neuronal activity in various areas, including

34. Ibid., p. 87.

35. For a discussion of this issue, see William C. Dement, "An Essay on Dreams," in Frank Barron et al., *New Directions in Psychology II* (New York, 1966), pp. 146–149. Hereinafter, this study is cited as "Dement."

36. REMs do not, however, accompany the EEG Stage I which signals the onset of sleep; they are normally associated only with subsequent ("emergent") Stage I occurrences.

37. Dement, pp. 153–155. However, William J. Baldridge points out that "heart rate is under the reflex influence of nearly every organ and system in the body, yet compensation has not generally been made for these effects." See his "Discussion" paper in Milton Kramer, ed., *Dream Psychology and the New Biology of Dreaming* (Springfield, 1969), p. 34.

38. Allan Rechtschaffen, "The Psychophysiology of Mental Activity during Sleep," in F. J. McGuigan and R. S. Schoonover, eds., *The Psychophysiology of Thinking* (New York, 1973), pp. 171–173. Hereafter cited as "Rechtschaffen."

39. Dement, p. 157. Since some of the REM correlates suggest a high degree of arousal, while the loss of muscle tension suggests the opposite, some researchers have labeled the REM phase "paradoxical sleep." At present there is no terminological uniformity in sleep and dream research, a point made dramatically by Michael Chase, ed., *The Sleeping Brain* (Los Angeles, 1972), esp. pp. 497–501.

the visual cortex.[40] As a result, researchers have been inclined
to view the REM period as a period of "definite conscious experience." [41]

Obviously, however, this conclusion has not been established
beyond all reasonable doubt,[42] even granting that the above-
mentioned correlations do lend it prima-facie plausibility. And,
given the current absence of a well-founded neurophysiological
theory which, for example, correlates mental states with specific sets of brain processes, it has been necessary to appeal to
other sorts of arguments. Several interesting studies have attempted to relate behavioral measures to dream content. In
their 1957 study, Dement and Kleitman awakened subjects either five or fifteen minutes after the beginning of an REM
period, and asked them to judge how long they had been
dreaming. With one exception, the subjects were able to make
the "correct" choice. Other experiments have tried to provide
temporal landmarks of conscious activity during sleep by modifying dream content through the introduction of external stimuli.[43] Finally, Dement has argued that "the most conclusive evidence that dreaming takes place during the REM period, and
further, that it is an ongoing phenomenon, is the demonstrable

40. Dement, pp. 159–160. This finding occurred in experimental studies of
the cat, and cross-species generalizations should of course be viewed with cir-
cumspection. For a discussion, see Frederick Snyder, "The Physiology of
Dreaming," in Kramer, *op. cit.*, pp. 14–15, hereafter cited as "Snyder." In fact,
even intraspecies generalizations have definite limitations, as contributors to a
recent symposium on dreaming emphasized. See "Dreams, Dream Content,
and Their Psychophysiological Correlates," in Chase, *op. cit.*, pp. 239–276, esp.
pp. 249–253.

41. The quoted phrase occurs in Ernest Hartmann, *The Biology of Dreaming*
(Springfield, 1967), p. 147, and seems to represent the view of many investigators.

42. In discussing the issue, for example, Snyder (pp. 17–18; 21) and Rechtschaffen ("Dream Reports and Dream Experiences," *Experimental Neurology*,
Supp. 4 [1967], pp. 4–15) pay brief homage to skepticism, but ultimately em-
brace the "conscious experience" view of dreaming.

43. See William C. Dement and Edward A. Wolpert, "The Relation of Eye
Movements, Body Motility, and External Stimuli to Dream Content," *Journal of
Experimental Psychology*, 55 (1958), esp. pp. 548–550. Matters have been compli-
cated, however, by the more recent evidence that dreaming may occur during
NREM sleep, along with the discovery that external stimuli are possibly capable
of being incorporated into NREM dreaming. See Rechtschaffen, p. 162.
(NREM dreaming will be discussed shortly.)

correspondence between the specific directional patterns of the REMs and the spatial orientation of events in the dream." [44] In one study, for example, given detailed dream reports, judges were able to deduce with seventy to eighty percent accuracy what the eye movements of the dreamer had been. [45] And, as Dement has recently demonstrated, judges dealing with *waking* subjects were unable to do appreciably better. [46] Unfortunately, however, not all researchers share Dement's optimism regarding the scanning hypothesis. In the first place, the original results have not been successfully duplicated. Furthermore, it has been pointed out that REMs occur in newborn infants and decorticate cats, the point being that "scanning" in these subjects is highly unlikely. There are also indications that REMs occur in subjects who are congenitally blind, although the issue is controversial due to the techniques of measurement employed. [47] In replying to some of these points, Frederick Snyder suggests "that all of the physiological features of REM states we are now aware of are probably much more fundamental than dreaming, yet this is not incompatible with the premise that higher central nervous activities, such as we assume to be involved in the physiology of perception, or thought or memory, have become integrated with this older mechanism in that complex psychic process (just as speech in its service to conceptual thought makes use of the ancient biological mechanism of respiration)." [48]

But it should be apparent that these considerations, even though they may be cited in support of the view that dreams are "definite conscious experiences," are still far from yielding a definitive resolution of the issue.

44. Dement, p. 173. Snyder expresses agreement with this outlook (Snyder, p. 22).

45. This study was originally reported by H. Roffwarg, W. Dement, J. Muzio, and C. Fisher, "Dream Imagery; Relationship to Rapid Eye Movements of Sleep," *Archives of General Psychiatry*, 7 (1962), 235–258; it is reviewed in some detail in Dement, pp. 174–180.

46. William C. Dement, *Some Must Watch While Some Must Sleep* (San Francisco, 1974), pp. 51–52.

47. For a discussion, see Rechtschaffen, pp. 178–180.

48. Snyder, pp. 22–23.

B. NREM Sleep and the Concept of Dreaming

Due perhaps to the initial emphasis placed by researchers on REM sleep, interest in the NREM period developed somewhat slowly. Dement and Kleitman, it will be remembered, suggested that dreaming is associated exclusively with REMs. In a paper published in 1962, however, W. David Foulkes reported that dream recall had been elicited from seventy-four percent of NREM awakenings.[49] And since this figure was almost the same in instances where there had been no recent REM period, it seemed quite unlikely that the subjects were recalling dreams from earlier REM sleep.

Foulkes' result illustrated how crucial an experimenter's *concept* of dreaming can be. Compare the following passages, the first from Dement and Kleitman, and the second from Foulkes:

The [subjects] were considered to have been dreaming only if they could relate a coherent, fairly detailed description of dream content. Assertions that they had dreamed without recall of content, or vague, fragmentary impressions of content, were considered negative.[50]

The following criteria (essentially those used by the subjects themselves) were used in classifying reports with some substantive content as dreams or thoughts: any occurrences with visual, auditory, or kinesthetic imagery were called dreams; phenomena reported to lack such imagery but in which the subject either assumed another identity than his own or felt that he was thinking in a physical setting other than that in which he actually was (i.e., the laboratory) were also classified as dreams; phenomena lacking sensory imagery (no imagery other than visual, auditory, or kinesthetic was ever noted) and changed identity or setting were classified as thoughts.[51]

49. W. David Foulkes, "Dream Reports from Different Stages of Sleep," *Journal of Abnormal and Social Psychology,* 65 (1962), 14–25. Hereafter cited as "Foulkes." Impressive as this figure is in the light of earlier studies, the question still arises why it was not higher. Possible influencing factors include (a) the relationship between experimenter and subject; (b) duration of NREM phase prior to awakening; (c) abruptness of awakening; (d) different kinds of failures to report a dream (See Donald R. Goodenough, "Some Recent Studies of Dream Recall," in Herman A. Witkin and Helen B. Lewis, eds., *Experimental Studies of Dreaming* [New York and Toronto, 1967], pp. 130–131). Each of these factors of course raises important methodological issues.
50. Dement and Kleitman, p. 82.   51. Foulkes, p. 17.

Investigators have recognized the problems that stem from such terminological variations,[52] but as yet no uniformity of nomenclature has been achieved. Some writers seem happy to speak of NREM dreaming, despite apparent differences in the *kind* of mental activity during REM and NREM sleep;[53] one scientist even suggested recently that "dreaming probably goes on even during the waking state";[54] and Dement has recently advocated restricting the term "dream" to mental activity which occurs during REM sleep.[55]

But the issue is not *just* a terminological one. If our concern is to discover the physiological correlates of *dreaming,* then we of course cannot allow entirely new concepts to be substituted for those used in formulating our concern. Still, there appears to be plenty of room to maneuver short of that extreme; Dement's proposal (discussed by Curley) represents just one possibility. Whether the final result will be appraised as a conceptual change, however, is a matter that cannot be anticipated here.

C. Cartesian Skepticism Revisited

Descartes' skeptical argument began with the claim that on past occasions he had been deceived while asleep. We have seen Norman Malcolm's challenge to this idea, along with some of the philosophical replies on behalf of Descartes, and, finally, the contributions from experimental studies of dreaming. It seems clear that Malcolm's view cannot be sustained on purely a priori grounds, and that Descartes' view has not received conclusive experimental corroboration. Nevertheless, Curley's paper brings out a further interesting respect in which recent research does bear on the Cartesian problem:

(a) [T]here are very great individual differences in the ability that people have to recall their dreams; and (b) the conditions under which we ordinarily try to recall our dreams are not optimal; most people who have been awakened from an REM-period in a sleep laboratory find

52. Hence, an eight-point scale for the evaluation of dream reports has recently been proposed. See Dement, pp. 190–191.
53. Cf. Rechtschaffen, p. 162: "Dreaming does seem to occur in NREM as well as in REM sleep."
54. This came from Carl A. Meier at the symposium summarized in Chase, *op. cit.,* p. 247.
55. Dement, pp. 210–211.

that they can recall much more detail than they ordinarily can. The experience seems to them to have been much more vivid. So what look like individual differences in dream vividness may be individual differences in dream recall. It may well be that each of us, every night, has dreams as vivid as those Descartes reports, without recalling them in the morning. And so Descartes may well be right about what many dreams are like as experiences.

This is, of course, an intriguing conjecture, but at present it is no more than that. In the meantime, lacking definitive empirical support for his premise, the skeptic may remind us that (*pace* Malcolm) it is not self-contradictory to suppose that we have been deceived by our dreams. And of course he is correct. But, for good or ill, skeptical claims based exclusively on the logical possibility of error do not currently generate much epistemological excitement.

1

O. K. BOUWSMA

Descartes' Skepticism of the Senses

One of the most famous of all puzzles in the history of philosophy is that generated by Descartes' famous argument concerning the senses. The conclusion of that argument is skepticism of the senses generally. The central puzzle may be expressed in the question: "Am I awake or asleep?" I want in what follows to show how this puzzle is generated, and to show in what the puzzle consists.

The argument is this: "But it may be that although the senses sometimes deceive us concerning things which are hardly perceptible or very far away, there are yet many others to be met with as to which we cannot reasonably have any doubt, although we recognize them by their means. For example there is the fact that I am here, seated by the fire, attired in a dressing gown, having this paper in my hands, and other similar matters. . . .

"At the same time I must remember that I am a man, and that consequently I am in the habit of sleeping, and in my dreams representing to myself the same things or sometimes even less probable things, than do those who are insane in their waking moments. How often has it happened to me that in the night I dreamt that I found myself in this particular place, that I was dresseed and near the fire, whilst in reality I was lying undressed in bed! At this moment it does indeed seem to me

Reprinted from *Mind*, 54 (1945), 313–322, by permission of the publisher (Basil Blackwell, Oxford).

that it is with eyes awake that I am looking at this paper. . . . But in thinking over this I remind myself that on many occasions I have in sleep been deceived by similar illusions, and in dwelling carefully on this reflection I see so manifestly that there are no certain indications by which we may clearly distinguish wakefulness from sleep that I am lost in astonishment, and my astonishment is such that it is almost capable of persuading me that I now dream." [1]

Descartes is considering a certain class of perceptions, namely, those concerning which it may be said that with respect to them "we cannot reasonably have any doubt." This class is distinguished from those perceptions of things "hardly perceptible or very far away" with respect to which "the senses sometimes deceive us." Concerning perceptions in the latter class, I take it that Descartes is saying that with respect to any member of this class we may "reasonably" have a doubt. The reasonableness of the doubt in any such case is based on the fact that the perceiver in question will in the past have been deceived in some perceptions of this class. Hence every member of that class is now under suspicion. Now it may be that with respect to any member of the first class, we may also have reasonable doubts, and for the same sort of reason, namely that one has at some time or other been deceived. Descartes might have said: Just as you once mistook a cow out there beyond the meadow for a pony, and so you cannot trust your eyes in distinguishing far away things, so too I remember your flicking your ashes into a bowl of soup which you mistook for an ash tray, and so you cannot trust your eyes to distinguish things near-by either. But Descartes does not say this. He does, of course, say that concerning the bowl of soup you may also have a reasonable doubt, but not because you have ever been deceived about a bowl or an ash tray. I want to notice closely just what in such cases does, according to Descartes, constitute the basis of a reasonable doubt.

Before I proceed, I should like to point out with respect to Descartes' argument, that if it is a good argument, it remains a good argument even though no man at any time has been

1. *Philosophical Works of Descartes*, trans. E. S. Haldane and G. R. T. Ross, 2 vols. (Cambridge: Cambridge University Press, 1912), I, 145–146.

deceived by the senses. The argument does not depend in any way upon any instance of deception. It's as though Descartes asked : And do the senses deceive us? To which the answer is: Never. He goes on: Are the senses then to be trusted? to which he answers: Certainly not. This illustrates the unusual character of his argument. It may be noticed too that if his argument holds for that class of perceptions by which we perceive things near-by, it holds equally for that class of perceptions by which we perceive "things hardly perceptible and far-away." No perception is to be trusted.

We have then to consider what fact it is, about all perceptions whatsoever, that constitutes a basis for reasonable doubt concerning any perception. Descartes starts out from what he describes as a fact. ". . . there is *the fact that* I am here, seated by the fire, attired in a dressing gown, having this paper in my hands, and other similar matters." It is important to recognize that this is introduced as a fact. Concerning this Descartes has no doubt, either reasonable or unreasonable. In contrast with this Descartes now recollects certain dreams of his. "How often has it happened to me that in the night I dreamt that I found myself in this particular place, that I was dressed, and near the fire, whilst in reality I was lying undressed in bed." Concerning this Descartes is also quite certain. These were only dreams. There are here then two facts which provide Descartes with the starting point of his argument. There is the fact "I am here, . . . etc.," and there is the fact that I dreamed that I was here, "seated by the fire . . . etc." It may be odd that Descartes should have dreamed what actually often happened, and odder still that he should have dreamed this often. If one is inclined to any reasonable doubt concerning this, at any rate one may admit all that is requisite to the argument. All that is necessary is that Descartes should have dreamed it once.

We might even admit that once upon a time Descartes was "here, seated by the fire, attired in a dressing gown, having this paper in (his) hands," and that he fell asleep and dreamed. And Descartes dreamed, and behold! he dreamed that he was "here, seated by the fire, attired in a dressing gown, having this paper in (his) hands." Descartes, having dreamed, awoke, and he recollected his dream, and it was so.

Now what strikes Descartes is the likeness of the fact to what he has dreamed. The description of the fact is identical with the description of what he dreamed. This disturbs Descartes, and the disturbance is obvious in the language which he now employs. "At this moment it does indeed seem to me that it is with eyes awake that I am looking at this paper. . . ." The assumption is, of course, that if it only seems "that it is with eyes awake," then, too, it only seems "that I am here, seated by the fire. . . ." The alleged fact from which the argument proceeded has begun to shake. But so far as I can see there is no corresponding concretion, substantiation, of the dream. The real shakes, but the dream remains a dream. There is no exchange of status. Descartes does not say: Well, maybe what I took to be the fact is a dream, and what I took to be a dream is the fact. It is the fact which dissolves under this inspection. Maybe everything is dreams. Curiously, however, dreams are still described as deceiving "by similar illusions." But in this case, what is deception and what is illusion?

I should like now to study this predicament more closely. Imagine yourself in a fixed position in relation to a garden and to a mirror reflecting that garden as perfectly as possible. Imagine further that the mirror is not distinguishable. There is no shimmer, no smoothly shining surface. Now then suppose further that before you were placed in this position you thought you knew which was the garden and which was the reflection, but immediately before you were placed in that position you were turned round and round, and made so dizzy that even when you had recovered you were unable to identify which was the garden and which was the reflection. Now the question is put to you: Which is the garden, and which is the reflection? And you must answer by way of inspection from that fixed position. You look, and bend your head, now this way, now that; you study the detail of each closely, but all in vain. By inspection you cannot make out which is which. If by this time you have recollected somehow, which of the two you would have identified as the garden, had you not previously been made dizzy, you may also have lost all confidence in your previous judgment. "It did indeed seem to me that that was the garden, but in thinking over this I can see how a mirror reflection may have deceived me." If you are bold these possibilities may now occur to you:

(a) One is a garden and one is a reflection, but there is no way of knowing which is which.

(b) There are two gardens.

(c) There are two reflections.

You may, of course, conclude that hunches are from God, and that God's hunches are good hunches. So you had better try to discover your hunch.

Now this is something like the predicament in which Descartes finds himself. He sets out confidently enough from "the fact that I am here" (the garden), and the dream that I am here (the reflection). But too much inspection, or the wrong question prompting the inspection, dizzies him. He loses his confidence. Is this the fact? How does one tell? It seems to me that this is the fact, but that other too seems to me to be the fact. If only facts were marked *F* and what is merely dreamed marked *D*, everything would be so simple. As it is there is no telling. There are in any case three possibilities:

(a) One is fact and one is dream.

(b) Both are facts.

(c) Both are dreams.

Descartes sets out confidently from (a), but loses that confidence, and relapses into (c). Curiously it does not occur to Descartes to suggest that both are facts.

I want now to trace the course of his loss of confidence. The facts involved, and the nature of Descartes' probing are clear enough. Just where now does the dizziness begin?

Let us recollect Descartes begins with "the fact that I am here, seated by the fire, etc." Now he asks: But am I here, seated by the fire? His response is: "At the moment it does indeed seem to me that it is with eyes awake that I am looking over this paper." Clearly Descartes thinks that if he can be sure that he is awake, then he can be sure that he is here, seated by the fire. Very well then: Am I awake? I can't tell. How can I tell? Well, if it seems to me that I am here and I really am here, then I am awake. But am I here? That is the question. Since now the only fact which remains is that it seems to me that I am here, and that fact is equally established for any case in which I dream that I am here, there is no way of telling whether I am awake or dreaming. "There are no certain indications by which we may clearly distinguish wakefulness from sleep." It follows, of course, that Descartes cannot tell whether he is here, seated by the fire, etc., or not. One might in play suggest that he try going to bed and try falling asleep. If he succeeds, he was awake, and then it will follow that he was here.

Now I want to notice the peculiar question which Descartes asks himself: Am I awake or am I asleep? This question is either a very peculiar question or it is readily answerable. In order to exhibit this I want to consider certain other questions which are very much like this.

Let us consider the question: Is he awake or asleep? We know very well how to go about finding out. Let us suppose he is lying down on a couch. Tip-toe up to him. Listen. You can tell by his breathing. Is he snoring lightly maybe? Is he talking incoherently perhaps as men do in their sleep? Look at him. Are his eyes open? Does he follow you with his eyes as you walk? Does he snuggle his head lower into the covers to avoid you as you approach? Are there lines on his cheek? Is his mouth open? Are there pouches under his eyes? Still you cannot tell? Well, talk to him, then, tell him his dinner is served or set the alarm clock at his head, and see how he re-acts. If you are still undecided, wait and when he gets up, ask him whether he was asleep. We know certainly how to find out whether he is asleep or not. And the same thing is true whether we ask as to whether he is now asleep or whether he was asleep.

We also have a use for the question: Are you awake? If one is awake, one may answer. The answer may then be "yes." If it turns out to be "no," there will be something suspicious about the answer. The "no" may be equivalent to yes, but I won't tell you, or may be uttered in sleep in which case the tone of the utterance may give evidence. In any case if the respondent is awake, he asks himself, "Am I awake?" and then gives the answer. I suppose that this is misleading actually. He does not ask himself since he knows and is not even curious. He simply is aware of what you want to know. On the other hand if he is asleep, your question is to be treated in the same way in which the question: Is he awake? was treated. Your asking the question, "Are you awake?" may serve in the way in which any other question or remark would serve. If there is no response or a sleepy one, then he is asleep, and you have the desired information.

The questions: Is he awake? and Are you awake? are accordingly readily intelligible. Now consider the question: Am I awake? There are certain kinds of experience, I think, in which this question is also intelligible. There is a rhetorical use of this expression with which we are all familiar, but in this use it is, of course, no longer a question. It serves in this instance simply to express one's usually grateful surprise. If today, walking along your street, you were to meet Mr. Stalin and you were at the moment convinced that this was Mr. Stalin, you might not then, as we say, believe your eyes. Your words might then be: Can this be? Am I awake or is this a dream? Your words would be Cartesian but your astonishment would be of a quite ordinary sort.

But there are also cases in which for a minute or for an instant we are genuinely puzzled and do ask: Am I awake or am I dreaming? There are experiences of waking out of a dream where the vivid peril of one's dream has not yet passed and when the safety of the real world is not yet clear, in which one may quite earnestly and fearfully and hopefully ask: Am I awake or dreaming? Then with great relief one may pat the pillow underneath one's head and greet the security of dawning light through the window. Such a question may indeed be asked with fear and trembling, and here too, fortunately, we also know how to distinguish the pit and the pendulum of our dreams from the refuge of a real bed and dear space. But notice that the question arises only when there is an awareness both of the strange encounter in the dream, and of something else vaguely distinguished in contrast with that encounter, and more definitely defined as one finds relief in one's answer. The identification of the pillow and of the familiar light through the window serve also to identify the horrors of the dream. It's like coming home after a journey, and enjoying the scene of one's habitual comfort.

There are no doubt other experiences, experiences of hallucination and delirium, in which we can well imagine questions very much like this. Macbeth's question:

> Is this a dagger which I see before me,
> The handle towards my hand?
>   . . . . .
> Art thou not, fatal vision, sensible
> To feeling as to sight? or art thou but
> A dagger of the mind, a false creation,
> Proceeding from the heat-oppressed brain?

is of this sort. Am I suffering an hallucination, or is this a real dagger? But once more the question is to be understood as arising from Macbeth's own recognition of a strangeness in this apparition in contrast with the familiar order of the furnishings of his affairs. And he makes up his mind in a moment:

> There's no such thing.

Macbeth does not treat the question as a philosophical puzzle. If he had, of course, there would have been no play. Had Macbeth cogitated further and concluded with: "At this moment it does indeed seem to me that it is with eyes awake that I am looking at this dagger. . . . But . . .," he would not have murdered sleep.

We are now prepared to examine Descartes' question: Am I awake or am I asleep? What prompts the question is first of all nothing like what prompts the question in any of these other cases. It isn't because he is lying down in a posture suitable to sleep that he becomes curious about himself, as though he wanted, for instance, to know so that he would not disturb himself with any noise. It isn't either that he has been asleep and has dreamed and has not fully recovered the assurance of his return to the substantial springs and mattress under him and the blue ceiling over him. There is no present fading dream, and no present emerging real world. And, of course, there is no vision, fatal or otherwise, that puzzles him. What, then, provokes the question? Nothing but the awareness of a certain fact, namely, that one may have dreamed something very much like what one now perceives to be the fact.

Now let us try the question in the ordinary sense to see how

Descartes might have gotten on with it. Either now Descartes is awake or he is asleep. Let us suppose first of all that he is awake. He is awake, sitting before the fire, etc., and he asks himself with a perfectly serious face: Am I awake? The question seems a little foolish, but let us treat it as though it were not foolish. By analogy with the question: Is he awake? he may try out the suggestions above. He may ask: Are my eyes closed? Am I snoring? Is my breathing like that of one asleep? etc. To all of these questions his answer is: No. Now if he is still uneasy he may call the landlady and ask her these questions. What she can discover will also be evidence. There is, in any case, no reason why Descartes could not answer his question. There is no puzzle. But if this will still not do, he may try the kinds of questions which the man waking from a dream tries: Is this the one-armed chair I always sit awake in? Of course. Is that the fireplace I throw twigs in? Throw a twig in. See it burn. If I shout will the landlady come in to bring me tea? Do. She did. And so on. It's the same old world, furnished with the same pleasant useful things. I am awake! Oh joy! Descartes is awake, and he knows it in the way in which we do discover facts of this kind.

Now let us suppose that Descartes is asleep. Now he asks: Am I asleep? It must be remembered, of course, that if he asks this, and is asleep, that he must be asking this in a dream, and must be asking this about what he is dreaming of. Accordingly he must be dreaming of himself as either awake or dreaming. But now obviously the nature of the test will not be different from the case in which he asked the question, being awake. Hence if Descartes is clearheaded as he asks the question and sets out in his dream to examine the Descartes he is dreaming of, that Descartes must furnish the evidence. Are his eyes open? Is he snoring? etc. We need not rehearse the nature of the relevant evidence. Everything depends upon the use of the expressions: Am I awake or asleep? and what one asks, being awake or asleep, will make no difference at all. It is clear then that if Descartes were using these expressions as they are ordinarily used, there is no reason why he should not readily find the answer to his question.

What I am mainly interested in pointing out is precisely that

Descartes' use of the expression: Am I awake or asleep? is not ordinary, and that his own unresolved puzzlement arises from this fact. The explanation is, I think, simple. It will be noticed that in all these common uses of this expression, the context in which the question arises involves the distinction of the real world, what Descartes introduced originally as the fact that I am here, etc. The question: Is he asleep? presupposes the real bulk of him prone on the couch, with eyes closed, a loose mouth, snoring facility, couch, pillow, etc.? The question: Am I awake? in the same way presupposes the familiar scene to be recognized, one's long snuggled pillow, the window and the peering light at the left, the swish of elm boughs outside, the screen, etc. How does Macbeth intend to test "the false creation"? By getting his hands on it. He is sure enough of his hands. His hands are not the stuff that dreams are made of. This, then, the real world, furnishes the criteria by which waking and sleeping are determined.

Doesn't Descartes then know all this? When Descartes asks: Am I awake? doesn't he know that open eyes are an indication that he is awake? Yes, he knows. This isn't news to him. He says "it does indeed seem to me that it is with eyes awake. . . ." The trouble now is that he cannot tell whether his eyes are open or not. True, they seem to be open, but that is not enough. Why then doesn't he throw a twig in the fire, finger his dressing gown, call the landlady? This won't help. For, for any test proposed, it will call forth the same story. "It does indeed seem to me" that I throw a chip on the fire, that this is my dressing gown, my fingers, and that the landlady said: Why, of course, Etienne (she never got my name right), your eyes are open. Clearly Descartes has abandoned the original distinction, the fact that I am here, etc., and the fact that I dreamed that I am here, etc., upon the basis of which he elaborated his argument. In order to find out whether he is awake or not, he must depend upon facts of the sort he began with. He continues however to use language which is significant only in terms of the distinctions which he has abandoned. The questions "Am I awake?" "Am I asleep?" are questions about bodies. Since he has ruled out bodies as within the range of the application of these terms, his language is now meaningless.

Had Descartes asked the question: Am I alive? or Am I dead? the same difficulty would have become evident. Am I alive? Feel of your heart. Breathe over a mirror. Walk. Talk. Still Descartes cannot tell. Why not? Because he cannot get at his heart. Mirrors are always behind seemings, and Descartes can never break through. He appears to walk and seems to talk, but real walking and talking are, if they are, beyond the veil. If Descartes had asked: Do I seem to be alive? he might very well have answered that question, but in the former case too he did not ask: Do I seem to be awake? or more precisely: Does the seeming I, seem to be awake? Here is another way of getting at the point. Descartes asks: Am I awake? The expression "awake" we have discussed. Now what does "I" apply to? If it applies to body, then the question presupposes what Descartes intends not to assert, namely the existence of body. But in that case, as has been pointed out above, the question can be answered easily enough. If on the other hand it refers not to body but to the self or mind, thinking substance, then what are the criteria of waking and sleeping thinking substances? Either the expressions employed here have no application, or once more the answers are easily forthcoming. Is a waking thinking substance, one which is active, asking such a question as: Am I awake? If so, Descartes is awake.

Descartes declared that he was lost in astonishment, and this is equivalent to saying that he was both lost and astonished. He writes as though he was lost because, the facts being what they are, he was incapable of distinguishing what he perceived and what was really so, from what he merely dreamed. Actually his starting point refutes this explanation. If Descartes was lost, this is rather because in thinking about "the fact" and his dream, he was misled into employing language under conditions stipulated by his own misgivings, such that the language so employed ceased to have any meaning. And this language is in this instance sufficient to give anyone a whirl. For the language itself is not at all suspicious. It is simple, ordinary language. "Am I awake or am I asleep?" But the condition defines the question in such a way that you must answer the question without employing the senses at all. You must not look or listen or ask anyone any questions. You must not suppose that there is any body to examine. Did the man commit murder? Oh, yes. And the body? There was none.

In what precedes, I have tried to discover what it is in Descartes' argument that makes it seem so convincing and yet convinces no one. My discovery then is this: What is crucial in the language of the argument has, by way of Descartes' philosophical misgiving, been cut off from all significance. Until this is understood, it may seem that Descartes' predicament is a predicament of ignorance, that he actually does not know whether he is awake or asleep. Once it is understood, however, one may also understand one's weakness, one's wilting, before this ghost question: Am I awake or am I asleep? and having recognized the ghost one may say: Booh! Then one may sit by the fire and twirl the tassels of one's dressing gown in confidence. It must be remembered that I have not dealt with the larger subject, skepticism of the senses. I have confined myself to a study of Descartes' argument.

2

MARGARET MACDONALD

Sleeping and Waking

"There exist", lamented Descartes, "no certain marks by which the state of waking may be distinguished from sleep." [1] This is disastrous because in sleep occur "those painted representations . . . in the likeness of realities" [2] which men call dreams and mistake for their originals. They finally discredit the plain man's belief in the existence of an external world which can be known by perception. Mistaken waking perceptions begin its discredit and the process of liquidation is completed by dreaming. Waking illusions and hallucinations deceive, but in dreams everything deceives. One, therefore, who dreams that he is in New York when he is, in fact, asleep in bed in London ought never to trust his senses again. It is useless for him to protest that after dreaming he wakes, for he must prove that he does not dream that he wakes and that what he perceives after waking is not another dream. Since he cannot do this, and, indeed, neither Descartes nor any other philosopher has given the slightest, intelligible hint of what would constitute such a proof, he is condemned to incurable scepticism of the senses.

I wish to challenge two assumptions in this slide. (1) The assumption that waking illusions and hallucinations constitute

Reprinted from *Mind,* 72 (1953), 202–215, by permission of the publisher (Basil Blackwell, Oxford).
1. *First Meditation. A Discourse on Method etc.* Everyman edition, p. 81.
2. *Ibid.*

with dreams a progressively degenerating perceptual series differing only in degree of deception. (2) The assumption that dreams are 'painted' or any other kind of representation of what is perceived or experienced when awake. I admit that, in some sense, these are both very natural assumptions. Indeed, the almost universal agreement of philosophical and other reflective literature on the question seems to show that there is a practically irresistible temptation to treat dreaming as a form of illusory perception and dreams, like illusions, as counterfeit physical realities. Both these assumptions are profoundly mistaken. They are excused by certain similarities in ordinary discourse about dream and waking experience. But these have been so stressed as to conceal far more important differences. I shall argue that neither the logic of discourse about waking realities and illusions nor that of their representations applies to dreams. Nor, in consequence, the distinction between 'appearance' and 'reality'; 'seems' or 'looks to be' and 'is' and the parallel distinction between 'good' and 'bad' imitation. In short, that none of the criteria appropriate to waking life apply to dreams. The failure to realise, or the ignoring of this by philosophers has caused much confusion of the Cartesian kind in the philosophy of perception. I shall, then, begin by discussing some important differences between waking illusions and dreams. I include among waking illusions both those perceptions of an object as it appears but is not and those completely hallucinatory. By "dreams" I refer only to what occurs during sleep. I exclude day dreams and waking imagery.

One glaring difference between dreams and waking illusions is that the latter, except perhaps for the totally insane, occur in a context of real objects with which they can be compared. Normally, not all waking experience is equally delusive. (It is because it is so for the completely insane that they must be protected.) The distant mountain looks small and blue through the haze, though it is over 4,000 feet high and covered with vegetation. To the right is something which may be a rock or a goat, I am not sure which. But at my feet is green grass, above hot sun and just ahead a tree which offers shade. About the existence and qualities of these objects there is no doubt. The stick *looks* but is not *really* bent in the water, but the water *is* and does not merely *feel* wet to an immersed hand. But may not the colours of all objects be distorted by wearing, e.g. brown spectacles? True, but their shapes, tactual and other qualities are unaffected. Similarly, the rattle of the train may compete for attention with the hallucinatory voices of imaginary persecutors. A real companion will confirm the first but not the second. The visionary Banquo is compared by the guilty Macbeth with his astonished flesh and blood guests, their abandoned meal and the familiar furniture of the banqueting hall. Moreover, an illusion or hallucination very often (though not, perhaps, always) fits into its context. The objects seen through brown spectacles are not all brown, but they all have some colour and it could have been brown. Either a rock or a goat might equally, well be in a field. There are bent sticks as well as straight sticks which look bent in water. Banquo might have entered alive, but battered, after fighting with his assailants. There could be a lake on the horizon though what is seen happens to be a mirage. From which it follows that the objects of illusory waking perception are, in some sense, located among the real objects which form their context. It is perfectly sensible to compare the apparent size of the distant mountain with the real size of the tree near at hand; to assert that the hallucinatory voices come from behind the victim or whisper in his right ear; that Banquo's ghost crossed the room and took his place at the table. True, there are differences. A camera will record the relative shapes and sizes of mountain and tree much as they are perceived; the bent appearance of the stick in water; the object which may be rock or goat, but it will not record Banquo's ghost. Nor will a microphone transmit the voices of imaginary persecutors. Nevertheless, whatever distinctions may be made between perceptual and physical space, or between different uses of the word 'place'; for the unsophisticated perceiver illusory objects certainly appear among and in spatial relations to other perceived objects.

None of this applies to dreams. The contents of dreams do not appear in a context of real objects, for there are none. It makes sense to say, "Banquo's ghost appeared at the banquet" but it would be nonsense to say "My dream of Westminster Abbey appeared between the window and the wardrobe". Correct expressions of such an experience would be, "I dreamed that Westminster Abbey was between my window and wardrobe" or "In my dream Westminster Abbey appeared there". For the contents of my dreams are not contents of my room. In fact, dreams are rarely of the place in which the dreamer is dreaming. But even when they are, they are not that place and their contents are not the objects nor in any spatial or other relation to the objects of that or any other place. 'In a dream' is a tricky phrase which helps to create this confusion. My wardrobe is in my bedroom; the stick looked bent, in a stream; the hallucinatory mouse ran, across a carpet. All these descriptions inform one of the whereabouts of certain perceived objects. But to the question, "Where did you meet Bernard Shaw?" the answer, 'in a dream' would be silly. It locates no meeting place. A dream is not a queer kind of stream, carpet or banqueting hall in which one may meet either real or illusory objects. No dream is a place. But neither is it not a place. 'In a dream' is not equivalent to 'No-where'. Rather is it nonsensical to ascribe the contents of a dream to a dream as their place. It is highly significant that for the adverbial phrase 'in a dream' one can always substitute some part of the verb 'to dream'. "I saw Westminster Abbey in a dream" is equivalent to "I dreamed that I saw Westminster Abbey". This sort of equivalence does not hold of proper adverbs of place. "I met him in Africa" cannot be alternatively expressed by "I Africa-met him". There may appear to be idioms which refute this. "I put the apples in a box" may, e.g. be expressed by "I boxed the apples". But then one will find that the verb disguises a reference to place. "I boxed the apples" means "I put the apples in a box" because 'boxed' = 'put in a box'. But "I dreamed" does not mean "I placed something in a dream". It does mean "I experienced something in a dream" or (another alternative) 'while dreaming'. These translations show that 'in a dream' is utterly different from 'in a place'. Similar differences exist for time references. When I dream (in April, 1952) that I win a fortune on the Derby (in June, 1952) do I win a fortune in April, when I dream, or in June, when the race is run? The answer is that neither makes sense. All that is true is that I have a certain dream on a certain date but that neither clocks nor fails to clock, its incidents. It is absurd to ask when they occur. Some people may prefer to say that the notions of space and time are very different in dreams and in waking life. So be it. I wish only to stress how very different they are. So different that 'I dreamed', 'in a dream', 'when dreaming', seem much more properly classified as indications of state than of place and time.

Dreams and waking illusions also differ in respect of confirmation. Not only are waking illusions compared with their neighbouring real objects but there are recognised ways of testing their character and when and where they exist. One removes coloured spectacles and sees the real colours of objects; walks to the mountain and finds its proper size; investigates the doubtful object and discovers whether rock or goat; tries, without avail, to strike the visionary Banquo; watches the cat sit down in the place in which the hallucinatory mouse appears; notices that the imaginary voices began again, as usual, at 9 a.m. In short, there are procedures for determining whether any waking perception is veridical or illusory. One perception is checked or corrected by others. These procedures may not have been precisely formulated, but neither are they haphazard and without any order or rule and they are constantly and deliberately employed when a perception is doubted. "Is this a dagger that I see before me? Let me try to clutch it. I cannot, so it is not." He tries to touch in order to prove that the object is, or is not, real. *This is logically impossible in a dream.* It is not that it is much more difficult to determine whether what is perceived in dream is real or illusory; that one is too tired, vague and confused; but rather that it makes no sense to assert that one could employ any confirming technique in a dream. For one would but dream such employment. It would be absurd to say, "I dreamed that I saw King's College Chapel but on looking more closely I discovered that it was really Westminster Abbey". What can be meant by 'looking more closely' and 'discovering' that one was mistaken in a dream? Only, surely, that one dreamed that one looked and discovered and a dream cannot bear witness for or against itself. The answer to this has always seemed obvious. Admittedly, while dreaming, one cannot confirm that Westminster Abbey and not King's College

Chapel was perceived but on waking up one finds that neither was present. What is perceived after waking proves the unreality of what is dreamed. "Thank goodness", we exclaim, on waking from nightmare, "it was only a dream". But I suggest that this obvious answer is wrong. For it assumes that 'waking up' is a method of proof, which is very queer. When was it learned and what are its rules? We learn from experience, example, tuition the procedures, already mentioned, for testing perceptual validity. These are refined upon in scientific theory and practice and chosen for their success as means to the end of obtaining empirical knowledge. But no one chose or was instructed by his teachers to wake up as the best method of making experiments. Waking up is not done by rule, in order to get information or for any other conscious purpose. "First make sure you are awake" does not occur on the first page of text books of methodology as a fundamental principle of scientific method. Waking, like sleeping, is a process of nature, not of logic. Indeed, how could 'waking up' be a procedure for testing perceptions? For such procedures are designed to show what exists and where, at the time of testing. Testing an illusory perception substitutes now the real for an apparent quality of an object; a real for an apparent object in the same context. The real colour, size, shape, etc. of an object *are,* now, roughly, where its apparent colour, size, shape, etc., *appear;* some other object *is* now where an illusory object *appears;* air, and not a dagger or ghost; sand, not water; carpet but no snakes. So it is perfectly sensible to say, "I thought the mountain could not be as low as it looked from a distance, so I went nearer and found that it was very high" [3] or "It looked like a dagger so I tried to grasp it but met only empty air" but it would be absurd to say "I dreamed that I saw the Eiffel Tower so I awoke and found it

3. I admit difficulties about some of these cases, especially about place and position. E.g., how can a high mountain be said to occupy the same place as that in which a low mountain appears? Does this not require a distinction between different kinds of space, e.g. physical and perceptual? I think, however, I may ignore these refinements for my present purpose. I will observe only that no-one would ordinarily say that the mountain was in a different place from that in which it differently appears. One approaches the same place from which it appears small and is found to be large. Nor does it move or would be said literally to grow (and so come to occupy a larger place) during this journey. No difficulties are solved by multiplying spaces.

was only the bedpost". For the bedpost was not being misperceived when I dreamed that I saw the Eiffel Tower, nor did the Eiffel Tower appear where the bedpost now *is*. The bedpost, as W. S. Gilbert might say, "has nothing to do with the case". The drunkard may console himself with "No, there isn't a real snake on the carpet, it is only one of my turns" but the dreamer cannot wake to exclaim, "Thank goodness, there isn't a real corpse on the floor". For the dream corpse never was on the floor to which he wakes and the murder may have been dreamed to occur ten years ago and not five minutes before he wakes on Friday, 18th April, 1952. So if there is no 'it' here and now of which one can say "It seemed to be something else" there is nothing which waking up can confirm. When a dreamer wakes his dream vanishes and its contents cannot, therefore, be checked for they no longer exist in any context for comparison. They may be remembered but not corrected. Dreams are thus incorrigible by waking experience. Since they are not corrigible by dream experience it seems to follow that they are totally incorrigible. But, again, what rather seems true is that dreams are neither corrigible nor incorrigible; the notion of corrigibility cannot significantly be applied to dreams. They neither conform nor fail to conform to criteria of physical reality. Consequently, they do not appear or seem to be what they are not and so do not qualify for the categories of either perceptual appearance or reality. In this dreams differ fundamentally from waking illusions which are opposed as appearances to physical realities. For one means by 'waking illusion' an object which is perceived to be or to be a quality of, a physical object and is found by subsequent experience to be a fraud.

This difference may be shown in reverse. A waking illusion is a perception which may lead to error. True, it need not always do so. One may become wary and refuse to be deceived. The experienced traveller and even the experienced drunkard cease to be taken in by mirages and pink rats. They are, so to say, disillusioned. But deception is always possible from the nature of what is perceived. It appears so like what it is not. Weaker, or less sophisticated, percipients succumb without resistance. Rash, foolish or prejudiced they fail to get the right answer they intend from experience. I did not want to take the wrong bus when too tired or lazy to distinguish '8' from '2'. I intended to get the right one and was shocked to find myself at Piccadilly Circus instead of Victoria. I should have known better and could have avoided my mistake and thus the inconvenience. Even when a mistake is not my fault, when an illusion is rare or unfamiliar to me, I wish I had been forewarned so that I could have guarded against error by being more alert, wary, dispassionate. To be deceived by a waking illusion is to be frustrated in a genuine attempt to know what exists. This cannot sensibly be said to occur in dreams. A dreamer is not trying, and failing, to be right about what he dreams. When he dreams that he sees, touches and even enters Westminster Abbey he is not failing, despite his best efforts, to achieve an intended visit to Westminster Abbey. He is not trying to do something right and getting it wrong. So he cannot be reproached for being so foolish as to imagine that he could visit Westminster Abbey in a dream. To dream what one dreams is neither wise nor foolish; successful nor unsuccessful. No precautions can be taken against it, except, perhaps, that of remaining permanently awake. According to Descartes a dreamer supposes that what he dreams are real objects and incidents and is thus deceived. But this is false. At most a dreamer may dream that he affirms the reality of what he dreams. But he is not deceived even in so doing since he cannot be undeceived. Nor can he be cautious and clever in guarding against error in his dreams nor lucky in being right without taking such precautions. Just as waking up is not a method of discovery, so falling asleep is not falling into error. "I dreamt that I dwelt in marble halls" does not imply "I then (or ever) did dwell in marble halls" but neither does it imply, still less mean the same as, "I mistakenly believed that I dwelt in marble halls". For, as in the converse situation of waking up, what rule has been broken, test omitted or misapplied which constitutes this mistake? When in waking life Macbeth believes that the visionary Banquo is real he believes that something which he sees could also be touched, fed, warmed, argued with and he is wrong. But no such tests can be applied in dreams and this is part of what is asserted by "I dreamt". This inability to apply tests is logical, not physical or psychological. But when it is logically impossible that tests which prevent or correct mistake should be applied then it is nonsensical to assert that mistake can occur. No-one can be deceived where no distinction can be made between what is and is not deceptive. A dreamer is thus neither correct nor mistaken about what he dreams. While dreaming, a dreamer cannot significantly be said to know or truly or mistakenly believe any proposition about the contents of his dreams. But a person can, and very often does, assert false propositions about his illusory waking perceptions.

I have indicated probably only some of the differences between dreams and waking illusions which could be unveiled. There are also many differences within waking illusions, to consider which would take me too far from my main task. Undoubtedly, the philosophical dump labelled 'Illusions' contains a great variety of displaced perceptions. This brief discussion has, however, I hope, shown that much which can be significantly said of waking illusions cannot be said of dreams and conversely. Or, in other words, that the use of 'dream' differs in ways important for philosophers to note from that of words for waking illusions. Indeed, it may be thought too much has been proved, too great difference shown. For, according to me, it is senseless to affirm that what is dreamed is either illusory or real or that one can or cannot be mistaken about it. This sounds a strange conclusion. One thinks, if I dream of a snake my dream must contain, if not a snake then an illusory or pretence snake. For do I not perceive something snake-like and is not this fact the reason for Descartes' doubt? My answer is that whether or not something is real depends upon what is meant by 'real'. There is nothing which is real in general. 'Real' by itself has no meaning. But there are significant, particular uses of this word and what does not conform to the criteria for these uses is, in relation to them, unreal. 'Snake' is used for a certain kind of physical object. What might, but does not, conform to the criteria of physical reality is not a real physical object, e.g. a real snake. It is, therefore, correctly termed an illusory, i.e. an unreal object of that kind. But none of the criteria of physical reality can sensibly be applied to dreams. In dreams anything may happen; nothing is ruled out. So the question whether what one dreams is a real or illusory physical object is quite unanswerable. The conditions for answering it do not exist. But, if so, how were philosophers, like Descartes, misled into classifying dreams with illusions? Why did it seem inevitable or even plausible, to conclude that though waking illusions discredit, dreams totally destroy the realiability of sense perception? How did anyone ever come to connect veridical perceptions, illusions, hallucinations and dreams? What could tempt philosophers to slide into total scepticism of the senses?

The main source of this temptation is contained in a previous question, "When I dream of a snake do I not perceive something snake-like?" It is due to the fact that many sentences which describe dreams resemble those which describe waking perceptions by sharing the common vocabulary of sensation-verbs; 'see,' 'hear,' 'touch,' 'smell,' etc. So that the following statements might all be true: "I saw a rabbit"; "I thought I saw a rabbit but found I was mistaken"; "I dreamed that I saw a rabbit." A subsidiary cause is the fact that, after waking, one can, and often does, remember dreams and compare these memories with waking perceptions. So, it is argued, if I sometimes perceive or seem to perceive a physical object and can remember and describe what I dream in perceptual terms then I must have been perceiving and perceiving some perceptible object when I dreamed. If not, why should I use the vocabulary of sensation? But if I was perceiving in dreams and find on waking that there was nothing to perceive how do I know that what I perceive when awake is not also a dream and so by what right do I ever trust my senses? Descartes' proof that the state of waking cannot be distinguished from sleep depends upon these facts (a) that dreams are remembered (b) that what is so remembered resembles an object or combination of objects perceived when awake.[4] Thus, noticing that it is in fact very difficult for him to doubt that he is sitting before a fire, clad in a dressing gown, writing the Meditations, he "cannot forget" that he has often believed in dreams that he was "in these same familiar circumstances" and woken to find himself deceived.[5] So, how can he be sure that he is not always deceived? The answer to part of this should now be plain. The criteria of 'real' and 'il-

4. *Loc. cit.*   5. *Ibid.*

lusory' physical object which apply to the perceptions of waking life do not apply to the contents of dreams. So that when "we, in dreams, behold the Hebrides", it is neither true nor false that the Hebrides exist. Nor are we being deceived or not deceived about them. Words which are the complements of sensation verbs function differently when used of dreams and of any objects perceived in waking life. But so also do the sensation verbs. From the fact that I saw the Hebrides in a dream it does not follow that I *saw* any more than that which I saw was the Hebrides. Nor does it follow that I seemed to see or thought I saw but later found that I was mistaken, found that I was having an image or some other sensation. For, as with the objects of a dream, no such correction can be made during or after dreaming. So that it makes no sense to say either that one perceives or does not perceive in a dream. Some people again may prefer to say that this shows only that sensation verbs and their complements are used differently of dreams and the objects of waking perception. For example, some philosophers will say that what I perceive when I dream that I see the Hebrides is a sense datum of or related to the Hebrides. They also say that whenever I perceive what I directly perceive or am acquainted with is a sense datum and that the difference between dreaming and other forms of perception consists in the difference of relation between dream and other sense data and physical objects. This relation, however, has never been explained. Or, they distinguish two senses of 'perceive,' *viz.* perceive$_1$ or "directly perceive" in which one perceives all sense data, including the contents of dreams, and perceive$_2$ in which one perceives physical objects and this will not apply to dreams.[6] But, again, apart from the fact that no one has yet clearly explained how perceive$_1$ applies to all perception, including that of physical objects, to suppose that it does so apply blurs too much the distinction between dreaming of and perceiving objects. It is very true that sensation verbs and their complements are used differently of dreams and in other contexts. But also the same words are used. The question is whether these uses can be more than exemplified, whether any attempt to characterise

6. Cf., for example, G. E. Moore, "The Status of Sense Data" and "Some Judgments of Perception", *Phil. Studies*, pp. 168, 220 ff.

them further results, in effect, in their assimilation to each other or to those of another type. Again, when Descartes asks how he can be sure he is not always dreaming he seems to ask for a crucial experiment to determine an infallible mark of separation between the states of waking and sleeping. But in what state is such an experiment to be performed? If in either that of waking or sleeping this presupposes that its result is already known. Descartes gives no hint of a possible third state. He is obviously operating with the model of an experiment in waking life to determine between two theories which appear to explain the same facts. But the analogy fails. For it is logically impossible to perform such an experiment in respect of the state in which and only in which all experiments whatever can be performed. He may also be interpreted as trying to identify the use of the sensory vocabulary for dreams with (a) its use for physical objects and waking illusions, (b) with idioms appropriate to pictures, stories, plays and similar forms of representation. For, he suggests, if what are perceived in dreams are not physical objects they must—like illusions—be shams, forgeries or fictions—'painted representations' of realities. I have tried to show that the first identification leads to nonsense. I will now discuss the second.

According to this, then, which is a very common interpretation and not confined to Descartes, if I did not behold the Hebrides in a dream and must have seen *something,* this could only have been a picture or likeness of the Hebrides. But, a fact which Descartes and others have tended to overlook, one is not always a passive spectator in dreams. One dreams of travelling, eating meals, holding conversations with others, engaging in many and often violent activities. Perhaps the relative immobility of philosophers when writing about perception has led them to treat dreams as sheer spectacles of which the only valid questions to ask are, "Is it a real scene?" or "Is it a fair copy?". But dreams are often more like dramas in which the dreamer plays a leading role than presentations which he contemplates. However, its defenders could accept this extension without substantially modifying their view that dreams are substitute or imitation realities. Dreams are a copy or enactment of the objects and incidents of waking life. Professor Ryle has pointed out that the 'copy' metaphor is inapplicable to waking imagery.[7] The grammar of 'picture', 'representation', 'fake', 'imitation', is quite different from that of 'image'. A picture, copy or any other kind of duplicate, however cleverly and carefully executed, can always be distinguished from its original or it would not be a copy but the original. Copies have their own peculiar characteristics. They are executed in a certain material, with paints on canvas, in plastic instead of leather, recorded on a wax disc, worm-holed by a gimlet and not by termites. None of these is a characteristic of images. To try to stretch the analogy by inventing an ethereal, mental material from which copies are produced by a ghostly artist is just to show that the analogy has evaporated and so to talk nonsense. This is also true of dreams. If "we are such stuff as dreams are made on" the poet does not disclose the nature of this material. The same lack of analogy also exists between dreams and the enactment of actual or imagined incidents from real life. Despite their feeling of activity dreams are no more dramas than pictures. Dream scenes are not pasteboard stage 'sets'; no lanthorn "doth the hornéd moon present". Dreams do not take place on a stage, in a theatre, nor are their participants, including the dreamer, performing players. These may be thought trivial objections. 'Drama' and 'dramatic performance' are vague terms applied to a widely varying family of histrionic forms. Surely one may compare dreams to dramas without requiring that they conform to all the paraphernalia of full-scale theatrical performance? I do not deny this, but my point is different and more general. The analogy attempted by all these comparisons is between dreams and, roughly, the arts and crafts. Pictures, plays, novels, even fakes and forgeries have to be made and some of them produced and performed. I have said that dreams do not conform to the standards of reality. But the arts also have their standards and canons. Even the expert forger prides himself on a decent job. But dreams are not produced by a dreamer trying to achieve artistic merit. They are not artefacts. Nor would it be appropriate to praise or condemn them by the canons of art criticism or craftsmanship. Most dreams, I suspect, would

7. Cf. *The Concept of Mind,* Chapter VIII.

hardly qualify as pictures for the walls of a village schoolroom or as theatre for the repertoire of the feeblest company of barnstormers. But even if they were as perfect as a Cézanne canvas or as a play of Racine performed by the stars of the Comédie Française they still would not fulfil nor fail to fulfil the conditions of art any more than those of reality. For they have neither function. One no more falls asleep in order to become an artist or craftsman than to become a scientist or ignoramus. Works of art, like Kubla Khan, may be suggested by dreams but they are not dream compositions. For to compose or create a work of art is to produce a certain result from deliberate intent with appropriate materials and in accordance with artistic criteria. Dreams may have subconscious causes; they do not have conscious aims. 'Bad dreams' are not bad because they are bad imitations or inferior works of art. Dreams have no standards. Or, rather, it is senseless to apply the notion of standards to dreams.

Another way of expressing the view here criticised might be to say that what happens in dreams is that one has images or imagines that one sees the Hebrides or takes part in a fight. Professor Ryle seeks to assimilate 'having images' to imagining, fancying, pretending rather than to looking at pictures.[8] It seems plausible to apply this to dreams. But though Professor Ryle's interpretation may be correct for waking imaging and day dreaming it is, nevertheless, not applicable to dreams. A person who dreams that he is climbing a mountain or seeing the Hebrides is not properly described as fancying, pretending or imagining that he is climbing a mountain or seeing the Hebrides. For it always makes sense to say that fancying, pretending, imagining, like producing or contemplating works of art, can be controlled. One may choose to begin or end them. An artist, like Leonardo da Vinci, may abandon most of his works before completion. Likewise, a person may 'shake himself out of' a day dream and start to do something more useful. True, he may not always succeed. If he is insane, neurotically obsessed, hysterical or, perhaps, in some very peculiar circumstances, like dangling from a parachute over a raging sea, he

8. *Loc. cit.*

may not, in fact, be able to control his imaginings any more than his terrors. But I think, though I am not absolutely certain of this, that it does make sense to say that he could control both, if he chose, and that it is *logically possible* that he should choose. Perhaps total insanity is an exception. But I am inclined to think that it is senseless to say that a person could choose to start or stop dreaming when he is asleep. My reason for this is the one which I have cited before, that once asleep, a dreamer can only dream that he makes such a choice. "I dreamed that I chose to dream or stop dreaming" does not, according to me, imply that I chose or that I did not choose but only that I *dreamed* that I chose, which is different. I admit that one sometimes dreams of saying "I will go on with this" and sometimes the dream continues or "I will stop this one" and the dream changes or one awakes. But these seem to me very different from deciding to continue or abandon a train of thought, a problem, a composition in waking life. No one is held responsible for dream choices, praised or blamed for them and their consequences. Suppose someone says, "I had a terrifying experience last night; I imagined (fancied) that I was falling (pretended to fall) down a precipice; it was horrible". One would be a little surprised, even contemptuous and might reply, "Well, why did you not stop fancying, imagining, pretending if it frightened you so much? Since you are not mad you were not obliged to continue." But he retorts, "You don't understand. I had a nightmare of falling." One would become much more sympathetic. "Why did you not say so at first? A nightmare is different. You can't help that and it may be terrifying. But you first said that you were only making believe." One normally thinks very differently of the day dreamer and the sufferer from 'bad dreams'. Not even a psycho-analyst expects a person wilfully to change or end his dreams. So far as is known, a dreamer will wake up when the dream has ceased to 'guard sleep' and that is not of his own free will. If this is so, it does indicate a fundamental logical difference between what can be said of dreams and of the fancies, imaginings and pretences which occur when awake. Moreover, "I imagined, fancied, pretended that p" implies that p either was or could have been discovered to be otherwise. But what is dreamed is not and cannot be later found otherwise than as dreamed. So on two counts, at least, dreaming must be distinguished from imagining, fancying and pretending.

To conclude. Philosophers have wrongly tried to assimilate dreaming to the waking perception of real and illusory physical objects; to the creation, construction and contemplation of pictures and other representations and to waking imaginative experience, though, perhaps, the last two are alternative expressions of the same state. All these identifications break down and lead to philosophical puzzles including that of scepticism of the senses which afflicted Descartes. What philosophers have overlooked is the peculiar significance of the verb 'to dream' which affects the logical status of all expressions used with it to describe what is dreamed. What is asserted by and is logically important in such statements as, "I dreamed that I perceived (did, chose, etc.) . . ." is not that I perceived, did, chose, etc. but that "I *dreamed* that. . . ." Philosophers have tended to emphasise the subordinate clause at the expense of the rest of the sentence. To shift the emphasis to the main clause may help to show that what is asserted by the subordinate statement when used independently is quite different from what is asserted when it is subordinated to any part of the verb "to dream" or is used with any cognate expression referring to a dream state. This is shown by differences in what is implied by each type of assertion. So that what can be significantly said of what is done outside dreams cannot be so said of what is dreamed even though similar expressions may be used of both. Having realised this, one may admit that dreams link up with waking states; that they occur to those who perceive physical objects and act and suffer in the external world, but their contents are not physical objects or states nor copies or reproductions of them nor anything else but *dreams.*

I have tried, then, to show some of the ways in which the use of 'dream' differs from that of other words with which it has been confused. I suggest that these differences destroy the need for Descartes' lament that "there exist no certain marks by which the state of waking may be distinguished from sleep." For if what is said of one state is nonsensical when applied to the other, then this provides at least one certain mark by which to distinguish between them. I have not attempted to give an exhaustive account of the grammar of any of these words nor completely to unravel their entanglement by philosophers of perception.

3

R. M. YOST, JR., *and* DONALD KALISH

Miss Macdonald on Sleeping and Waking

Since the publication of Descartes' *Meditations,* many writers
on epistemology have claimed that the phenomena of dreams
compel us to believe that some sensa do not belong to physical
objects. The surface of a dream hand, they would say, is not
part of the surface of any physical object, and it is not a mental
state; physical objects and minds do not exhaust the particulars
of the world. In recent times the claim has been reflected in the
view that a physical-object language will not allow us to talk
about dreams, and that this defect can be remedied only by
supplementing a physical-object language with a sensum-
language. No one has welcomed this doubling-up of things and
languages. Those who have thought it necessary have regarded
it as a necessary evil. It is not surprising, therefore, that there
have been persistent efforts to find a way of talking about
dreams without having to assume the existence of vagrant
sensa and without having to use a special sensum-language.
During the past two years, some drastic measures have been
proposed as a means to this end. For example, Miss Margaret
Macdonald has advanced the view, if we understand her correctly, that although a dream is an experience, it is as different
from any waking experience as seeing is from hearing.[1] And if

Reprinted from the *Philosophical Quarterly,* 5 (1955), 109–124, by permission
of the authors and the *Philosophical Quarterly.*
1. 'Sleeping and Waking', *Mind,* April, 1953. [All page numbers refer to
Chapter 2 above—ED.]

we have understood Professor Karl Britton correctly, he has suggested that dreaming is not an experience at all, that there are only tales about dreams, but no dream experiences.[2] Proposals like these seem to be gaining acceptance.[3] If any of them is correct, sensum 'theories' will have lost one of their chief remaining supports. In our opinion, however, none of them is correct, and some other way of finishing off sensum 'theories' will have to be found. Because of the revival of interest in the relevance of dreams to epistemological problems, we have thought it worthwhile to examine one of these proposals in detail and to show precisely why, in our opinion, it is untenable.

For this purpose we have chosen to consider Miss Macdonald's view, which she set forth in a recent article entitled 'Sleeping and Waking'. Her article is especially suitable for two reasons. It is worked out in considerable detail. And it illustrates, so it seems to us, a way of philosophizing that is rather widespread today, particularly in England. Miss Macdonald philosophizes in a tradition whose chief representatives have been Professors G. E. Moore, L. Wittgenstein, John Wisdom, and G. Ryle; and like these philosophers, she is opposed to sensum 'theories'. We feel that if our comments on her article are correct, they will have some bearing on the work of authors who philosophize as she does.

In the opening lines of 'Sleeping and Waking', Miss Macdonald recites one of the sceptical conclusions of Descartes' *First Meditation,* which may be put as follows: In any single experience one may justifiably believe that perhaps one is dreaming and that none of the sensory contents of the experience is real. She then tries to show not only that Descartes failed to prove this conclusion, but also that the conclusion is false. The most important point in her refutation is the assertion that Descartes, and most of his successors, misunderstood the grammar, or 'logic', of the word 'dream'. It is our belief that Descartes did not misunderstand the 'logic' of the word 'dream', and that in spite of her efforts she has not destroyed the grounds of Car-

2. See *Proceedings of the Aristotelian Society,* Supplementary Volume XXVI, 1952, 'Symposium: Seeming', p. 208.

3. For example, see L. E. Thomas' article 'Waking and Dreaming' in *Analysis,* Vol. 13, No. 6, June, 1953, pp. 121–127.

tesian scepticism of the senses. We can best present our specific reasons for this belief by first restating Descartes' argument and Miss Macdonald's refutation of it in our own words.[4]

I. Reconstruction of Miss Macdonald's Argument

We shall put Descartes' case by means of an example. While seated in his study Descartes had an experience that led him to believe the statement 'This is a real hand' to be true. But he then recalled that while asleep the night before he had had a very similar experience, which had led him to believe the statement 'This is a real hand' to be true. But the statement he believed true while asleep was false. He was mistaken when he believed it to be true. And no matter how hard he searched his present experience and the memory of his sleeping experience, he could find no marks in them that would infallibly show which of the statements was true and which false. Moreover, while seated in his study he believed that all the contents, or objects, of his experience were real. But he again recalled that while asleep the night before he had believed that all the contents, or objects, of his sleeping experience were real; yet none of them was real. Again, his total present experience and his total sleeping experience were extremely similar, and each of them was void of any distinguishing mark that would infallibly show which of them was real. And so even though he was seated in his study, Descartes concluded that he could justifiably believe that perhaps none of the contents, or objects, of his present experience was real, that he might be mistaken in believing any of them to be real, that he might be dreaming.

Three of the premises of Descartes' argument are impugned by Miss Macdonald; they are:

(1) While dreaming, Descartes mistakenly believed the statement 'This is a real hand' to be true.

(2) His waking experience while seated in his study was *very* similar to the experience he had the night before while dreaming.

4. Miss Macdonald writes subtly and amply, and we do not presume to restate her thoughts bluntly and sparsely without some fear that we have failed to catch the drift of her refutation. All page references are to her article 'Sleeping and Waking'.

(3) In any given experience, there is no certain mark by which he could discover whether he was awake or dreaming.

If any of these premises is false, then even if Descartes' argument is valid, it does not support his sceptical conclusion. Miss Macdonald first argues that (1) is false, and then among her arguments for the falsity of (1) she finds grounds for concluding that (2) and (3) are false. We will explain her arguments against (1), (2), and (3) in that order.

1. The argument against (1) depends in large measure on the 'logics' of the three verbs 'dream', 'believe', and 'test', which will be explained in that order. It seems to us that the most important premises in her vision of the 'logic' of 'dream' are the following:

(A-   Any sentence of the form
      X dreamt that he . . . O
      where 'O' refers to part of the contents of the dream, and the blank is to be filled by a transitive verb, implies the corresponding sentence of the form

      1a) while dreaming, it is logically impossible that X . . . O
           or of the form

      1b) it is nonsensical to say of X that while dreaming he
           . . .O.[5]

(A-2) The contents of a dream do not appear in a context of real objects.

(A-3) The contents of a dream do not survive the dream in which they occur.

Miss Macdonald nowhere explicitly asserts (A-1a, b) in the generalized form presented here. She does say, however, that if one is dreaming it is logically impossible for him (nonsensical to say he is able) to touch anything,[6] to look more closely at anything,[7] to affirm anything,[8] or to choose anything.[9] We feel that she does not intend each of these remarks to be an indepen-

---

5. In her exposition Miss Macdonald seems to use 'nonsensical' and 'logically impossible' interchangeably. (See, e.g., the first passage quoted below.) Thus, to facilitate our statement of her argument we formulate (A-1) as two statements, (A-1a) and (A-1b), and in our criticism of her argument (See (II) below) attempt to determine whether (A-1a) and (A-1b) are two independent premises or two ways of saying the same thing.

6. See page 68, lines 25 and 26.   7. See page 68, lines 34–37.
8. See page 71, lines 22 and 23.   9. See page 78, lines 5–7.

dent premise, but that she would rather regard them all as special applications of (A-1a, b). She very nearly says as much in the following two passages:

'Is this a dagger that I see before me? Let me try to clutch it. I cannot, so it is not.' He tries to touch in order to prove that the object is, or is not, real. *This is logically impossible in a dream.* . . . it makes no sense to assert that one could employ any confirming technique in a dream. For one would but dream such employment.

When in waking life Macbeth believes that the visionary Banquo is real he believes that something which he sees could also be touched, fed, warmed, argued with and he is wrong. But no such tests can be applied in dreams, and this is part of what is asserted by 'I dreamt'. This inability to apply tests is logical, not physical or psychological.

Miss Macdonald's acceptance of (A-2) is embodied in the passage:

The contents of dreams do not appear in a context of real objects, for there are none. It makes sense to say, 'Banquo's ghost appeared at the banquet" but it would be nonsense to say 'My dream of Westminster Abbey appeared between the window and the wardrobe'.

And her acceptance of (A-3) is embodied in the passage:

When a dreamer wakes his dream vanishes and its contents cannot, therefore, be checked for they no longer exist in any context for comparison. They may be remembered but not corrected.

Judging from the contexts from which all these passages were taken, we should say that none of them is offered as a consequence of anything that has gone before, and hence that Miss Macdonald intended them to be premises.

The relevant point in the 'logic' of 'belief' need not be stated with respect to all kinds of beliefs but only with respect to those that are expressed by such sentences as: 'This is a real hand', 'This is Banquo', 'This is green', etc. Given that S is a sentence of this kind, the relevant point in the 'logic' of 'belief' is given by the assertion: [10]

(B) Any sentence of the form
    X believes S

10. This is how we interpret Miss Macdonald's statement on page 71, lines 39 ff.

implies the corresponding sentence of the form
    S is testable.

If one identifies meaningfulness with testability, as is usually done in the so-called "verifiability theory of meaning," then (B), if generalized for any empirical belief, asserts that one cannot believe meaningless statements.

We come now to the 'logic' of the word 'test.' Miss Macdonald often speaks of testing, or checking, the contents of experiences, whether waking or dreaming; but we take this to be an abbreviated way of discussing the testing, or checking, of statements about the contents of experiences. And we limit ourselves, as before, to statements like 'This is a real hand', 'This is Banquo', 'This is green', etc., where in each case 'this' refers demonstratively to an experienced object. As shorthand let us say that S is any statement of this kind, X is the person who utters or considers S, and O is the object of experience to which X refers demonstratively by means of 'this'. Having allowed ourselves these aids and delimitations, we can now state what seems to us to be Miss Macdonald's chief premises concerning the 'logic' of the word 'test'.

(C- S is testable only if the following conditions hold:

1) When X considers S, say at t (which may be regarded as the beginning of the test), O appears to him in a context of real objects.

2) During a short interval t-t' (the duration of the test) X is able to perform and perceive certain real confirmatory activities, and performs these activities purposely and according to appropriate rules derived from common sense or scientific manuals.

3) At t' (when the outcome of the test occurs) either O again appears to X in a context of real objects, or X perceives the real place where O appeared to him at t.

It seems to us that the requirements (C-1) through (C-3) are implied by the following passages:

Not only are waking illusions compared with their neighbouring real objects but there are recognized ways of testing their character and when and where they exist. One removes coloured spectacles and sees the real colours of objects; walks to the mountain and finds its proper size; . . . tries, without avail, to strike the visionary Banquo.

[Procedures for testing perceptions] are designed to show what exists and where, at the time of testing. Testing an illusory perception substitutes now the real for an apparent quality of an object; a real for an apparent object in the same context. The real colour, size, shape, etc. of an object *are*, now, roughly, where its apparent colour, size, shape, etc., *appear;* some other object *is* now where an illusory object *appears;* air, and not a dagger or ghost; sand, not water; carpet but no snakes. So it is perfectly sensible to say, 'I thought the mountain could not be as low as it looked from a distance, so I went nearer and found that it was very high' or 'It looked like a dagger so I tried to grasp it but met only empty air' . . . So if there is no 'it' here and now of which one can say 'It seemed to be something else' there is nothing which waking up can confirm.

Now that we have stated our understanding of the 'logics' that Miss Macdonald adopts for the words 'dream', 'believe', and 'test', let us formulate the argument in which she employs them. If (1) is true, then while dreaming Descartes considered the sentence 'This is a real hand'. In fact, anyone who held (1) could not object to the claim that a dreamer may consider any sentence normally used to express judgments of perception such as 'This is Banquo', 'This is green', etc. As before, let S be a sentence of this kind, considered while dreaming. To refute (1) Miss Macdonald wants to show that even if a dreamer did consider S, he could not believe it, either truly or mistakenly. The scheme of her argument is the following: If a dreamer believes S to be true, then S is testable; if S is testable, then either it is testable during the dream or it is testable after the dreamer wakes up; but it is not testable during the dream, and it is not testable after waking up; hence, the dreamer cannot believe S to be true, and *a fortiori* he cannot mistakenly believe S to be true. The important steps in this argument are established by applications of the 'logics' of 'dream', 'believe', and 'test'.

The first step in the argument

(4) If a dreamer believes S to be true, then S is testable

follows immediately from (B).

The next important step

(5) S is not testable during the dream

takes a little longer to establish. The dreamer believes S to be true of a certain object O that he is experiencing. O is part of the contents of his dream. If S is testable during the dream, then by (C-1) O must appear to the dreamer in a context of real objects. But by (A-2) O does not appear in a context of real objects. Furthermore, if S is testable during the dream, then by (C-2) the dreamer must be able to perform and perceive real confirmatory activities. But he is only dreaming that he perceives and performs such actions. From this and (A-1a) it follows that it is logically impossible for him to perceive at all or to perform any real confirmatory activities. Hence, (5) is true.[11]

The most difficult step in her argument is the proof of

(6) S is not testable after the dreamer wakes up

which proof falls into two parts. First, S is not tested by the event of waking up; for waking up is not done on purpose or according to appropriate rules, and therefore, by (C-2) waking up cannot be a test of any statement.[12] Secondly, S is not testable by anything that happens after the event of waking up. For suppose that the duration of the test period, t-t′, extended beyond the event of waking up. It would then be completed by some perception at t′. This perception could have a real thing or place as its object, but the thing could not be O and the place could not be the place where O appeared at t, for by (A-3) none of the dream-contents survives the dream experience. Thus, although this terminal perception might reveal the nature of some object at t′, it cannot reveal, directly or indirectly, the nature or place of O. And thus by (C-3) it cannot be a test of S.[13] Since S is tested neither by waking up nor by anything that happens after the event of waking up, (6) is true.

The steps (5) and (6) yield immediately

(7) S is not testable.

Step (7) along with (4) implies that the dreamer in question did not believe S to be true, and hence, *a fortiori,* he did not mistakenly believe S to be true. Therefore, (1) is false; that is to say, Descartes was wrong when he asserted that while dreaming

---

11. See pages 66–69 for these arguments.
12. See page 69 for this argument.   13. See page 70 for this argument.

he mistakenly believed the statement 'This is a real hand' to be true.

2. We now turn to Miss Macdonald's argument that (2) is false, that is, to her argument that no dream experience can be *very* similar to any waking experience. As we understand it, her argument depends on either (A-1b) or (A-1a), on (7), and on some points in the 'logics' of 'test', 'significant', and 'nonsensical'; these points can be expressed by the assertions:

(D-1) If a sentence is not testable, then its predicate is not significantly applicable to the thing referred to by its subject.

(D-2) If a sentence contains a non-applicable predicate, then it is nonsensical.

(D-3) If a property characterizes two different things, then it is significant to say to each that it has that property.

We now outline our interpretation of her argument.

When people talk about dream experiences they tend to use the same sentences that they use when talking about waking experiences. For example, persons often say that a dreamer did see something instead of saying that he dreamt that he saw something. That is to say, when people talk about dreamers and their experiences, they often assert sentences of the form 'X . . . O'—where the blank is filled with a transitive verb such as 'saw', 'touched', 'affirmed the reality of', and where 'O' refers to an object—instead of asserting the corresponding sentence of the form 'X dreamt that he . . . O'. But if an instance of the second form is true then by (A-1b) the corresponding instance of the first form is nonsensical. In short, sentences with verbs such as 'see', 'touch', 'affirms', etc., are nonsensical when asserted of dreamers.[14] This conclusion could also be derived as an extension of the argument used in refuting (1). For it was shown there that when sentences such as 'This is Banquo', 'This is green', etc., are asserted of the contents of dreams, they are not testable. By the same argument, *mutatis mutandis,* sentences of the form 'X . . . O' are shown to be non-testable when asserted of dreamers. It follows from this and the premises (D-1) and (D-2) that such sentences are nonsensical. In this second

14. See page 68 for an argument of this kind.

way of deriving the conclusion (A-1a), but not (A-1b), occurs as a premise.[15]

Further, when talking of a dream experience, people often say that the *object* of a dream experience, or part of its contents, was green, instead of saying that a dreamer dreamt of a green thing. That is, one often asserts a sentence whose subject denotes the object of a dream experience but whose predicate is applicable to the objects of waking experiences. If S is a sentence of this kind whose subject is a demonstrative, there could be a corresponding sentence S' whose subject is a descriptive phrase. For example, if S is 'This is green', then S' could be 'Part of the contents of the dreamer's experience was green'. We have outlined the argument that led Miss Macdonald to conclude that S is not testable; this argument, if sound, would even more readily prove that S' is not testable. Thus any sentence whose subject refers to the object of a dream experience and whose predicate is applicable to the objects of waking experiences is non-testable. Given (D-1) and (D)-2), it follows that such sentences are nonsensical.

Thus, all sentences in which certain waking verbs are applied to dreamers are nonsensical, and all sentences in which waking adjectives are applied to dream objects are nonsensical. There may be other kinds of sentences whose subjects refer either to dreamers or to the objects of dream experiences. But anyone who has agreed with Miss Macdonald so far would probably be willing to concede that after she had examined such sentences it would turn out, generally, that

(8) What can be significantly said of what is done outside dreams cannot be so said of what is dreamed [16]

and, we suppose, conversely. From (8) Miss Macdonald seems to infer that

(9) [dream] contents are not physical objects or states nor copies or reproductions of them nor anything else but *dreams*.[17]

Presumably, this conclusion follows by *modus tollens* from (8) and (D-3). We understand (9) to assert, despite its tautological appearance, that dream experience and waking experience

---

15. See page 74 for an argument of this kind.   16. Page 79.
17. Page 79.

must be *very* dissimilar, as dissimilar, say, as colours and sounds. Thus (9) is incompatible with (2), and if Miss Macdonald has demonstrated its truth she has proved another of Descartes' premises false.

3. Miss Macdonald's argument that within a single experience there is a mark by means of which one can tell whether he is dreaming or waking—that is, her argument that (3) is false—is based on (8). For suppose that a sentence about an experience E is properly formulated in the language for talking about waking life. It follows from (8) that E is a dream experience if the sentence is nonsensical, a waking experience if the sentence is significant. Presumably there is such a sentence for each experience. Thus, there is at least one mark that is common and peculiar to dream experiences and there is at least one mark that is common and peculiar to waking experiences. This point is expressed by Miss Macdonald in the following passage:

> For if what is said of one state is nonsensical when applied to the other, then this provides at least one certain mark by which to distinguish between them.

If all has gone well until now, Miss Macdonald has shown that three of the key premises in Descartes' argument cannot be maintained; if Descartes' sceptical conclusion can be established at all, it must be based on a set of premises that does not include either (1), (2), or (3).

II. Criticism of Miss Macdonald's Argument

We have done our best to understand Miss Macdonald's refutation of Cartesian scepticism. And we have now completed our attempt to say what we think it is. The reader may well wonder why we have presumed to substitute our pedantic outline for Miss Macdonald's spirited prose. We have done so because we think that our objections to her refutation can be stated most clearly if it is reduced to bare and labeled bones. We shall first point out some blemishes in the over-all structure of her argument, and then with regard to each of Descartes' premises (1), (2) and (3), we shall try to show that her specific argument against it fails either because it has some false premises or because it is invalid.

Miss Macdonald's exposition is somewhat marred, and the structure of her argument somewhat confused, by her failure to distinguish sharply between the meanings of 'nonsensical' and 'logically impossible'. The term 'logically impossible', as ordinarily understood, applies to a supposed object or event whenever the sentence referring to the object or event is logically false. For example, one says that it is logically impossible to square the circle, for the sentence 'With ruler and compass one can construct a square and a circle with equal areas' is self-contradictory. What is logically false, however, is not nonsensical for a nonsensical sentence is neither true nor false. For example, the sentence 'C-sharp is red' is neither true nor false, but nonsensical; its predicate is not applicable to that to which its subject refers. Thus, it is nonsense to say of C-sharp that it is red, but is not nonsense to day that C-sharp is C-flat even though it is logically impossible that C-sharp be C-flat.

To see that Miss Macdonald intends the usual distinction between the nonsensical and the logically impossible let us reconsider in its broadest outline her arguments against (1). Let S be a sentence, considered while dreaming, whose subject refers to a dream object and whose predicate is applicable to the objects of waking experience. Miss Macdonald argues that it is logically impossible to test S, that is, she argues that 'S is tested' is self-contradictory. But if S cannot be tested, then it is neither true nor false and hence, she concludes, it is nonsensical. Given that S is nonsensical, she can assert that Descartes was incorrect in assuming that he mistakenly believed S to be true. But in order for her to conclude that S is nonsensical it is essential that a sentence such as 'S is confirmed' is not nonsensical, but logically false; that is to say, it must be logically impossible that S is confirmed, not nonsense to say that it is confirmed. Further, in order to conclude that Descartes could not mistakenly believe S to be true, S must be nonsensical but not logically false. Thus, we conclude that Miss Macdonald's argument requires her to distinguish sharply between the meanings of 'nonsensical' and 'logically impossible'.

Once it is established that 'nonsensical' and 'logically impossible' have their ordinary meanings, then it is clear that (A-1a) and (A-1b) are not two ways of asserting the same premise. In

fact, not both of them can be true, for the same sentence cannot be both nonsensical and false. And hence, Miss Macdonald
must reject one or the other. There are two good reasons for
preferring (A-1a) to (A-1b). First, with the former alone Miss
Macdonald is able to give her refutations of (1), (2) and (3).[18]
Secondly, (A-1b) makes her argument seem trivially circular,
for it assumes exactly what she later proves. She postulates, as
an instance of (A-1b), that it is nonsensical to say that anything
is perceived in a dream, and then six pages later draws this
conclusion.[19] On the other hand, there is a strong argument
for preferring (A-1b) to (A-1a), for the latter implies its own
negation. (A-1a) postulates, for example, that if X dreamt that
he perceived a dagger, then it is logically impossible that he did
perceive a dagger. But (A-1a) in conjunction with the other A
and C premises implies that it 'makes no sense to say either that
one perceives or does not perceive in a dream'.[20] A nonsensical
sentence, however, cannot be a self-contradictory sentence, and
hence it is not logically impossible to perceive a dagger during
a dream.

Miss Macdonald's own argument has shown us that (A-1a) in
conjunction with some of her other premises implies its own
negation. We will now show that it alone is sufficient for the
refutation of (1), (2) and (3). She seems to be aware that (A-1a)
has the remarkable power of implying directly the negation of
(1). For in one place she says that the reason why a dreamer
cannot affirm the reality of what he dreams is that 'at most a
dreamer may dream that he affirms the reality of what he
dreams'.[21] Let us paraphrase her point as follows: a dreamer
cannot believe true a sentence about the contents of his dream,
for a dreamer may at most dream that he believes true such a
sentence. We have here an instance of (A-1a); the blank has
been filled by 'believes to be true' and 'O' has been replaced by
the sentence 'This is a real hand'. Given this instance of (A-1a)
and the fact that Descartes did dream that he believed the sen-

18. In our outline of Miss Macdonald's arguments (A-1b) is employed only
in a step toward the rejection of (2), and an alternative argument for that step
based on (A-1a) is given. See pages 89–90.
19. See page 68, lines 29–31, and page 74, lines 14–15.
20. Page 74.   21. Page 71.

tence 'This is a real hand' to be true, it follows that, while dreaming, it is logically impossible that Descartes believed the sentence 'This is a real hand' to be true; that is to say, it follows that (1) is false.[22] Thus, we maintain not only that (A-1a) is a necessary premise in Miss Macdonald's argument against (1), but also that it is sufficient.

Now let us show that (A-1a) is itself sufficient to establish the negation of (2). Dreaming is a real experience. And since dreams can be remembered, they must be conscious experiences. Just as it is correct to say that a dreamer really dreams and does not merely dream that he dreams, so it is correct to say that a dreamer is really aware of the contents of his dream and does not merely dream that he is aware of them. Miss Macdonald herself seems to hold that within a dream experience there is a distinction to be drawn between the contents, or objects, of the experience and the dreamer's awareness of them. Now to be aware of a colored object is to see it, to be aware of a sound is to hear it, to be aware of a tactile surface is to touch it, etc. But it follows from (A-1a) that in a dream one never sees, hears, touches, etc. Hence, whatever it is that one is aware of in a dream, it cannot have any quality falling under the determinables of color, sound, touch, etc. Therefore, the determinables under which the qualities of dream-contents do fall must be different from any of the determinables met with in waking life. The contents of a dream experience must be at least as different from the contents of waking experiences as colors are from sounds. If this is so, the contents of Descartes' dream experiences could not have been at all similar to the contents of his waking experiences; that is to say, (2) is false.

Finally, let us deduce the negation of (3) from (A-1a). If (A-1a) is true, then there is no certain mark by which Descartes could discover while dreaming that he was dreaming; for if (A-1a) is true, no one could discover anything, etc. On the other hand, if Descartes is awake, he can discover that he is. For if he

---

22. If one is not satisfied with this argument on the grounds that 'believes true' is not a transitive verb, he may put 'considers' in its place. Then the conclusion that it is impossible for Descartes to have considered the sentence in question follows, and hence, *a fortiori*, he could not have mistakenly believed it to be true. A similar argument can be constructed with (A-1b) yielding as a conclusion not that (1) is false, but that it is nonsensical.

is awake he can notice that he is seeing or hearing or touching or otherwise perceiving, and it follows from (A-1a) that he can do these things only while he is awake. But (3) claims that in *no* experience is there a mark by which he could tell whether he was awake or dreaming. (3), therefore, must be rejected if (A-1a) is true.

This completes our comments on the formal structure of Miss Macdonald's argument against Descartes' premises. Its most pervading defect is its inelegance, for of all the assumptions to which we assigned numbers—much of the 'logic' of 'dream', and the 'logics' of 'belief', 'test', and 'significant'—only (A-1a) is necessary to her argument. Now we want to show that (A-1a) is unacceptable. There is doubtless no such thing as *the* 'logic' of 'dream' that everybody always uses, either consciously or unconsciously. But a 'logic' of 'dream' containing (A-1a) fails to fit too many actual cases where 'dream' is commonly used, and it would fail to fit some important hypothetical case where we think 'dream' would be used.

If we are right, (A-1a) implies that dream experiences and waking experiences are radically dissimilar, as dissimilar as colors and sounds. This consequence is incompatible with the plain testimony of *our* memories of dreaming and waking. Nor is this an idiosyncrasy of ours. While trying to recall the past, people are commonly unable to decide whether they are remembering a dream or a waking experience. This often happens to people who have been drunk, utterly exhausted, terrified, etc., the night before. And primitive people are often convinced that certain remembered dreams are really remembered waking experiences. Sometimes the conviction is so strong as to lead to marital complications, suits for compensation, etc. Miss Macdonald attempts to account for such facts by saying that since people describe dreams and waking experiences by means of the same words, they are invariably—until quite recently—deceived into believing that dreams and waking experiences are qualitatively alike.[23] We think that this is putting the cart before the horse. In waking life we apply the same word to two things *because* they are qualitatively similar. With

23. See last paragraph beginning on page 73.

this habit firmly established in waking life, it seems incredible that in the case of dreams we should first apply waking words to them and then, *because* of this, fall into the erroneous belief that they are qualitatively similar to waking experiences. Her way of explaining the matter would be hard to accept even if dreams and waking experiences were only moderately dissimilar. But it follows from (A-1a) that they are as dissimilar as colors and sounds. And it is utterly incredible that people could be made to confuse colors and sounds by making them apply color-words to sounds or sound-words to colors.

(A-1a) also implies that none of the contents of a dream can be veridical. But this is contrary to what many, perhaps most, of us would say about a large class of dream situations. For example, asthma sufferers often dream that they are suffocating, and upon awakening discover that they are suffocating. Their dreams of suffocating are very vivid and fantastic; they are unquestionably dreams. Yet the feeling of suffocation that they have in a dream seems most powerfully to continue one and the same after they wake up. And most of them would say that however fantastic and non-veridical the visual part of the dream was, the feeling of suffocation was veridical and in no way different from the veridical feeling of suffocation they have upon awakening. The reader can probably think of many other and pleasanter cases of this kind.

So much for the conflict of (A-1a) with the use of 'dream' in actual cases. Let us now construct a hypothetical case where, we think, the most common use of 'dream' would conflict with (A-1a). Suppose that hereafter all dreams led people to make successful predictions after they awakened. If a person in California were to dream that the Washington Monument was being painted blue, he could successfully predict upon awakening that a telephone call to the Capitol would bring word that the Monument was indeed being painted blue. If he were to dream that Westminster Abbey was on fire, then, after awakening, he could confidently expect that motion pictures of the fire would soon be shown at the local cinema. And generally, no dream from now on would conflict with any subsequent waking experience. If this were to happen, we should certainly be perplexed for a while. Some might say, 'After all their wayward years, dreams have now become veridical'. And some might say, 'Instead of having dreams, we now have paranormal but veridical perceptions while asleep; I wonder what the explanation is?' But if anyone had formerly been inclined to accept (A-1a) and the entailed radical dissimilarity of dreams and waking experiences, he would surely abandon it now. He would want to say now that while he was asleep the Washington Monument did really look blue to him, did really appear to him in a context of real objects, etc. He would totally reject the claim that while he was asleep he did not see anything blue, but only experienced a content whose qualities fall under a determinable that is never met with in waking life. And he would say that he was mistaken when he formerly believed that a dreamer could not see, touch, hear, etc.

For the above-mentioned reasons we cannot accept (A-1a). In the 'logic' of 'dream' we would substitute for (A-1a) the rule: To say that one dreams is to say that one sees, hears, touches, etc., while asleep. We should then say that *in fact* all visual contents of dreams are non-veridical. Perhaps all auditory and most tactual contents of dreams are non-veridical. But they all *could be* veridical. On the other hand, the internal, visceral, or kinesthetic sensations, such as the sensation of suffocation, are quite often veridical while occurring in a dream. And as regards the so-called mental operations, we should maintain, with Descartes, that if anyone dreams that he believes, doubts, expects, desires, etc., then he really does. According to the rule we would substitute for (A-1a), it is logically possible for a dream to be a veridical but paranormal perception. Our rule can be made to fit wherever (A-1a) fits, but it will also fit many cases that (A-1a) does not. And so we would substitute it for the rule which we have rejected.

In the space still left to us we shall criticize each of Miss Macdonald's specific arguments against (1), (2) and (3). We shall reject each of them either because we cannot accept all the assumptions on which it is based or because it does not proceed validly to its conclusion.

Let us begin with her argument against (1). In this argument she tries to show us that if S is used by a dreamer, it is not testable during the dream (5), or after the dream (6), and hence it is not testable at all (7); and that since all sentences believed to be true, whether correctly or mistakenly, and testable (4), Descartes, while dreaming, could not have mistakenly believed S to be true. In order to establish (5), (6) and (7), she employs the assumptions (A-1a), (A-2), (A-3), (C-1), (C-2) and (C-3). In our opinion, all of them except (C-2) are false.

We have already given our reasons for rejecting (A-1a), and in its place we have offered our own rule for the use of the clause 'X dreamt that . . . O'. If our rule is accepted, a dream could be a paranormal perception that occurs during sleep; dream-objects *might be* veridical. For example, if one dreams he perceives the Washington Monument, he *might be* perceiving the Washington Monument, and it *might* appear to him in a context of real objects. Further, after a dreamer wakes up, the object of his dream *might* continue to exist, just as the object of a waking perception continues to exist after one turns his head or closes his eyes. Thus, if our rule is correct, (A-2) and (A-3) are false, for taken together they say that the contents of a dream could not appear in a context of real objects or survive the dream-experience.

Turning now to her assumptions about the 'logic' of 'test', we shall try to show that (C-1) and (C-3) are not tenable. Given that S expresses a judgment of perception about O, (C-1) states that a test of S can be *started* only if when S is asserted O is perceived in a context of real objects. (C-3) states that such a test can be *completed* only by perceiving O again in a context of real objects or by again perceiving the real place where O appeared when S was asserted. We present our case against (C-1) and (C-3) in the form of a counter-example. Suppose X, a man in California, dreams of the Washington Monument. According to our rule for 'dream' people can really believe sentences to be true while they are dreaming. And so we may suppose further that while dreaming of the Washington Monument, X considers the sentence 'This is the Washington Monument' and believes it to be true of O, part of the contents of his dream experience. Finally, although our rule for 'dream' permits all the contents of a dream-experience to be veridical, we shall suppose that in this example none of them is. O does not appear in a context of real objects, and neither it nor its context survives the dream. (C-1) states that a test of the sentence about O could never get started; (C-3) states that a test of the sentence about O could never be completed. We think, however, that a test of the sentence could get started during or after the dream, and that it could be completed during or after the dream. Let us consider first the case in which the test is started and completed after the dreamer awakens. After awakening, X could remember that while dreaming he had believed O to be the Washington Monument. But even though he could not see O or its place again, he could still find good evidence for rejecting the belief he had while dreaming. For he could discover that when he dreamed of the Washington Monument he was in bed asleep some three thousand miles away from it, that there very likely is no paranormal perception, and so on. All of this would make it highly unlikely that O was the Washington Monument.

Our reasons for maintaining that a test of the sentence could be both started and completed during the dream are, as might be expected, more complicated. If our rule for 'dream' is correct, a dreamer could consider a sentence such as 'This is the Washington Monument' and believe it to be true. We think that in fact many dreamers do this. Also, if our rule is correct, a dreamer who is inspecting one dream-field could predict and expect certain later dream-fields; and when they occur he could recognize them to be or not to be the ones he predicted while inspecting earlier dreamfields. Some persons claim that they in fact do this in dreams, but perhaps most people would not make this claim. Suppose, as in our example, the dream-field in which O occurs leads X to believe that O is the Washington Monument. And suppose that it is followed by a dream-field exactly like it except that in place of O there is an element that would normally lead X to believe he was seeing a gigantic snake standing on its head in Washington, D.C. As a predicting, expecting, recognizing, and remembering dreamer, X *might* then decide that he had mistakenly believed O to be the Washington Monument; and if he had in mind the general plan of consistency and congruency that underlies our concept of the real world, he might even come to believe that he was dreaming. The mere fact that during the dream he does not go closer, touch, use instruments, etc., does not prevent him from testing. A passive observer of the passing scene, whether the scene is dream-stuff or real-stuff, could still predict and test. The role of the observing, predicting, and testing dreamer would be analogous to that of the early stargazers who worked out the first rough star-charts. While awake we can review in retrospect our past experiences, and by applying in thought certain schemes of consistency and congruency we can sort out the dreams from the waking experiences. If our rule for 'dream' is correct, there is no reason why we *could* not do this while dreaming, even if it were never done in fact. And so, even on the assumption that O never appears in a context of real objects, S is still testable; hence, (C-1) and (C-3) are false.

We have now given our reasons for rejecting (A-la), (A-2), (A-3), (C-1) and (C-3). If they are good reasons, then Miss Macdonald has not proved (5), (6) or (7). Further, in rejecting her assumptions we have provided positive grounds for showing that (5), (6) and (7) are false; that is to say, we have attempted to show that S is testable. But if S is testable, then it is believable; and if believable, mistakenly believable. Contrary to Miss Macdonald we find no good reason for denying (1).

Our objection to Miss Macdonald's argument against (2) can be given more briefly. For that argument depended upon (7) and we have already explained why we think (7) is false. Moreover, in presenting our case against (A-la), we provided strong positive grounds for believing that (2) is true, that is, for believing that the contents of dream experiences and those of waking experiences are qualitatively very similar. It may be that if we had anything worth saying on this head, we have already said it. Yet we venture to give one more objection to Miss Macdonald's argument against (2). This objection may be telescoped into the following brief implication: If none of the contents of an experience is a real object, then from her premises it follows that the experience is wholly dissimilar to any waking experience. Now there are or could be total waking hallucinations none of whose contents is a real object; an experience all of whose contents consists entirely of entities like Banquo's ghost, the drunkard's pink rats, etc. The totally insane are supposed to have experiences of this kind. If Miss Macdonald's argument against (2) is sound, then such experiences are totally dissimilar to other waking experiences. We find it difficult to accept this consequence of her argument.

We come finally to a consideration of Miss Macdonald's argument against (3). Here again, we think some of its premises are false. This, however, is not our main objection to it. Even if all its premises were true it would not be grounds for rejecting (3), for its premises do not imply the negation of (3). As we have formulated (3), it states that in any given experience there is no certain mark by which one can *discover* whether he is awake or dreaming. What Miss Macdonald has proved, given that (8) is true, is that there is a common and peculiar mark of waking experiences. For (8) states that certain sentences properly formulated in the language of waking experience are significant if and only if they are applied to the contents of waking experience. But in any given experience no one could *discover* by means of this mark whether he is awake or dreaming.

To show that Miss Macdonald's mark will not enable one to discover whether or not he is dreaming, the epistemological order as well as the logical relations of statements must be considered. She gives us the following logical relationship: judgments of perception such as 'This is green', 'This is C-sharp', etc., are nonsensical if and only if asserted of dream experiences. Given that one knows either terms of the bi-conditional to be true, he can then assert the other is true. But what is the order of knowledge in this case? Clearly it is from knowledge that a judgment of perception is significant to knowledge that one is not dreaming. But what are the marks by which one discovers that a judgment of perception is nonsensical or significant? If the demonstrative in a judgment of perception is merely an ellipsis for 'this dream experience' or 'this waking experience', then the 'logics' of 'dream' and 'wake' enable one to discover whether or not the sentence is significant. But to know that the demonstrative is an ellipsis for 'this dream experience' or 'this waking experience' is to reverse the epistemological order. On the other hand, for those cases in which the subject of the judgment of perception does not implicitly contain the term 'dream' or 'wake', Miss Macdonald has given no criteria for discovering whether or not the statement in question is significant other than that its subject refers to a dream or to a waking experience. Again, the epistemological order has been reversed. In short, we can find in Miss Macdonald's arguments no means for knowing that a judgment of perception such as 'This is green', 'This is C-flat', etc., is nonsensical or significant - other than that of first discovering whether it is asserted of a dream or of a waking experience.

In fact, given Miss Macdonald's thesis concerning the language of dreams we can reinstate Descartes' lament at the language level. In his *First Meditation* Descartes lamented that he could find no certain mark by which to distinguish dreams from waking experiences. Miss Macdonald claims that he could have found such a mark.[24] In any given experience Descartes had merely to say something in waking language about an object of his experience, e.g., 'This is a real hand', and then determine whether what he said was sense or nonsense. But by what certain marks could Descartes discover whether what he said was sense or nonsense? We ask Miss Macdonald for such a mark. If none can be produced, she has not destroyed the grounds of Cartesian scepticism of the senses, but merely shifted it from experience to language.

24. We cannot forbear adding that in the concluding paragraph of the *Sixth Meditation* Descartes himself indicates marks, though not infallible ones, that would enable one to discover whether he is awake or dreaming. Thus, he did not believe as Miss Macdonald says, that he had condemned us 'to incurable scepticism of the senses'.

4

NORMAN MALCOLM

Dreaming and Skepticism

In the *First Meditation,* Descartes represents himself as at first having the thought that surely it is *certain* that he is seated by the fire, and then as rejecting this thought in the following remark: "I cannot, however, but remind myself that on many occasions I have in sleep been deceived by similar illusions; and on more careful study of them I see that there are no certain marks distinguishing waking from sleep. . . ." [1] I believe that it is worth while reflecting on his assertion that he has often been *deceived* when asleep. In his reply to the objections against the *Meditations* raised by Hobbes, he repeats this assertion in the form of a rhetorical question: "For who denies that in his sleep a man may be deceived?" [2]

—Descartes is clearly implying that while a man is asleep a certain thought may occur to him or he may come to believe something or to affirm something. And there is no doubt that he held this to be so.[3] In the *Fifth Meditation* he says that "once I have recognized that there is a God, and that all things depend

Reprinted with minor changes from the *Philosophical Review,* 64 (1956), 14–37, by permission of the author and the *Philosophical Review.*
1. Norman Kemp Smith, *Descartes' Philosophical Writings* (London, 1952), p. 198; hereafter cited as *DPW.*
2. E. Haldane and G. Ross, *The Philosophical Works of Descartes* (Cambridge, 1934), II, 78; hereafter cited as HR.
3. Other philosophers have held it too. Aristotle, in a short paper on dreams, says: "It is . . . a fact that the soul makes . . . assertions in sleep" (*De Somnis,* in *The Basic Works of Aristotle,* ed. by R. McKeon [New York, 1941],

on Him, and that He is not a deceiver, and from this, in turn, have inferred that all things which I clearly and distinctly apprehend are of necessity true," then no grounds remain for doubting any of the things that he remembers as having been previously demonstrated—for example, the truths of geometry. He continues:

Will it be said that perhaps I am dreaming (an objection I myself raised a little while ago), that is, that all the thoughts I am now entertaining are no more true than those which come to me in dreams? Even so, what difference would that make? For even should I be asleep and dreaming, whatever is present to my understanding in an evident manner is indisputably true. [*DPW*, 247]

Descartes thinks that a man might have thoughts and make judgments while sleeping, and if those thoughts are "clear and distinct" they are true, despite the fact that he is sleeping. This doctrine is plainly set forth in his reply to the Jesuit, Bourdin: ". . . everything which anyone clearly and distinctly perceives is true, although that person in the meantime may doubt whether he is dreaming or awake, nay, if you want it so, even though he is really dreaming or is delirious" (HR II, 267). In Part IV of the *Discourse,* Descartes remarks that "whether awake or asleep, we ought never to allow ourselves to be persuaded save on the evidence of our reason" (*DPW*, 146). Here he implies that a man can reason, can be persuaded, and can resist persuasion—though all the while he is asleep!

His view is that when we sleep the same *kinds* of mental states and mental occurrences are present in us as when awake; the difference is that, as a general rule, our minds don't work as well when we are asleep.[4] But they work. Indeed, they *must* do so; for the "essence" or "principal attribute" of mental sub-

---

p. 618). Kant, in *An Inquiry into the Distinctness of the Principles of Natural Theology and Morals,* says: "In deepest sleep perhaps the greatest perfection of the mind might be exercised in rational thought. For we have no reason for asserting the opposite except that we do not remember the idea when awake. This reason, however, proves nothing" (Immanuel Kant, *Critique of Practical Reason and Other Writings in Moral Philosophy,* ed. L. W. Beck [Chicago, 1949], p. 275).

4. As Gilson puts Descartes' view: "Sleep does not constitute in itself a state of error, but simply, because of physiological conditions, a state less favorable than waking to the free exercise of thought" (E. Gilson, *René Descartes: Discours de la Méthode:* Texte et commentaire [Paris, 1930], p. 366).

stance is consciousness, and so long as a mind exists there must exist "modes" of that essence, i.e. states of consciousness, mental occurrences, mental acts. As Descartes says in a letter:

I had good reason to assert that the human soul is always conscious in any circumstances—even in a mother's womb. For what more certain or more evident reason could be required than my proof that the soul's nature or essence consists in its being conscious, just as the essence of a body consists in its being extended? A thing can never be deprived of its own essence.[5]

Descartes conceives of a dream as being a part of this continuous mental life. The thoughts of a dream are real thoughts. The feelings in a dream are real feelings. Descartes holds that to be frightened in a dream is to be frightened in the *same* sense as that in which I should be frightened now if half of the ceiling were suddenly to fall. He holds that the proposition "In my dream last night I was frightened" *entails* the proposition "Last night I was frightened." He holds that if in my dream I thought someone was at the door, then I had this thought, while asleep, in the very same sense as that in which I should have it now were I to hear the doorbell. It is only because Descartes conceives of a dream as composed of thoughts and sensations, in the same sense that a period of waking life is, that he is able, in the *First Meditation,* to derive a ground for doubting his senses from the fact that sometimes he dreams. According to his conception, the identical thoughts and sensations that you had when you were wide awake could have occurred to you when you were asleep. The *content* of a dream and of a waking episode could be the same. From this it follows "that there are no certain marks distinguishing waking from sleep." I will try to show that this conception is mistaken.

I

To begin with, I should like to call attention to the familiar distinction between being *sound* asleep and being *half* asleep. It is noteworthy that in American colloquial speech the phrase "dead to the world" is a synonym of the phrase "sound asleep"

5. C. Adam and P. Tannery, *Oeuvres de Descartes* (Paris, 1899), III, 423; trans. E. Anscombe and P. Geach, *Descartes: Philosophical Writings* (Edinburgh, 1954), p. 266.

and not, of course, a synonym of the phrase "half asleep." If a man is half asleep he is also partly awake but not "clear" awake. Many different degrees of being asleep fall under the heading "half asleep." The criteria we commonly use for determining whether another person is or was sound asleep are different from the criteria we use for determining whether he is or was half asleep. It would seem that the former criteria are of two sorts: (1) a "present-tense" criterion, and (2) a "past-tense" criterion. We use the "present-tense" criterion to determine whether someone *is* (not was) sound asleep. It consists of things of this kind: that his eyes are closed, his body inert, his breathing rhythmical, and (more important) that he is unresponsive to questions, commands, and stimuli of moderate intensity. (Example: The sleeper does not react in any way when the carpenter begins hammering in the next room. In contrast, he might have rolled over and muttered a sleepy protest against the noise.) The "past-tense" criterion is used to determine whether a person *was* (not is) sound asleep, and it can be satisfied only when he is awake. It applies when the present-tense criterion has not been fulfilled in such a way that all question is removed as to whether the person is or is not sound asleep. We wait until he is awake and then find out whether he has any knowledge of what transpired in his vicinity while he was asleep: if he has none it is confirmed that he was sound asleep. (Example: He is surprised to learn that there was hammering close by while he slept: he has no recollection of any noise.) These two sorts of criterion can combine or conflict in many ways. It is possible that there should be cases in which there is no correct answer to the question "Was he sound asleep?"

The criteria of someone's being half asleep would seem to fall into the same two categories. The main difference between the present-tense criteria for being sound asleep and for being half asleep is that if someone is merely half asleep he will be in some degree responsive to questions, commands, and disturbances, although only sluggishly or groggily so. The main difference in the past-tense criteria for these two conditions is that if someone was only half asleep then he will be able to produce, when fully awake, some account of what took place in his immediate vicinity while he was half asleep, an account that will, however, be hazy and incomplete.[6] (A refinement of this last difference, pertaining to dreaming, is mentioned in footnote 9.)

II

In the next place, I wish to compare the following two sentences:
(1) "I am sound asleep."
(2) "I was sound asleep."
Although (1) and (2) differ grammatically only in tense, (1) is seen, straight off, to be a queer sentence, but (2) is not. Wherein lies the oddity of (1)?

Let us say that when a person utters or writes a sentence he can *use* the sentence to claim or affirm or assert something. It will depend on circumstances whether one has used a sentence to claim something, or whether one has merely uttered the sentence in order to call attention to the sentence itself, as I might utter (1) merely to call attention to it. (Also, of course, a sentence may be used to give a command or to put a question, and so on.) Now it is obvious that sentence (2), "I was sound asleep," can be and is used to claim or affirm or assert something. I shall express this by saying that it can be "used as an assertion."

The question now is whether (1) can be used as an assertion. It is not hard to see that there would be an absurdity in attempting to so use it. Suppose that I am in bed and that you come and shake me and ask "Are you asleep?" and that I reply "I am sound asleep." It would be amusing if you took me as claiming that I am sound asleep and then concluded from this that I am sound asleep. ("He says that he is sound asleep, and he ought to know.") The absurdity that would lie in the use of the sentence "I am sound asleep" as an assertion consists in this: if a person *claims* that he is sound asleep then he is *not* sound asleep. Notice that "claims" is a stronger verb here than

6. The psychoanalyst Lawrence Kubie remarks that "sleep is a psychologically active state, and we are never completely asleep, nor completely awake" (E. Hilgard, L. Kubie, and E. Pumpian-Mindlin, *Psychoanalysis as Science* [Stanford, 1952], p. 95). One wonders whether Kubie is so using the words that no one *could* be "completely awake" or "completely asleep."

"says." There is *a* sense of "says" in which a person says whatever words come out of his mouth. In this sense a man who is sound asleep can say things: he may talk in his sleep. He could say, in this sense, "I am sound asleep"; but this would not prove that he is not sound asleep. He is not claiming that he is sound asleep.

The absurdity that I am trying to describe does not lie in my uttering the words "I am sound asleep" but in my claiming or affirming or asserting that I am sound asleep. Whether I make the claim by using spoken or written words or by any other audible or visible signs is, therefore, irrelevant. If I use no physical signs but merely affirm in my mind that I am sound asleep (as I might affirm in my mind that my companion is a bore), it follows that I am not sound asleep.

The matter can be put by saying that the *assertion* "I am sound asleep" would be, in a certain sense, self-contradictory. The sentence "I am sound asleep" does not express a self-contradiction in the way in which the sentence "A is taller than B and B is taller than A," expresses a self-contradiction. If the latter sentence were written down in front of you, you could straight off deduce a proposition of the form "p and not-p." You cannot do this with "I am sound asleep." But as soon as you bring in the notion of a person's *asserting* or *claiming* that he is sound asleep then you get a kind of self-contradiction. It would be an assertion of such a nature that *making* the assertion would contradict the *truth* of the assertion. The proposition "I am sound asleep" (if it can be called a "proposition") does not entail the proposition "I am not sound asleep." But if I am asserting that I am sound asleep then I am not sound asleep. If I am asserting that I am sound asleep someone else is entitled to say of me "He claims that he is sound asleep." And this latter proposition, "He claims that he is sound asleep" (if it can be called a "proposition"), entails the proposition "He is not sound asleep." Thus the first-person assertion "I am sound asleep" and the related third-person proposition "He claims that he is sound asleep" may each, with propriety I think, be called "self-contradictory," although in somewhat different senses. In neither case, of course, is it that "strict" kind of self-contradiction that is illustrated by my "taller" sentence: for the latter expresses something from which there follows a proposition of the form "*p* and not-*p*"; whereas neither from "I am sound asleep" nor from "He claims that he is sound asleep" does there follow any proposition of that form. The kind of self-contradiction is this: if someone claims that he is sound asleep then it follows that he is not what he claims. It is an assertion that would necessarily be false each time it was made.

Not only is there a kind of self-contradiction in claiming or affirming that one is sound asleep; there is the same kind of self-contradiction in wondering or conjecturing whether one is sound asleep, or in being in doubt about it. The proposition "He wonders whether he is sound asleep" is absurd in the same way that the proposition "He claims that he is sound asleep" is absurd. From either of them equally there follows the proposition "He is not sound asleep." So not merely is the *assertion* "I am sound asleep" self-contradictory: the *question* "Am I sound asleep?" is self-contradictory in the same sense. And if the *thought* should occur to you that you are sound asleep it would be a self-contradictory thought. And if you should be under the *impression* that you are sound asleep it would be a self-contradictory impression: for the proposition "He is under the impression (it seems to him) that he is sound asleep" entails the proposition "He is not sound asleep."

Finally, it should be mentioned that the proposition "He knows (he realizes, he is aware) that he is sound asleep" is a self-contradictory proposition in the "strict" sense. Therefore, a person who is sound asleep cannot know, realize, or be aware that he is.[7]

Of course, a person can *dream* that he is sound asleep and can *dream* that he *knows* that he is sound asleep. It can be said of a person who dreamt either of these things that "he knew in his dream" that he was sound asleep. What my argument proves is

7. A proposition of the form "He knows that *p*" differs from a proposition of the form "He claims (thinks, conjectures, doubts) that *p*," in the respect that the former entails "*p*," the latter not. Therefore, "He knows that he is sound asleep" is self-contradictory in the "strict" sense: for, like propositions of the latter form, it entails "He is *not* sound asleep"; and, unlike those of the latter form, it entails "He *is* sound asleep."

that knowing-in-your-dream that you are sound asleep is not knowing that you are sound asleep.

III

So far I have called attention to the fact that if a person affirms, doubts, thinks, or questions that he is sound asleep then he is not sound asleep—and also to the fact that a person who is sound asleep cannot know that he is. But now it is important to see that if a person affirms, doubts, thinks, or questions *anything whatever* (and not merely that he is sound asleep) then he is not sound asleep. No doubt all of those verbs have "dispositional" senses: for example, you can truly say of a man who is in fact sound asleep that he affirms that war will break out within the year. But it is not that sense of those verbs to which I am referring. If we take "He affirms that there will be a war" in the sense in which it means "At this very moment he is affirming that there will be a war," then it entails "He is not sound asleep." In this "non-dispositional" sense of those verbs, "He is affirming (doubting, thinking, questioning) that *p*" entails "He is not sound asleep," *regardless* of what proposition is substituted for "*p*." Surely it is obvious that if "He is claiming that he is sound asleep" entails "He is not sound asleep," then also "He is claiming that someone is at the door" entails "He is not sound asleep." And likewise, if the thought has struck him that there might be someone at the door, or if he wonders whether there is, or if he doubts that there is, or if it seems to him that there is, or if he is afraid that there is—then he is not sound asleep. To state the principle for which I am arguing in its most general form: if a person is in *any* state of consciousness it logically follows that he is not sound asleep. The proposition with which I started my argument—namely, the proposition that "He claims that he is sound asleep" entails "He is not sound asleep"—is a special case of this general principle, which may be expressed in Cartesian terms as follows: *Cogito ergo non dormio.*

When Descartes declared, in the course of his *Reply* to Gassendi's objections to the *Meditations,* that "when we sleep we perceive that we are dreaming" (HR II, 212), he was mistaken if he meant that when we are *sound* asleep we perceive that we are dreaming.[8]

The fact is that if someone is in bed with his eyes closed, whatever serves as a criterion for saying that just now he is thinking that so-and-so is the case, or is wondering or doubting whether it is, or perceives that it is—also serves as a criterion for saying that he is not sound asleep.

And if one cannot have thoughts while sound asleep, one cannot be *deceived* while sound asleep.

IV

There will be a temptation to conclude that, if all the foregoing is true, then clearly a person cannot *dream* when sound asleep. But this would be a mistake. Our normal criterion for someone's having had a dream is that, upon awaking, he relates ("tells") a dream. Suppose that the present-tense and past-tense criteria of sound sleep were satisfied in the case of a certain person—i.e. his body was inert, his breathing was heavy and rhythmical (perhaps he even snored); he did not react to moderately loud noises or to occurrences in his immediate vicinity that would have provoked his lively interest had he known about them: furthermore, when he woke up he had no suspicion that those noises and incidents had occurred. Also suppose that on awaking he related a dream. It would have been established both that he slept soundly and that he dreamt.[9]

8. Note the following consequence drawn by Freud from his theory of dreams: "Throughout the whole of our sleep we are just as certain that we are dreaming as we are certain that we are sleeping" (*The Interpretation of Dreams,* in *The Basic Writings of Sigmund Freud,* ed. A. A. Brill [New York, 1938], p. 513).

9. The proposition "I was sound asleep" has, on my view, the nature of an inference. I conclude that I was sound asleep from things that I notice or learn after or as I wake up. For example, I find out that while I slept for the past hour a heavy tractor was making an uproar a hundred feet away, yet I have no recollection of hearing any noise. I infer that I was very soundly asleep.

I must mention here a complicating subtlety. Suppose, in the above example, I *dreamt* that I heard a roaring and clanking (like that of a nearby tractor) and dreamt that this noise was made by a dinosaur. I believe we should be inclined to say that I *heard* the tractor *in my sleep,* although I had no suspicion, upon awakening, that there had been such goings-on, until I was told. I think we should also be inclined to say that my sleep was not completely sound, that I was not utterly "dead to the world." I think that in general a certain degree of

V

I will anticipate, at this point, a very general sort of objection to the manner in which I argue. It will be said that I am assuming throughout that there are *criteria* for determining whether a person other than myself is or was thinking, or frightened, or awake, or asleep; i.e. I am assuming that I have criteria for the existence of particular sorts of mental occurrences and states of consciousness in other persons, those criteria being of such a nature that if they are fully satisfied the existence of those occurrences and states is established beyond question—whereas, the objection runs, there are no such criteria and could be none: at best I only have *evidence,* which makes the existence of those mental states and occurrences in others more or less probable. It is true that I make this "assumption." I believe that to deny it leads one to the view that each person *teaches himself* what fright, doubt, thinking, and all other mental phenomena are, by noting his own fright, doubt, etc.: each person "knows from his own case" what these things are. And this view leads to the untenable notion of a language that "I alone *can* understand." I will not attempt here to show either that the denial of the above "assumption" has this consequence or that it is untenable. I believe that both of these things have been established by Wittgenstein in his *Philosophical Investigations.* A

---

similarity between the events of a dream and the events occurring within normal perceptual range of the sleeper counts in favor of saying both that the sleeper faintly perceived the latter events and that his sleep was not an absolutely deep sleep. This would be so even if the sleeper had no idea, after awaking, that the events in question had occurred. I doubt that there is any way of specifying what the degree of similarity must be. I will comment briefly on two examples adduced by R. M. Yost, Jr., and Donald Kalish in their paper "Miss Macdonald on Sleeping and Waking" (*Philosophical Quarterly,* April 1955) [Chapter 3 above]. One is of an asthmatic who dreams that he is suffocating and finds on awaking that he is suffocating. The right thing to say here, I think, is that his dream was partly a perception of the reality, and also that it was not a dream of perfectly sound sleep. The other example is that of a person in California who dreams that the Washington Monument is being painted blue. A dream with such a content would not count against the dreamer's having been sound asleep, even if the Monument were being painted blue at the time he slept. What would indicate that a dreamer's sleep was not a very deep one would not be that his dream was veridical, but that the content of the dream suggests that he was to some extent perceptive of things that he would probably have perceived clearly, located as he was, had he been awake.

rough guide to some of his thoughts on this topic may be found in my review of that book (*Philosophical Review,* October 1954).

VI

Let us consider again Descartes' famous remark: "I cannot, however, but remind myself that on many occasions I have in sleep been deceived by similar illusions; and on more careful study of them I see that there are no certain marks distinguishing waking from sleep." Of course, if by "sleep" he means sound sleep, then it is false that in sleep he could ever have been deceived by any illusions whatever. But I want to pay particular attention to the idea that there are no certain marks distinguishing waking from sleep, an idea that has been commonly entertained and accepted by philosophers. Socrates put to Theaetetus the question:

What evidence could be appealed to, supposing we were asked at this very moment whether we are asleep or awake—dreaming all that passes through our minds or talking to one another in the waking state?

To which Theaetetus replied:

Indeed, Socrates, I do not see by what evidence it is to be proved; for the two conditions correspond in every circumstance like exact counterparts. The conversation we have just had might equally well be one that we merely think we are carrying on in our sleep; and when it comes to thinking in a dream that we are telling other dreams, the two states are extraordinarily alike.[10]

Bertrand Russell says the following:

I dreamed last night that I was in Germany, in a house which looked out on a ruined church; in my dream I supposed at first that the church had been bombed during the recent war, but was subsequently informed that its destruction dated from the wars of religion in the sixteenth century. All this, so long as I remained asleep, had all the convincingness of waking life. I did really have the dream, and did really have an experience intrinsically indistinguishable from that of seeing a ruined church when awake. It follows that the experience which I call "seeing a church" is not conclusive evidence that there is a church, since it may occur when there is no such external object as I

10. F. M. Cornford, *Plato's Theory of Knowledge* (London, 1935), p. 53.

suppose in my dream. It may be said that, though when dreaming I may *think* that I am awake, when I wake up I *know* that I am awake. But I do not see how we are to have any such certainty. . . . I do not believe that I am now dreaming, but I cannot prove that I am not. I am, however, quite certain that I am having certain experiences, whether they be those of a dream or those of waking life.[11]

This manner of comparing dreaming and waking inevitably results in the skeptical question: "How can I tell whether at this moment I am awake or asleep?" and in the skeptical conclusion: "I *cannot* tell." The conception that underlies the comparison is the following: "Take any sequence of sensations, thoughts, and feelings. That same sequence could occur either when you were awake or when you were asleep and dreaming. The two conditions, being awake and being asleep, can have the same *content* of experience. Therefore, you cannot tell from the sensations, thoughts, and feelings themselves, at the time you are having them, whether you are awake or asleep."

If, however, we state the problem in terms of *sound* sleep, and bear in mind my preceding argument, then we see at least one respect in which this conception is mistaken. When a person is sound asleep he cannot have any sensations, thoughts, and feelings at all; sound sleep cannot, in *this* sense, have any "content of experience." This is so regardless of whether or not the sleeper dreams. Therefore it is not true, but senseless, to say that sound sleep and waking are "indistinguishable" from one another, or that they are "exact counterparts." For the meaning of this philosophical remark is that identically the same sensations, impressions, and thoughts could occur to one in either condition. But one might as well assert that a house and the mental image of a house could have the same weight; it is as meaningless to attribute sensations, impressions, thoughts, or feelings to sound sleep as to attribute weight to a mental image.

It is undoubtedly an ordinary use of language to call a dream an "experience": one may say of an unpleasant dream "I hope that I won't have that experience again." In this sense a man can have experiences when sound asleep. But this use of the

11. Bertrand A. W. Russell, *Human Knowledge* (New York, 1948), pp. 171–172.

word "experience" should not mislead us. In his dream a man may see, hear, think, feel emotion. To say that "in his dream" he thought his bed was on fire and was frightened, is equivalent to saying that he dreamt that he thought his bed was on fire and dreamt that he was frightened. The fallacy I am warning against is to conclude "He was frightened" from "He dreamt that he was frightened," and "He thought his bed was on fire" from "He dreamt that he thought his bed was on fire." The experience of thinking your bed is on fire and (if you are sound asleep) of thinking in your dream that your bed is on fire are "experiences" in different senses of the word.

VII

In the notion of the dream of sound sleep there is no foothold for philosophical skepticism. It is an error to say that a person *cannot tell* whether he is awake or sound asleep and dreaming. For this implies (a) that he might *think* he was awake and yet be sound asleep—which is impossible. And it implies (b) that he might think he was sound asleep and yet be awake. Now (b), unlike (a), is not impossible: but the thought that the man has—namely, that he is sound asleep—is self-contradictory (in the special sense that I explained), and a little reflection could teach him that it is. Whether or not a particular person would see this point of logic, in any case no general ground for skepticism is provided.

But it is also an error to say that a man *can* tell whether or not he is sound asleep. For this would imply that he had some criterion or test at hand for determining the matter, and there is an absurdity in this idea—for he could not even *use* a criterion unless he were *not* sound asleep, and so nothing could turn on the "outcome" of using it. Therefore, it is wrong to say *either* that you can tell or cannot tell (in the sense of *determine*) that you are sound asleep and dreaming, or that you are awake.

There is a temptation to object to the preceding argument in the following way: "even if I cannot have thoughts and sensations during sound sleep, yet when I dream during sound sleep it seems to me that I am having thoughts and sensations, and so there remains the problem of determining, at any given time,

whether I am having thoughts and sensations or merely seeming to have them." [12] The pretty obvious answer to this is that
to a person who is sound asleep, "dead to the world," things
cannot even *seem*. He cannot hear the telephone ring nor can it
seem to him that it rings. Suppose that A is apparently sound
asleep, but that B makes the following report to C: "It seems to
A that he hears the telephone ringing." C's natural reply would
be: "Why, I thought that he was sound asleep!" Whatever
movements, gestures, or utterances of A's indicate that it seems
to him that the telephone is ringing, also indicate, to an equal
degree, that he is not sound asleep.

Another objection to my argument is the following: "Granted
that while a person is sound asleep he gives no indication of
having any thoughts or of being conscious of anything, nevertheless upon awaking he might testify that such and such a
thought had occurred to him while he slept. Likewise, nothing
in the demeanor of the man who is quietly smoking his pipe
reveals that the thought of resigning his government post has
just occurred to him; but afterwards he may declare that it did
first occur to him then. You would accept his testimony! Now,
why shouldn't you accept it in the other case too? Since the
cases are similar it is merely dogmatic and unreasonable to
reject his testimony there while accepting it here."

It is true enough that a man's declaration that a certain
thought passed through his mind on a particular occasion in
the very recent past is used by others as a criterion of that
thought's having passed through his mind on that past occasion, even though his behavior at the time gave no indication
of it. Similarly, someone who is calmly discussing something
with you and giving no indication of physical discomfort, may
later declare that he felt slightly ill just then; and you will probably use his declaration as a criterion of his having felt slightly
ill just then, even though he gave no sign of it. But note that we
have said that he did not, in fact, give any sign of it. He *could*
have done so. Whereas it is false that a man who is sound
asleep could, while he is sound asleep, give any signs or indica-

12. Socrates in the *Republic* asks: "Does not dreaming, whether one is awake
or asleep, consist in mistaking a semblance for the reality it resembles?" (F. M.
Cornford, *The Republic of Plato* [New York, 1945], p. 183).

tions that a certain thought was occurring to him or that he was experiencing some sensation.[13] For any sign of this would also be a sign that he was at least partly awake.

If a man were to get up from an apparently sound sleep and declare that while he was lying there a certain thought had occurred to him we might conclude that he was about to tell us something that he had dreamt; or we might conclude that, despite appearances, he had not been sound asleep; or we might conclude that he had awakened *with* that thought. Famous men testify to having solved difficult problems in their sleep. This can seem a paradox until we understand what it means: namely, that they went to sleep without a solution and woke up with one. But if a man, who knew English as well as anyone, declared that a certain thought had occurred to him while he was *sound* asleep, and insisted that he did not mean that he dreamt it or that he woke up with it, but that it had occurred to him in the same literal sense in which thoughts sometimes occur to him when he is drinking his coffee or weeding the garden—then I believe that in ordinary life we should not be able to make head or tail of his declaration.

VIII

It will appear to some that there is a contradiction in maintaining, as I have, that it is true that someone who is sound asleep can in a dream think it is raining and in a dream seem to hear thunder, and yet that it is not true that he thinks it is raining or seems to hear thunder. One wants to argue: "In your dream you thought such-and-such. Dreams take place during sleep. Therefore, in your sleep you must have thought such-and-such." I have no objection to the conclusion if it merely means that I dreamt that I thought such-and-such: for this

13. [Footnote added 1966] I was assuming here the following principle: If there is a certain state, S, such that it is *logically* impossible for a person in state S to give any *signs* of thinking or having experiences, then it is logically impossible for a person to think or to have experiences while in state S. Unfortunately this principle is not true. One can define a state (e.g. *total* paralysis) such that by definition a person in that state could not give any *signs* of thinking or experiencing: yet it would not follow that a person in that state could not think or have experiences. This problem is treated with greater sophistication in my monograph *Dreaming* (New York: Humanities Press, 1959). My argument there does not assume the foregoing false principle.

repeats the first premise and nothing is proved. It is only when the "argument" is taken, not as platitudinous and redundant, but as proving something, that I wish to attack it: when, that is, it is understood as proving that during a period of sound sleep I could have thoughts, sensations, impressions, and feelings in the *same* sense as that in which I have them during a half-hour of waking reverie.

Consider the second premise: "Dreams take place during sleep." Looked at in one way it is a tautology; looked at in another way it is a dubious proposition. It is a tautology in the sense that the inference from "He had a dream last night" to "He got at least some sleep last night" is valid. It is a dubious proposition when a dream is conceived of as an occurrence during sleep in the sense in which breathing is, or as an occurrence during the night in the sense in which a fright or a toothache can be. What is dubious about it? Well, let us take note of the fact that we have no way of determining *when* a dream occurred or *how long* it lasted. Of course it occurred "while he slept": but *when* while he slept? Some psychologists have conjectured that dreams occur, not during sleep, but during the period of *awaking* from sleep. Our feeling that it is impossible to decide whether this is so or not shows that we have no *criterion* for deciding it—shows that there is no sense in the question "When, while he slept, did he dream?" as there is in the questions "When, last night, did his headache begin?" or "When did his fright occur?" There is a similar lack of any criterion with respect to the duration of dreams: when should you say of a sleeping person, "Now he has begun to dream," "Now he has stopped dreaming?" We know what it means to find out whether someone has had a dream: he tells us a dream on awaking, or tells us he had one. (This concept of verification does not apply, of course, to small children or dogs. Just how much sense is there in the familiar half serious "conjecture" that the dog whose feet are twitching is dreaming of rabbits? And where this concept does apply—namely, to people who can tell dreams—there is much indefiniteness; e.g., a man says, on awaking, "I don't know whether I had a dream or not: perhaps I did." Does it make any sense to insist that either he had a dream or he didn't have one, *regardless* of whether he knows anything about it?) In the way that we find out whether someone had a dream, we sometimes also find out that it was a long dream: i.e. he *says* it was a long dream. But what is the duration of a "long" or "short" dream in "objective" time?

We can imagine the discovery of a uniform correlation between the occurrence of a specific physiological process during sleep and the subsequent reporting of a dream.[14] This correlation might be so impressive that scientists would be tempted to adopt the occurrence of the physiological process as their criterion for the occurrence of a dream. Let us imagine that it even became the criterion in ordinary life. There would then be such a thing as *proving* that a man had dreamt, although on awaking he honestly reported that he had not; and the duration (three minutes, say) of the physiological process, and its time of occurrence, could be made the criterion of the duration and time of occurrence of the dream. It would even have sense to say of someone "He is halfway through his dream!" All of this would amount to the adoption of an extremely different use of the word "dreaming." Its meaning would have to be *taught* differently; and all sorts of remarks would make sense that at present do not.

As things are, the notions of duration and time of occurrence have no application in ordinary discourse to dreams. In *this* sense, a dream is *not* an "occurrence" and, therefore, not an occurrence during sleep. The proposition "Dreams occur during sleep" can now be seen to be a curious one. It is important to ask *why* we say such a thing. The answer, I believe, is not hard to find. When someone "tells" a dream he talks in the *past* tense: after sleeping he relates how he *did* this and *saw* that (none of which is true). It is this peculiar phenomenon of speaking in the past tense after sleep, the phenomenon called

14. There is some evidence in favor of there being a positive correlation between the occurrence of strong electrical currents in the bodies of sleeping persons and their subsequently reporting that they dreamt. The experiment in which this evidence was obtained is summarized in *Recent Experiments in Psychology,* by Crafts, Schneirla, Robinson, and Gilbert (New York, 1938), pp. 377–384. I quote: "In 33 cases, series of intense action currents . . . were recorded during sleep. After the action currents had been in progress a short time, but before they had disappeared, the subjects were awakened. In 30 of the 33 cases, subjects reported that they had just been dreaming" (p. 380).

"telling a dream," that provides the sense of the proposition that dreams occur during sleep.

One would like to object here that a person who is telling a dream speaks in the past tense *because* he is reporting something that took place in the past while he slept, namely, his dream. The objection rests on the idea that his report corresponds to his dream in the same way that my report of yesterday's events corresponds to them. This is wrong. It is senseless to suppose that his dream differed from his report of it unless this means that he might change, add to, or contradict his report. No one knows what it would mean to "verify" his report. Others use his report as their criterion of what his dream was. In contrast, no one uses my report of the events of yesterday's robbery as his *criterion* of what actually happened: there are familiar ways of confirming or disconfirming my report, independently of my inclination or disinclination to amend or contradict it. If you take seriously the idea that the two reports correspond with reality, or fail to, in the *same* way, then you are confronted with the disturbing "possibility" that there are no dreams at all! I am guided here by Wittgenstein's remarks:

> People who on waking tell us certain incidents (that they have been in such-and-such places, etc.). Then we teach them the expression "I dreamt," which precedes the narrative. Afterwards I sometimes ask them "did you dream anything last night?" and am answered yes or no, sometimes with an account of a dream, sometimes not. That is the language-game. . . .
> Now must I make some assumption about whether people are deceived by their memories or not; whether they really had these images while they slept, or whether it merely seems so to them on waking? And what meaning has this question?—And what interest? Do we ever ask ourselves this when someone is telling us his dream? And if not—is it because we are sure his memory won't have deceived him? (And suppose it were a man with a quite specially bad memory?—) [15]

Perhaps when people give accounts of their dreams these accounts correspond to nothing at all! Perhaps it only *seems* to them on awaking that they dreamt!

I hope that I will not be misunderstood. I am not claiming that there are no dreams or that they do not occur in sleep—

---

15. *Philosophical Investigations* (New York, 1953), p. 184.

nor that these are genuine possibilities: of course they are not! If someone talks in a certain way after sleep then we say "He dreamt such-and-such while he slept." That is how the words are used! What I am trying to show is that *if* one thinks that a man's account of his dream is related to his dream just as my account of yesterday's happenings is related to them, one is in a hopeless difficulty: for then it *would* appear that our ostensible remembering that we dreamt such-and-such could be mistaken, not just once but all the time. If the report of the dream is "externally" related to the dream, then it may be that we are always only under the *illusion* of having had a dream, an illusion that comes to us as we awake. Trying to look at the matter in this way, we see that the notion that dreams really take place during sleep would become senseless: we should have no idea as to what would go to prove that they do.

We get out of this impasse only by realizing that there is nothing to be proved. If after sleep a person relates that he thought and did and experienced such-and-such (all of this being false), and if he is not lying, pretending, or inventing, then we say "he dreamt it." "That is the language-game!" That he really had a dream and that he is under the impression that he had a dream: these are the same thing.

There is a sharp break between the concept of "remembering a dream" and the concept of remembering what happened downtown yesterday. If a man confidently relates that he witnessed such-and-such happen in the street the day before, it can turn out that it didn't happen that way at all: it merely seems to him that he remembers such-and-such. When he gives an account of his dream there is no sense in supposing that it merely seems to him that he dreamt such-and-such. In the case of remembering a dream there is no contrast between correctly remembering and seeming to oneself to remember—here they are identical! (It can even appear surprising that we should speak of "remembering" a dream.) ·

IX

I have put forward an argument intended to prove that a person who is sound asleep cannot have any thoughts or impressions or sensations. Many persons will not be convinced by this argument, which is perfectly sound, one reason being that they tend to misapprehend the concept of the dream. They think: You can dream in sound sleep (which is true enough); in your dream you can have various thoughts, impressions, sensations (also true); therefore, while you are sound asleep you can have thoughts, etc. (which is false, unless it is the redundant conclusion that *in the dream* you have in sound sleep there can be thoughts, etc.).

The inclination to draw the false conclusion comes from the mistake of thinking that someone's report that in his dream he was, say, afraid of snakes is a report that he was afraid of snakes *in the sense* in which his report that he was afraid of snakes when he was in the woods an hour ago is a report that he was afraid of snakes. But if his demeanor and behavior when he was in the woods expressed fearlessness of snakes, this would be in conflict with this report and would make its truth at least doubtful. Similarly, if in the woods he did show fear of snakes this would fit in with and confirm his report.

The logic of the matter is entirely different in the case of the report of a dream. If when he was in bed he had, by utterances and behavior, expressed a fear of snakes, this would have no tendency to confirm his report that he dreamt that he was afraid of snakes. Quite the opposite! It would tend to establish that he had *really* felt fear of snakes and not dreamt it at all! It would also tend to establish, in the same degree, that he had not been asleep, or at least not sound asleep, not "dead to the world." It is a logical impossibility that he should, when sound asleep, express fear or fearlessness or any other state of consciousness.

If a man declares that he was in a certain state of consciousness, what would count against his assertion would be evidence that he was, at the time referred to, either in an opposite state of consciousness or else not in any state of consciousness. Evidence that he was sound asleep would be evidence for the latter. His assertion that he dreamt last night that he was afraid of snakes (an assertion that could be true even though he slept soundly) does *not*, therefore, imply the proposition that in the night he was afraid of snakes, *in the sense* of this proposition in which it would be confirmed by his having manifested a fear of snakes in the night. And that is the normal sense of the proposition! When we say "He was afraid of snakes last night" we usually mean something that would be confirmed by the fact that during the night he expressed, by some demeanor or behavior of his, a fear of snakes. When we say "He dreamt last night that he was afraid of snakes" we do not mean anything of the sort. The latter proposition, therefore, does not imply the former one. In general, and contrary to Descartes, the proposition that a certain person had in his dream last night various thoughts, sensations, impressions, or feelings does not imply the proposition that last night he had those thoughts, sensations, impressions, or feelings, in the normal sense of the latter proposition.

X

So far I have discussed the notion of dreaming only in relation to sound sleep. The concept of dreaming when partly awake is different. A person who is partly awake can have thoughts (however groggy and confused) and so can be deceived. But he does not *have* to be deceived. He is not "trapped in a dream." If it seems to him that he is sailing in the air high over green meadows he can decide to investigate—for example, to open his eyes and see where he is. The person who is sound asleep, in contrast, cannot *decide* to do anything; he can only dream that he decides; and, unlike the man who is half asleep, he cannot *find out* anything but can only dream that he does.[16]

16. A. Baillet, in his *Vie de Descartes* (Paris, 1691), Bk. II, ch. i, pp. 81–86, gives an account of the famous three dreams that apparently had an important influence on Descartes' life. In the third dream a man and a book appeared before him and then suddenly disappeared. I quote: "What especially calls for remark is that in doubt whether what he had just seen was dream or actual vision, not merely did he decide in his sleep that it was a dream, but proceeded to interpret the dream prior to his awaking" (translated by Norman Kemp Smith, *New Studies in the Philosophy of Descartes* [London, 1952], p. 36). If my argument is correct either Descartes was not sound asleep or else he *dreamt* that he decided and interpreted.

Miss Margaret Macdonald, in her paper "Sleeping and Waking" (*Mind*, April 1953) [page numbers refer to Chapter 2 above], observes that "it makes no sense to assert that one could employ any confirming technique in a dream. For one would but dream such employment" [p. 68]; that a person who is asleep cannot choose to do anything, e.g. to stop dreaming, for "once asleep, a dreamer can only dream that he makes such a choice" [p. 78]; that if I saw the

He who is sound asleep cannot realize that he sleeps; but neither can he mistakenly think he is awake. He who is half asleep *can* mistake the sights and sounds that he "dreams" for real sights and sounds; but the concept of half sleep does not *require* that he make this mistake.

A consequence of my argument is that there is no room left for the skeptical question (a) "How can I know whether I am awake or sound asleep?"—for the question is absurd, since if I raise it I am not sound asleep. It is still possible, however, for a philosopher to be troubled by the question (b) "How can I know whether I am fully awake or only partly awake?" This cannot be disposed of in the same way, and I do not try to deal with it in this paper. I will only remark that it is in essence the

---

Hebrides in a dream it does not follow either that I saw them or seemed to see them or thought I saw them [p. 74]; and that dreaming is neither a form of perception nor of illusion (*passim*). Assuming that she refers to dreaming in sound sleep, I am in agreement with these contentions although her method of argument does not resemble mine. Unfortunately Macdonald seems to have made a blunder. After noting important distinctions between the concepts of sleeping and waking, she adds, "I suggest that these differences destroy the need for Descartes' lament that 'there exist no certain marks by which the state of waking may be distinguished from sleep.' For if what is said of one state is nonsensical when applied to the other, then this provides at least one certain mark by which to distinguish between them" [p. 79f]. From the fact that there are differences between the concepts of the two states it does not follow that I can tell whether I am in the one state or the other. I have argued (Sec. VII *supra*) that the notion of a person's determining whether he himself is awake or sound asleep is senseless. Macdonald is attacked on the above point by M. J. Baker ("Sleeping and Waking," *Mind,* October 1954).

Yost and Kalish (*op. cit.*) give an elaborate analysis of Macdonald's paper. Some of their critical remarks are in disagreement with what I have contended: e.g. "to say that one dreams is to say that one sees, hears, touches, etc., while asleep" [p. 97 above]; "And as regards the so-called mental operations, we should maintain, with Descartes, that if anyone dreams that he believes, doubts, expects, desires, etc., then he really does" [p. 97]; "People can really believe sentences to be true while they are dreaming" [p. 98]; "A dreamer who is inspecting one dream-field could predict and expect certain later dream-fields; and when they occur he could recognize them to be or not to be the ones he predicted while inspecting earlier dream-fields" [p. 99]. Apparently there is *a* sense of "dream" (dreaming when partly awake) in which it is possible for a dreamer to do the above things or at least some of them. But since there is another sense of "dream" (dreaming when sound asleep) in which none of them are possible, it follows that the general statements, "To say that one dreams is to say that one sees, hears, touches, etc., while asleep," and "If anyone dreams that he believes, doubts, expects, desires, etc., then he really does," are false.

same as the question (c) "How can I know whether I am having an hallucination?" That questions (a) and (c) have a very different status is in itself a point of considerable interest.

XI

One result of the preceding treatment of the notions of sound sleep and dreaming is to show that Descartes' own solution of his problem of skepticism of the senses is untenable. In the *First Meditation* he observes that "there are no certain marks distinguishing waking from sleep." But after he has proved that God exists and is no deceiver, he goes on to declare, in the *Sixth Meditation,* that he ought

to reject as hyperbolical and ridiculous all the doubts of these past days, more especially that regarding sleep, as being indistinguishable from the waking state. How marked, I now find, is the difference between them! Our memory can never connect our dreams with one another and with the whole course of our lives, in the manner in which we are wont to connect the things which happen to us while awake. If, while I am awake, someone should all of a sudden appear to me, and as suddenly disappear, as happens in dreams, and in such fashion that I could not know whence he came or whither he went, quite certainly it would not be unreasonable to esteem it a spectre, that is, a phantom formed in my brain, rather than a real man. When, on the other hand, in apprehending things, I know the place whence they have come, and that in which they are, and the time at which they present themselves to me, and while doing so can connect them uninterruptedly with the course of my life as a whole, I am completely certain that what I thus experience is taking place while I am awake, and not in dreams. And if after having summoned to my aid all my senses, my memory and my understanding, in scrutiny of these occurrences, I find that none of them presents me with what is at variance with any other, I ought no longer to entertain the least doubt as to their truth. God being no deceiver, it cannot be that I am here being misled. [*DPW*, 264–265]

Descartes is undoubtedly intending to point out a criterion for distinguishing waking from sleep (although I do not believe that he is rejecting what he *meant* when he said in the *First Meditation* that there is no criterion): and undoubtedly this is intended to be a criterion that will enable me to tell whether *I* am awake or asleep, and not merely to tell whether some other person is awake or asleep. In the sentence "Our memory can

never connect . . ." he is surely implying that if I cannot "connect" the things that I experience with one another and with
the whole course of my life then I ought to *conclude* that I am
asleep and that these things belong to a dream. To this there is
the conclusive objection that in regard to a person who is sound
asleep (and sound sleep has to come into the question here)
there is no sense in speaking of his making a connection or
drawing a conclusion. Similarly, in the sentence "When, on the
other hand . . . ," Descartes is implying that if I do not know
where the things I apprehend come from and cannot connect
them with the course of my life as a whole, then I am justified
in *concluding* that I am asleep and dreaming. This involves the
same absurdity. Descartes' criterion is identical with the principle of "coherence" or "consistency" that Leibniz,[17] Russell,[18]
and others offer as a principle for distinguishing waking from
sleeping. If my argument is correct, there cannot be such a
principle.

17. E.g. see Leibniz' paper "On the Method of Distinguishing Real from
Imaginary Phenomena," *New Essays concerning Human Understanding,* trans.
A. G. Langley (La Salle, Illinois, 1949), pp. 717–720, esp. pp. 718–719.
18. E.g. see Russell's *Our Knowledge of the External World* (Chicago, 1914),
p. 95.

5

A. J. AYER

Professor Malcolm on Dreams

In a book on *Dreaming,* which he has recently contributed to Mr. R. P. Holland's series of *Studies in Philosophical Psychology,* Professor Norman Malcolm sets out to challenge the received opinion that dreams are conscious experiences which are enjoyed during sleep. His aim is to refute philosophers like Descartes and Russell, who draw sceptical conclusions from what they regard as the fact that our waking experiences are not intrinsically distinguishable from the delusive experiences that make up our dreams. Against them, Professor Malcolm argues that our dreams are not delusive experiences, because they are not experiences at all.

He begins by considering a remark of Aristotle's that the soul makes assertions in sleep. The example which Aristotle gives is that of a man who dreams that "some object approaching is a man or horse" or that "the object is white or beautiful." But, says Professor Malcolm, if a man can make assertions in his sleep then he can presumably assert among other things that he is asleep. And since he is in fact asleep this assertion would be true. But the fact is that if he did make this assertion it would be bound to be false. For the expression "I am asleep" does not have a use which is homogeneous with that of "he is asleep." "He is asleep" can at any time be asserted, truly or falsely, of any man other than oneself; but "I am asleep" can be

Reprinted from the *Journal of Philosophy,* 57 (1960), 517–535, by permission of the author and the Editors of the *Journal of Philosophy.*

asserted only falsely, since from the fact that someone made an assertion it follows that he is awake. To say "I am asleep" is like saying "I am unconscious" or "I am dead" in that the falsity of what is asserted is a necessary condition of the assertion's being made. But this means for Professor Malcolm that these are not genuine assertions; for he takes it to be the mark of a genuine assertion that it is at least theoretically possible that it should be made with truth.

This argument turns on the assumption that to make an assertion of any kind is logically incompatible with being asleep, and I shall argue presently that this assumption is false. But setting this aside for the moment, it is clear that Professor Malcolm has not refuted Aristotle. For what Aristotle meant, as his examples show, is that people make judgments during sleep. And even if Professor Malcolm were right in what he says about assertions, it might still be the case that a sleeping man could make judgments. And in that event might he not make the true judgment that he was asleep?

Professor Malcolm considers this objection and makes three answers to it. In the first place, he remarks that he does not see how one can be able to judge what one cannot assert. Secondly, he points out that in order to prove that one was asleep one would have to understand the use of the expression "I am asleep" or some equivalent expression, and he thinks there is a difficulty in the question how the use of such expressions could ever be learned. And, thirdly, he maintains that if we are to credit a sleeping man with the ability to judge that he is asleep, we must ourselves have reason to suppose that he understands the content of this judgment; we must be able to verify the claim that he knows the meaning of such an expression as "I am asleep." But, Professor Malcolm argues, in order to do this we should have to be able to determine that the man applied the words to himself at the right time. For if he used them to say what "was always or usually false one would have reason to think that he did not understand the words in the required sense." [1] And since Professor Malcolm holds, for reasons which we shall presently examine, that there could be no way of dis-

1. *Dreaming*, p. 9.

covering that a sleeper ever truly judged that he was asleep, he concludes that we are not entitled to assume that the expression "I am asleep" is one that anybody understands.

The only comment that I wish to make at this point is that all three answers are easily rebutted. To say that it is impossible to judge what one cannot assert is in this instance to beg the question. For if we define "assertion" in such a way that in order to make an assertion it is necessary to be awake, we thereby make room for the possibility of judging what one cannot assert; it may be held to be possible just in those cases where the person who makes the judgment is asleep. It may also be held that there could not be such cases; but this must then be established on other grounds. As for the argument that one could not teach another person the use of the expression "I am asleep" or ever discover that he had succeeded in understanding it correctly, the fallacy should be obvious. For the argument assumes that the only way in which we can teach someone the use of a sentence, and also be sure that he has learnt his lesson properly, is to train him to use it in the presence of the fact which it expresses. But to see that this is wrong we have only to remark that a great many sentences, which are successfully taught and known to be understood, are never used in the presence of the facts which they express, simply because there are no such facts: this happens in every case in which a sentence serves only to state what is false. But it would be absurd to suggest that there is no means of telling that sentences of this kind are ever understood.

What has misled Professor Malcolm here is the fact that one's using a sentence to state what is false may in certain circumstances be a sign that one does not understand it. For example, if someone kept on saying "I am asleep," with every appearance of believing it, at times when he was manifestly awake, we might reasonably conclude that he did not understand what he was saying. But the mere fact that he failed to use this sentence during his waking moments would prove rather that he did understand it than that he did not. Neither can anything be inferred about one's understanding of a sentence from the fact that one fails to assert it when the assertion would be true. For there are a great many sentences which are perfectly well understood, and yet may not be asserted because the facts which they express are considered to be boring, or embarrassing, or obscene, or just because it never occurs to anyone to assert them. It may indeed be argued that the sentence "I am asleep" falls into a special category, inasmuch as it does not merely happen not to be asserted when its assertion would be true, but logically could not be, since the making of the assertion would falsify it. But the answer to this is that it has yet to be proved either that the use of the sentence is in this way self-defeating or that if it were self-defeating it would not still make sense.

Returning to the main argument, let us now imagine that we are listening to someone who is talking in his sleep and that one of the things we overhear him saying is "I am asleep." Why should we not conclude that he was making a true judgment? Professor Malcolm's answer to this is that "in order to know that when a man said 'I am asleep' he gave a true description of his own state, one would have to know that he said it while asleep *and* that he was *aware* of saying it." [2] But this, he argues, would be impossible, for "whatever showed that he was aware of saying that sentence would also show that he was not asleep." [3] But might there not be indirect evidence? Suppose that when the man wakes he tells us that he remembers thinking that he was asleep? Again Professor Malcolm has his answer ready. If the sentence "I am asleep" has no legitimate use, there can be no such thing as thinking that one is asleep, and consequently no such thing as remembering that one had thought it. Neither, he adds, can one remember being asleep, for what would be the content of this memory? That one had one's eyes shut and was breathing stertorously? But such manifestations of sleep can be observed only by others, not by the sleeper himself.

Professor Malcolm concludes that there are not outward criteria by which one can determine that someone is aware of being asleep, and this leads him to contrast the sentence "I am asleep" with sentences like "I am in pain." Both might be held to be reports of inner experiences, but only the second is so, for we have it on the authority of Wittgenstein that an inner

2. Page 10.   3. Page 10.

process stands in need of outward criteria. And it is this same alleged absence of outward criteria that leads Professor Malcolm to conclude that there is no meaning in the suggestion that someone may be aware of saying to himself that he is asleep.

An obvious objection to the view that the sentence "I am asleep" is meaningless is that its negation is unquestionably significant. But this does not worry Professor Malcolm. He gives as an analogy the example of a roll-call, where to answer "here" is proper and significant, but to answer "not here" would be an abuse of language. In fact, surely, it would be an abuse of discipline rather than of language. It would at worst be false and in the case of a powerful ventriloquist might even be true. In the same way, Professor Malcolm argues that to ask someone if he is asleep is not to put a genuine question but merely to make a noise to test his wakefulness, and *a fortiori* that it is impossible to put such a question to oneself. People are indeed known to say such things as "Am I dreaming?" or "I must be dreaming," but these are no more than exclamations of surprise.

It is now time to examine the whole argument, so far as it has gone. There are three different questions which Professor Malcolm does not sufficiently distinguish. The first is: Can one understand the sentence "I am asleep"? The second: Can one correctly use this sentence to express a proposition which one believes? And the third: Can one correctly use it to express a true proposition? Since Professor Malcolm answers No to the first question, the second and third do not arise for him; but the least implausible of his reasons for answering No to the first question is, if anything, a reason for answering No to the third.

In fact it seems to me quite clear the proper answer to the first question is Yes. A simple proof of this is that someone who is feigning sleep may say to himself of those whom he is deceiving, "They believe that I am asleep." Now there is no question but that this sentence is intelligible. But in that case the sentence "I am asleep" must also be intelligible; for, if it were not intelligible, how could one significantly credit others with believing the proposition it expresses? Against this, all that Professor Malcolm really has to urge is that it is unverifiable, in the sense that the subject himself cannot test it, if what it states is true. But this is to take an unduly narrow view of verifiability. For the proposition which the sentence expresses is one that other people can test, whether it is true or false: the subject himself can test it if it is false, assuming, that is, that he can know that he is awake; and he can subsequently test it even if it is true by relying, if not on his memory, at least on the testimony of others. Furthermore, it has yet to be established that its truth would prevent the subject from testing it at the time. It does sometimes happen that people wake with the memory of having dreamt that they were sleeping. Professor Malcolm would deny that this was any indication that they had been aware of being asleep, or indeed that they had been aware of anything. But insofar as this denial rests merely on the assumption that the sentence "I am asleep" is unintelligible, we have seen that it is unwarranted.

The answer to our second question is also Yes. No doubt, as Professor Malcolm says, such expressions as "I must be dreaming" are very often, perhaps normally, used as exclamations of surprise. But he is not entitled to infer from this that it is impossible really to wonder whether one is dreaming, and so asleep, or even to believe it. Consider the story of Hassan, the barber of Baghdad, who was taken one night by the Caliph and introduced to such phantasmagoric scenes of luxury that neither at the time nor subsequently was he ever sure that it was not a dream. In such a situation a man might very well decide, at the time that he was having these experiences, that they were dreams, and infer from this that he was asleep. His belief in this instance would be false; but this is not to say that he could not seriously hold it.

There remains the third and more difficult question. Given that it is possible to believe that one is asleep, might not the belief be true? The ground for saying that it could not be true is that its truth would be inconsistent with its being held. It is alleged that if I am really to believe the proposition that I am asleep, or indeed any other proposition, I must first be awake. But why need this be so? The criteria which Professor Malcolm gives for a man's being asleep are first his behavior, the fact that his eyes are closed, that his breathing is regular, that he seems unaware of what is going on around him and so forth; and secondly his testimony, or rather the lack of it, the fact that he is unable later to report what was going on around him while he slept. Of these the first is the more important; indeed it is doubtful if the second should be included at all since there are cases, such as those of persons who have been hypnotized, where a man is able to give some report of what went on while he was sleeping and can still correctly be said to have been asleep. But now why should the fact that a man's eyes are closed, that he does not react in the normal way to his environment, and all the rest of it, make it impossible for him to be aware of anything at all, or to entertain any belief? A man who is lost in a day-dream may not react in the normal way to his environment; yet we do not for this reason say that he cannot be aware that he is day-dreaming, or know what he is day-dreaming about. Why should the question whether his eyes are open or shut, or the rate of his breathing make so radical a difference?

But how could we find out that the sleeper was aware of anything? Well, how do we find out? Most commonly, by questioning him when he wakes. But then we should have no way of corroborating his report. Neither as a rule do we have any way of corroborating the day-dreamer's report; but this does not prevent us from attaching a meaning to it, or even from accepting it as true. Besides, there might be corroboration. People talk in their sleep; sometimes when people have fallen into trances they engage in automatic writing. I see no logical reason why someone should not acquire the habit of writing down his dreams, automatically, as they occurred. Suppose, then, we found that his waking report agreed with what he had written down or, to take the less fanciful case, with what we had overheard him saying in his sleep, would not this be corroboration? And might not one of the statements which was so corroborated be that he thought he was asleep? There is also the case where the sleeper has been hypnotized. We know little enough about the machinery of hypnotism. But surely we are not bound to say that the sleeper who obeys the hypnotist's orders does not hear them.

Professor Malcolm does consider these objections and his

way of meeting them is to say that the sleeper who talks, or responds to the hypnotist, or in any way behaves as though he were conscious, is to that extent not fully asleep. But this is a mere evasion. Certainly, if you choose to define the state of being fully asleep in such a way that it is incompatible with any manifestation of consciousness, you can safely conclude that someone who is fully asleep will then give no outward signs of being aware of anything. But nothing is gained by this except the power to make a verbal point. It does not dispose of the examples in which the sleeper's subsequent report of what he thought or imagined in his sleep does receive corroboration; and if we are entitled to believe him in this case, why should we not also accept the similar reports that he gives us on waking from a less troubled sleep?

I conclude, then, that Professor Malcolm's argument fails on all counts. He does not show that the sentence "I am asleep" is unintelligible: he does not show that the proposition which it expresses cannot then be believed by the person to whom it refers; and so far he has given us no sufficient reason for thinking that, when this proposition is so believed, it cannot be true.

II

Having proved to his own satisfaction that it is impossible for any sleeper to make the judgment that he is asleep, Professor Malcolm generalizes his argument to cover all judgments. He relies, as before, on a strict application of the verification principle. To talk of our making judgments during sleep must be meaningless because this involves two propositions which cannot be conjointly verified. The sleeper cannot observe that he is sleeping and others who can observe that he is sleeping cannot observe that he is then making any judgment.

But could there not be indirect verification? If the sleeper tells us on waking that such and such thoughts occurred to him during sleep, why should we not believe him? The answer, according to Professor Malcolm, is that no one, including the sleeper, can be in a position to know that when the thought occurred to him he really was asleep.

To this there are a number of possible answers which Professor Malcolm tries to deal with. For example, there might have been a storm while the subject was observed to be asleep, and he might report on waking that certain thoughts were occurring to him at the same time as he heard the thunder; but Professor Malcolm's answer to this is that if he heard the thunder he was not fully asleep. Or again, the subject may claim that he remembers making a certain judgment and remembers also that he did not make it either before he went to sleep or after he woke up. But perhaps, says Professor Malcolm, he only imagines that he made it; there is no independent way in which his claim to remember making it can be checked. In the same way Professor Malcolm argues that the fact that people appear to solve problems in their sleep is no proof that their minds were working on them while they were sleeping. The facts may simply be that they fall asleep with the problem unsolved and wake knowing its solution, without any conscious process intervening. Finally, he considers the possibility of physiological evidence. It might be that a connection could be established between the occurrence of certain thoughts and some physiological condition of the thinker. If a sleeping person were observed to be in this condition, would this not be evidence that he was thinking the thoughts in question? Professor Malcolm's answer to this is that if such a connection could be discovered at all, it could experimentally be found to apply only to waking people: there would be no warrant for assuming that it also held good for those who were asleep.

This set of arguments adds nothing new. Professor Malcolm still relies entirely on Wittgenstein's dictum that an inner process stands in need of outward criteria, which he interprets as meaning not only that it is senseless to credit anyone with private thoughts or feelings unless they are in some way given public expression, but even that the man's own testimony, which is a form of public expression, is not to be accepted unless it can be independently checked; without this independent check the testimony is not to be regarded even as significant. Now I do not know whether Wittgenstein would himself have agreed with this interpretation of his oracular saying, but, whether he would or not, the result seems to me quite clearly wrong. If we have reason to think that a man is generally truth-ful, then we may be able to believe his word when he tells us what he has been thinking, even though in this instance his word is unsupported by any other evidence, and so far as this goes it makes no difference whether he claims to have been awake when the thought occurred to him or asleep.

Professor Malcolm's position is all the less defensible in that he admits that the subject's testimony may in fact be supported by other evidence. He tries, however, to neutralize this evi-dence either by the device of saying that it proves the subject not to have been fully asleep, or by explaining it away in some other fashion. Now the evidence is by its nature not demon-strative, so that if one has decided from the start that it is im-possible for people to have thoughts of any kind while they are asleep, one may always be able to find some theory, however unconvincing, to dispose of the indications that they do have them. But this will be a highly arbitrary procedure. If the evi-dence is considered dispassionately it points the other way.

It is easy to see that the same technique can be employed to show not only that a sleeping man can make no judgments but that he can suffer no sensations, feel no emotions, and have no images. The conclusion being in each case supposed impos-sible, there can be no question of accepting any evidence which would tend to prove it true. In this way Professor Malcolm manages to satisfy himself that sleep is so effectively "the death of each day's life" that it excludes our having any form of con-scious experience.

III

What, then, are dreams? Surely if a man is dreaming, and it is not a day-dream, it follows that he is asleep. Professor Mal-colm admits this, but meets the difficulty by denying that peo-ple are conscious of their dreams; or rather, to put his point more fairly, by denying that dreams come into the category of things of which one can be conscious. Dreams are connected with sleep, not as being experiences that we enjoy while we are sleeping, but simply in the sense that reporting a dream is somehow the result of having been asleep. "The criterion of someone having had a dream," says Professor Malcolm, "is that upon awaking he tells the dream"; [4] and one test of its being a dream is that the events which make up its reported content did not in fact occur.

This is very like a suggestion once made by Professor Wisdom: we do not dream but only wake with delusive memories of experiences we never had; though Professor Wisdom meant it as a joke. Professor Malcolm does not in fact go so far as to identify dreams with such delusive memories; he does not give any account of what he thinks dreams are: no doubt he considers this an improper question. What he does say is that a person's conscious report of his dreams determines whether he dreamt or not and what it was that he dreamt. Thus dreams and the waking impressions which furnish the descriptions of dreams are said to be "two different things but not two logically independent things." [5] What this means is not made clear, but I take it to imply that the existence of the waking impression is at any rate a necessary condition for one's having had a dream, and further that if the subject's account of the dream is sincere, in the sense that it is a faithful record of his waking impression, there can be no question of its being either true or false. The reason for this is that there is nothing for it to be true or false of. On this theory a man who recounts his dreams is like a writer of imaginative fiction: we cannot significantly say of his story that it corresponds, or fails to correspond, with fact.

A consequence of this, which Professor Malcolm heroically accepts, is that dreams do not occur in physical time. We are naively inclined to think that people dream while they are asleep, but this is not true in any straightforward sense. Since dreams do not literally occur at all, they no more occur when the dreamer is asleep than when he is awake. It is, however, a convention that dreams are to be spoken of as though they occurred during sleep, and indeed on particular occasions of sleep. One says "I had such and such a dream last night" or "this afternoon," and what one is supposed to mean by this is that it is last night's sleep or this afternoon's sleep that has set up one's disposition to tell such and such a fairy story. At least this is the most plausible interpretation that I can put upon the

4. Page 49.   5. Page 60.

theory. All that Professor Malcolm himself can find to say on this point is that it is improper to ask why people relate their fairy stories in the past tense: it is just the way in which this language game is played. But in the first place this is not even a correct description of the language game: it is not the events which make up the content of a dream that are assigned, in retrospect, to a particular period of sleep, but the process of dreaming about them. These are no more to be identified than are the dates of the events recounted in a history book with the date at which the book is written. And, secondly, it is not at all improper to ask why the language game, if you must call it that, takes the form it does. If saying "I dreamed that . . ." were merely a way of saying that the story which follows is not to be regarded as a record of fact, why should we speak of dreaming as a process that occurs within a given period of time? To say that this is just part of the ritual is no answer at all.

In other ways, too, Professor Malcolm's account of dreams is stranger than he seems to realize. He treats them as though they posthumously masqueraded as waking experiences. Thus he says that "to find out that one dreamt an incident is to find out that the impression one had on waking is false" [6] and this leads him to suggest that statements of the form "I dreamt so and so" are always inferential. "If a man wakes up with the impression of having seen and done various things, and if it is known that he did not see and do those things, then it is known that he dreamt them." [7] The objection that by no means every statement which helps to compose the story of a dream is false, that the persons and places about which one dreams may well be credited in the dream with properties which they really have, can perhaps be met by saying that the cardinal feature of the waking impression is that it purports to be a record of the subject's own experiences; so that, just as a work of fiction may contain true statements without thereby ceasing to be a work of fiction, the story of a dream is false as a whole because the subject did not have the experiences it attributes to him. Thus, in

6. Page 64.   7. Page 66.

this special case in which the subject remembers, or rather seems to remember, dreaming that he was asleep, the statement to be considered is not the true statement that he was asleep but only the statement that he thought he was asleep; and we have seen that this statement is held by Professor Malcolm to be false, just because the other is true.

But even if this objection can be met, a more serious difficulty remains. It may be that children pass through a stage of being unable to distinguish dreams from waking experiences, and even when one has learned this distinction, there may be occasions when it takes one some time to realize that some incident of which one wakes with a strong impression was "only a dream"; but in the normal way people do not fall into this confusion. When they remember their dreams they do not remember them as waking experiences. Yet this is what they are required to do by Professor Malcolm's theory. For if, as he holds, to tell a dream is to give a fictitious report of one's past experiences, and if, as he also holds, experiences can be significantly attributed only to those who are awake, it follows that the report of a dream is the report of waking experiences that one never had. But as an account of the ordinary run of dreams, this is simply incorrect. When I relate my dreams to my friends, or to a psycho-analyst, my intention is not to tell them falsehoods about my waking experiences: it is to tell them the truth about the experiences I had while I was asleep. Admittedly, I do not claim that these experiences were veridical, that I really did all or even any of the things that I dreamt that I was doing. But neither am I reporting that I woke up with the impression that I had really done them. What I am reporting is that it seemed to me that I was doing them, and that I had this impression while I was asleep.

But this means, on Professor Malcolm's theory, that we are even more grievously deluded than he thinks. For, if I am right in my account of what dreams are taken to be, we constantly wake with the belief that we have achieved something which he holds to be impossible. That the process of emerging from sleep should produce in us a flock of illusions about our past would be mysterious enough; but that it should subject us to an overwhelming impulse to accept and assert meaningless statements is stranger still. Yet this is what Professor Malcolm's theory leads to when it is adapted to the facts.

Still, we must not be slaves to common sense. However odd a theory may seem, it may still be acceptable if it is supported by very strong arguments. It is disappointing, therefore, to find that Professor Malcolm has nothing better to offer us by way of argument, than his old dogma that an inner process stands in need of outward criteria. We must be mistaken in identifying our dreams with experiences that come to us during sleep, because we must be mistaken in supposing that we have any experiences whose existence is not vouched for by physical signs. If dreams were inner states, says Professor Malcolm, how could one ever tell that different people meant the same thing by dreaming? In one's own case, how could one tell that the state which one called a dream-state was the same each time? Just as we acquire the concept of pain not just through feeling pain but through being told that we are in pain when we display the appropriate physical signs, so "the concept of dreams is derived, not from dreaming, but from descriptions of dreams, i.e., from the familiar phenomenon that we call 'telling a dream.' " [8] The dream itself is no more logically separable from the telling of it than is the pain in a sore foot from the behavior which shows others that one has the pain. To assume in either case that there was an "inner" phenomenon which was connected only factually with the behavior which made it known to others would, in Professor Malcolm's view, be self-contradictory; for without physical criteria for the existence of the inner phenomena such empirical conclusions could never be established.

But even if it is true that the concept of a dream, or that of any other inner state or process, is acquired only through the association of what falls under it with certain physical events, it by no means follows that this association is not empirical; it does not follow that the extension of the concept must comprise these physical events. One might as well argue that the concept of memory is derived from the physical process of

8. Page 55.

relating one's memories, and that therefore no claim that one remembers anything can be either true or false. Neither am I impressed by the argument that if a word referred to an inner state, one could never tell that it was used with the same meaning by different people, or by oneself on different occasions. For how can one tell that this is true of a word which refers to a physical event? Only by noting that the different occasions of its use, by oneself or by others, are the same in the relevant respect. And how does one tell that they are the same? Only in the end by identifying some recurrent feature of one's experiences. And why should not pain be such a recognizable feature? Or, for that matter, the memory of a dream?

Thus, even if it were true that, apart from the reports of dreams, there was no physical evidence of their existence, I still should not regard Professor Malcolm's case as proved. But in fact it is not true: there is quite a lot of physical evidence. As we have already remarked, people talk in their sleep; and what they then say may be found to tally with the account they subsequently give of their dreams. When people have nightmares they may sweat and tremble and cry out in fear. Sometimes we can account for some detail of a dream in terms of the physical stimuli to which the sleeper has been subject; a familiar example is the way in which the sound of an alarm-clock may be woven into the last stages of a dream. There is even thought to be physical evidence that dogs have dreams, though they do not report them. Finally, there is the fact that, under hypnosis or when questioned by a psycho-analyst, people revise their accounts of their dreams; they recall incidents, perhaps entire dreams, which they had not previously been able to remember. This does not accord very well with the idea that there is nothing to which reports of dreams can correspond. Or are we to say that all that the hypnotist, or psycho-analyst, achieves is to cause the patient to remodel his fairy stories or to acquire a fresh set of delusions about his past?

Professor Malcolm makes an effort to deal with these facts, but the results are not happy. In the case where we hear someone talking in his sleep, and infer from this that he is dreaming, he says that our statement that the man is dreaming has no clear sense. The fact is that it has a perfectly clear sense, which cannot be accounted for on Professor Malcolm's theory. In the case where some reported detail of a dream can be connected with a physical stimulus, he falls back on his old device of saying that the subject cannot have been fully asleep. And when it comes to nightmares, he goes even further. The state of a man who is struggling in a nightmare is "so unlike the paradigms of normal sleep that it is at least problematic whether it should be said that he was 'asleep' when these struggles were going on." [9] I leave this argument to speak against itself. As for dogs, their dreams have no content, which appears to mean only that they do not report them. But can Professor Malcolm allow that they dream at all? Perhaps he holds that they dream in some special sense, like the patients who go to psycho-analysts. For they too fall under the same blunt axe: their reaction in replying to the analyst "is so dissimilar to the normal phenomenon of telling dreams that it is better, I think, to say that in psycho-analysis there is a different concept of dreaming, than to say that in psycho-analysis one finds out what one really dreamt." [10]

But surely one of the main points about psycho-analysis is that it does not introduce a new concept of dreaming. The analyst tries to elicit and interpret the dreams that people normally have. What reason has Professor Malcolm for saying otherwise? The same as he has for doubting whether people whose sleep is troubled by nightmares are really asleep. He is convinced of the truth of his theory; so the facts which go against it must have been wrongly described. He sees it, therefore, as his duty to bring them into line.

There are times, however, when the effort is too much for him. Thus he remarks at one point that "if I had a dream in which I heard a crash, and then found on waking that a vase fell in the night, I might make the conjecture 'I must have heard the crash' meaning that the noise probably caused me to hear a crash in my dream." [11] Now on the normal assumption that Professor Malcolm was literally dreaming at the time the crash occurred, this makes perfectly good sense. But what does it come to on his own theory? That the falling of the vase caused him, several hours later, to make the false report that

9. Pages 62–63.   10. Page 57.   11. Page 99.

he heard a crash, when in fact he heard nothing at all. Well, perhaps this could be explained physiologically, but if so Professor Malcolm does not try to tell us how. The truth is that he has forgotten his own theory and is using the expression 'hearing in a dream' in the way that I think it normally would be used: to imply that the dreamer does have an auditory experience, not that he does not.

A more striking example, perhaps, is to be found in a passage where he refers to Pharoah's dream, as recorded in Genesis. "Behold in my dream I was standing on the banks of the Nile; and seven cows fat and sleek, came up out of the Nile and seven other cows came up after them, poor and very gaunt and thin. . . ." [12] Professor Malcolm remarks, truly though perhaps not quite consistently, that if Pharoah had really believed that he had gone to the banks of the Nile during the night and had there seen seven fat and seven lean cows, he would not, or at any rate should not, have used the expression "in my dream." But then he adds, suppose that instead of saying "in my dream" Pharoah had merely said that "it seemed to him" during the night that he stood on the banks of the Nile and so forth, and suppose that there was independent evidence that this was so, that he talked aloud in his sleep, for example, and told the story about the cows; then, says Professor Malcolm, he would not have been dreaming but having an hallucination, and the statement which he made on waking that it had seemed to him that cows came out of the Nile and all the rest of it, would have been true.

Now this is surely very strange. For there might easily be a convention by which we always described our dreams by saying that it seemed to us during the night that such and such things were happening to us, and if these statements can be literally true when expressed in this form, it would appear that we are after all permitted to look upon dreams as conscious experiences, provided only that we do not describe them as dreams. This prohibition may seem a little arbitrary to Professor Malcolm's opponents, but it should not greatly worry them; for in allowing that we can have hallucinations during sleep he con-

12. Genesis XVI, 17–44; quoted by Malcolm, p. 67.

cedes the main point at issue. Admittedly, he would insist that a belief in the existence of such hallucinations must always be backed by physical evidence, and I suppose he would also say that when this condition is satisfied the subject is not fully asleep. But we have already met with these provisos at other stages of the argument and we have seen that they do not save his case.

But if we reject Professor Malcolm's theory, as it would now seem we must, does this not commit us to holding that reports of dreams are liable to error, and does not this raise difficulties? As Wittgenstein put it: "Must I make some assumption about whether people are deceived by their memories or not; whether they really had these images while they slept, or whether it merely seems so to them on waking? And what meaning has this question? And what interest? Do we ever ask ourselves this when someone is telling us his dream? And if not, is it because we are sure his memory won't have deceived him? (And suppose it were a man with a quite specially bad memory?)" [13] But the answer to this is that it has as much meaning as the question whether someone really had the thoughts or feelings that he claims to remember having in a waking state. And as for its interest, might not the fact that a person unconsciously, or even consciously, suppresses or distorts the recollection of his dreams be of great psychological importance? Neither does it seem at all absurd to suggest that people should be better or worse at remembering their dreams, as they are at remembering other things. There is in fact reason to believe that this is so.

But how could we ever find out that someone had given a false, or for that matter, a true report of his dreams? Well, I have already suggested various ways in which this might be done. The most effective, in the present state of our knowledge, would be to compare his unsolicited report with that which he gave when under hypnosis or when questioned by a psycho-analyst. But supposing they are in conflict; why are we bound to accept the revised version? The answer is that we are not bound to accept it, but there might well be independent

13. *Philosophical Investigations,* p. 184; quoted by Malcolm, pp. 55–56.

reasons for our doing so. For instance, it might have been established that his memory of events, which we could check, consistently improved when he was hypnotized. But perhaps this does not apply to his dreams. What reason is there to suppose that it does not? Or again, one version or the other might be in some degree corroborated by his behavior during sleep. Or there might be physiological evidence. Of course there will be an enormous number of cases in which we have to allow reports of dreams to go untested; and our tendency will be to accept them in default of any reason why we should not. But this applies equally to the reports of experiences which people claim to remember having while awake. There is no reason, so far as this goes, for putting reports of dreams into a different category.

IV

I conclude then that Professor Malcolm's own account of the nature of dreams is not satisfactory, and that what he calls the received view can be defended against his and Wittgenstein's arguments. But this means that he has also failed in his object of providing a check to Cartesian scepticism. If we can have experiences while we are asleep, and if these hallucinatory experiences, which we call our dreams, are not intrinsically distinguishable from the veridical experiences which we have when we are awake, how can we ever be sure that we are not dreaming? How can we ever know that the experiences which we take to be veridical really are so?

The usual answer is that we make sure that we are not dreaming in exactly the same way as we make sure that some waking experience is not hallucinatory. The test which a perception has to pass in order to qualify as veridical is that the information which it seems to yield shall fit in with that which is obtained from the vast majority of our other perceptions. So the unreality of dreams is not due to their occurring while we are asleep but simply to their failure to satisfy this condition. As Russell succinctly puts it: "Objects of sense, even when they occur in dreams, are the most indubitably real objects known to us. What, then, makes us call them unreal in dreams? Merely the unusual nature of their connection with other objects of sense." [14] And again: "It is only the failure of our dreams to form a consistent whole, either with each other or with waking life, that makes us condemn them." [15] This principle of coherence, as Professor Malcolm calls it, was also adopted by Leibniz and Descartes.

He maintains, however, that as a method of finding out whether one is awake or dreaming it is open to "a simple but devastating objection." "The objection," he says, "that should occur to anyone is that it is possible a person should *dream* that the right connections hold, *dream* that he *connects* his present perceptions with 'the whole course of his life'. The coherence principle tells us that we are awake if we can make these connections and asleep in a dream if we cannot; but how does the principle tell us whether we are noting and making connections, or dreaming that we are? It seems to me that obviously it cannot and therefore the principle is worthless." [16] His own solution is not that there is some better principle but that there is no need for any principle at all. For he holds that the question "How can I tell whether I am awake?" is senseless.

Now I think Professor Malcolm's argument has this much force, that it is indeed possible to have a dream in which one raises the question whether one is dreaming, applies the coherence test, and wrongly concludes that one is not. I do not think, however, that this makes the test worthless. What it does show is that it is not conclusive. Even if my present experiences seem to pass the test, it remains conceivable that further experiences will lead me to think otherwise. In fact I am quite convinced that I am not now dreaming, that I am really engaged in writing this paper; but this does not exclude the possibility that in the next moment I shall undergo the experience of waking up and, finding the paper still unwritten, conclude that I had only dreamt that I was writing it. Still, so long as this does not happen, the fact that my experiences continue to be entirely consonant with my having written these words may surely be taken as evidence that I really have written them. But suppose that I do have the experience of waking up. Might not that be the

---

14. *Our Knowledge of the External World,* p. 85; quoted by Malcolm, p. 107.
15. *Our Knowledge of the External World,* p. 95.   16. Page 108.

one which is delusive? Might not my finding the paper unwritten be part of an anxiety dream? Again, this is possible. And again, it is for further experience to decide. In taking it for granted that I am not now dreaming, I am taking it for granted that my present experience is in the main veridical; and the test for this is that further experience confirms it. In making this claim upon the future, I am indeed not betting on a certainty; but this is not to say that the claim has no support at all.

Apart from his objection to the coherence principle, Professor Malcolm's only reason for holding that it is senseless to ask for any sort of proof that one is awake is that he thinks it meaningless to say that one is not awake. "Our investigation proves," he says, "that nothing counts for or against the truth of 'I am not awake' and so nothing counts for the truth of 'I am awake.' " [17] On his own principles, he ought to conclude from this that the sentence 'I am awake' itself is meaningless, instead of maintaining, as he mostly does, that it expresses a significant statement, which has no significant negation. He does, however, also make the suggestion that one uses this sentence not to report or describe anything but simply to show that one is awake. So Professor Malcolm says 'I am awake' and thereby reports nothing. He merely uses the sentence to show something which he describes by saying 'I am awake.' But 'I am awake' describes nothing. So nothing is stated by these means and nothing is shown.

Happily, Professor Malcolm's investigation does not prove even that it is meaningless to say 'I am not awake,' and he himself tacitly acknowledges this. He remarks, for example, that someone who sought to prove that he was awake might try to use the following argument: "I am perplexed as to whether I am awake or dreaming in sleep. But it makes no sense to suppose that I should be perplexed while asleep. Therefore I am awake." [18] But this, he thinks, is open to the objection, which was suggested to him by Mr. Warnock, that the man might be only dreaming that he was perplexed. If he really was perplexed then it would follow that he was awake; but because he can always invoke the possibility that he is dreaming, there is

17. Pages 115–116.   18. Page 17.

no way of forcing the sceptic to admit that he really is per-plexed. But, whatever may be Mr. Warnock's views on the sub-ject, this is not a rejoinder that Professor Malcolm can accept. For if 'I am dreaming' makes no sense then 'I am dreaming that I wonder whether I am dreaming' makes no sense either. In allowing this refuge to the sceptic, Professor Malcolm im-plies, quite correctly, that these expressions do make sense. He makes a valiant effort to abide by the consequences of his misguided views, but now and again the truth breaks through.

The failure of Professor Malcolm's argument leaves us, so far as I can see, with no alternative to the classical theory. Dreams are experiences. They are mostly illusions and are found to be so by the same criteria as apply to illusions in general. Their peculiarity, by definition, is that they occur to us only when we satisfy the physical conditions of being asleep. But with respect to their status as illusions this is logically irrelevant.[19]

19. In fairness to Professor Malcolm, I should add that he did not consider that this essay gave an adequate account of his views. His comments on it and my rejoinder to them are to be found in the *Journal of Philosophy*, vol. LVIII, no. 11.

6

John V. Canfield

Judgments in Sleep

In his recent book, *Dreaming*, Norman Malcolm offers a proof of these two statements:

(1) "I am asleep" is a senseless statement,

and

(2) No one can ever judge that he is asleep.

I shall show that Malcolm's proof of these is inadequate. They may appear obviously true and in little need of proof, but certain considerations indicate that their denial retains at least some preanalytic plausibility.

The experience, for example, of being aware while dreaming that one is dreaming is a fairly common one, and has often been reported. More accurately, although on analysis it may turn out that it is illegitimate to say that one is aware of anything while asleep (and hence while dreaming), it is a fact that people do say this.[1] Since we shall take it as given that a person can dream only in his sleep,[2] and since it follows that "I am dreaming" entails "I am asleep," if one could think the former, he could, presumedly, think (or judge) the latter. And if the

Reprinted from the *Philosophical Review*, 70 (1961), 224–230, by permission of the author and the *Philosophical Review*.

1. Note that the reported experience is not "In my dream I was aware of dreaming" nor, what is equivalent to this, "I dreamt that I was aware of dreaming." These two reports are not equivalent to the one given above; to dream of being aware of dreaming is certainly not to be aware of dreaming. See *Dreaming* (London, 1959), p. 112. All page references are to this book.

2. Following Malcolm. See p. 41.

former makes sense, so does the latter. Thus to deny (1) and (2) is not utterly implausible.

Let us, then, examine Malcolm's argument. After noting that it is impossible to *assert* "I am asleep" (p. 7), Malcolm considers the possibility that one might be able to *judge,* or say to oneself, "I am asleep." But that "the very notion of such a judgment is absurd," he says, can be seen as follows:

> The absurdity comes down to this, that for the judgment to be *true* the person who made it would have to be asleep. The fact . . . that there could not be a criterion for the correct use of the words "I am asleep" depends on that: for to know that a person uses those words correctly we should sometimes have to observe him judging that he is asleep *while* he is asleep. And that is the absurdity [p. 35].

This is a summary and incomplete statement of the argument, which can be spelled out more fully as follows.

The argument is developed in two phases. In the first Malcolm tries to show that it is impossible for Jones to verify the supposed fact that Smith, while asleep, made the judgment "I am asleep." Having established this, Malcolm shows that Smith himself could never verify that he made the judgment while asleep. Thus it is shown that it is "theoretically impossible" for anyone to verify that Smith, while asleep, made the judgment "I am asleep." It is precisely in this way that "I am asleep" is a senseless statement. It is senseless in that no one could verify it: "nothing can count in favour of either its truth or its falsity" (p. 37). And if it is senseless, then (2) follows: no one can ever judge that he is asleep.

Let us examine the first phase of this argument more closely. "I am asleep" cannot be asserted or communicated.[3] Malcolm notes that "there is something dubious in the assumption that there can be a true judgment that cannot be communicated to others" (p. 9). For he says that although there is a difference between the *truth* and the *correctness* of an assertion, we cannot say that a person uses a sentence correctly unless he usually uses it to say something true. Since on Malcolm's view to understand a sentence is to know how to use it correctly, we can say:

3. See pp. 5–7. "I am asleep" when said to someone is either a humorous way of saying "I am awake" or else means something like "I am trying to go to sleep, don't bother me."

(a) A person understands a sentence ϕ *only if* for most of the times that he says ϕ, ϕ is true.[4]

Thus Malcolm writes, "You would have no right to say that someone understood the sentence 'He is asleep' unless, for the most part, when he applied those words to some person that person was indeed asleep" (p. 10).

Given (a) it follows that for Jones to verify that Smith understands the locution "I am asleep," Jones must discover that Smith makes the judgment when Smith is in fact asleep. But, Malcolm points out, Jones could never make this discovery. For anything about Smith's behavior that indicated that he was making a judgment would necessarily indicate also that he was not asleep.[5] Thus, if Smith makes the judgment "I am asleep," he must be aware of making the judgment. But any evidence that Smith is aware of making a judgment—his wearing a thoughtful look, for example, and mumbling the judgment to himself—is at the same time evidence that he is not sleeping.

The first phase of the argument, however, is not yet complete. For we must consider the possibility that Jones verifies that Smith judged truly "I am asleep" by simply having recourse to Smith's testimony that he had so judged. Here in full is Malcolm's argument on this point:

It may be thought that we could appeal to the sleeper's testimony after he awakened. Suppose he told us that he had said "I am asleep" while he was asleep. But this report would presuppose that he already knew when to say "I am asleep," and so it could not be used to establish the point at issue without begging the question. That is to say, his claim that he said certain words *while asleep*, implies that he was *aware* of being asleep and so implies that he knows how to apply the sentence "I am asleep." If he does not, his report is worthless. If we have no way of establishing that he knows how to use the sentence *other* than by appeal to his testimony, then we cannot appeal to his testimony [p. 11].

This argument seems to rest on the last sentence quoted, which instantiates the general principle:

(b) If we have no way of establishing that a person knows

4. We restrict the range of ϕ to descriptive statements of the form ". . . is. . . ."
5. Malcolm says, "It would be self contradictory to *verify* that a man was both asleep and judging that he was, because whatever in his behavior showed he was making the judgment would equally show he was not asleep" (p. 36).

how to use a sentence *other* than by appeal to his testimony, then we cannot appeal to his testimony.

It is obvious that if (b) were false, the argument, in the form just quoted, would collapse.

It now follows, Malcolm believes, that no one can ever verify that someone else judges truly "I am asleep." From this it follows, given (a), that no one can ever verify that another person understands the sentence "I am asleep." The second phase of the argument, as we have noted, will attempt to show that the person himself cannot verify that he knows how to use correctly the sentence "I am asleep." Given these two proofs, it will follow that "I am asleep" is senseless in that no one can ever verify that it is used truly, and also in the sense that no one can verify that it is used correctly.

This first part of Malcolm's argument is, I believe, inadequate in two ways. First, the principle (a) to the effect that a person can be said to understand a sentence only if he usually uses it to say something true seems false. There seem to be a host of counterexamples to (a). Consider the sentence "I am 32 years old," asserted through the years by a vain woman. It will often be the case that although such a woman understands the sentence perfectly and uses it on many occasions, she never uses it to say something true. It may be objected that she is lying, and that (a) is not meant to apply to such cases. Then consider the following example. The foster parents of a foundling never tell him that he is not their child. The boy, when grown up, has many occasions to say, "This is my father." Here he certainly knows what the sentence means, yet he never uses it to make a true statement. Such examples are easily multiplied. They indicate clearly that (a) is no necessary condition for saying that someone understands a sentence.

However, even if we grant (a) and thus the corollary that for Jones to verify that Smith understands "I am asleep" it is necessary that Jones discover instances where Smith uses the sentence to say (to himself or others) something true, I do not think Malcolm's argument will work. For consider the sentence:

(3) I am sitting perfectly still

meaning that none of the now voluntarily controllable muscles of my body are moving. Now this makes perfect sense, and is used to make a true judgment whenever anyone sits quietly and says (3) to himself. Furthermore, there seem to be ways of verifying that someone understands (3). But it can be easily shown, I think, that if Malcolm's argument works for "I am asleep," it also works for "I am sitting perfectly still." (3) is like "I am asleep" in that it cannot be asserted.[6] (This shows the incorrectness of Malcolm's statement that there is something dubious about a true sentence that cannot be communicated.) It is also like "I am asleep" in that we can never verify that someone else is making the judgment "I am sitting perfectly still." Whatever would indicate that the person is making this judgment would indicate also that he is not sitting perfectly still. For Smith, when sitting still, certainly need not be making the judgment that he is sitting still. The only way we have of deciding that at any given time he did make this judgment while sitting still (and thus that he made a true judgment using the sentence "I am sitting still") is by reliance on his testimony. Thus, on Malcolm's view, the only way we have of knowing that Smith understands the sentence "I am sitting perfectly still" is to ask Smith if he thought the sentence while he was indeed sitting perfectly still. But since this would be the only way of verifying that he understands it, by Malcolm's dictum (b) there is no way of verifying that he understands it.[7] We can know that he knows how to use the sentence only by appealing to his testimony; therefore, by (b), we cannot appeal to his testimony. Hence, using exactly the same arguments used by Malcolm to show that we cannot verify that someone else understands the sentence "I am asleep," we have shown that it is impossible to verify that someone else understands the sentence "I am sitting perfectly still." But the conclusion thus derived from Malcolm's premises is false. Everyone who understands English understands the sentence "I am sitting perfectly still." Is there any difficulty in verifying that some person understands it? There does not seem to be, especially when it is remembered that we are not looking for absolute verification, but only for some evi-

6. In the sense of "assert" used by Malcolm, where to assert x is to communicate (or attempt to communicate) x.

7. Here we assume, as Malcolm would, that if a person does not know how to use a sentence correctly, he does not understand it.

dence that "can count in favor of its truth or falsity" (p. 37). One method of verification would be simply to ask the person to describe the circumstances under which he would apply the sentence to himself. If he answered, "I would say to myself 'I am sitting perfectly still' provided I were seated and none of the (voluntarily controllable) muscles of my body were moving," then we would say without hesitation that he understands the sentence and we would have, in his testimony, evidence in favor of the hypothesis that he understands the sentence.

Before we can count the example of the sentence "I am sitting perfectly still" as a *reductio* of the first part of Malcolm's argument, however, there is an important objection that must be met. We noted that if someone could describe circumstances under which he would say to himself (truly) "I am sitting perfectly still," we would count this as a verification of the hypothesis that he understood the sentence. It might be replied that this description would not be enough, and that the person would have to describe a criterion by which he could recognize that he is sitting still. One might say further that the criterion would have to be such that it is possible for the person, when sitting still, to recognize that the criterion is being met. And one might say, finally, that although we can give such a criterion for the use of "I am sitting perfectly still," we cannot do so for "I am asleep." The usual criterion for saying that someone is asleep is that he is lying quietly, breathing slowly, is impervious to light sounds, and so forth. Obviously a person could not use this criterion to tell that he is asleep, since if he could recognize that these conditions held, he would not be asleep. Furthermore, it seems unlikely, as Malcolm argues, that there could be any criterion by which a person could decide that he is asleep when he is asleep.[8] To escape the *reductio* argument built on the example "I am sitting perfectly still," then, it can be argued that even though we can only rely on Smith's testimony to discover that he understands the locution "I am sitting perfectly still," his testimony is acceptable because he does have a workable cri-

---

8. Malcolm argues against the possibility of a criterion for the use of "I am asleep" in the second part of his argument, when he is trying to show that Smith could not know that he made the judgment "I am asleep" when he was asleep (pp. 12–13).

terion for the application of the sentence. Because there is no such criterion for the sentence "I am asleep" Smith's testimony cannot be relied on to show that he understands the sentence "I am asleep."

The difficulty with this objection is its assumption of the necessity of a criterion for the use of the sentence "I am asleep." At this stage of the argument, if it can be shown that there is no need for a criterion for the use of "I am sitting perfectly still," then it will have been shown that a similar criterion for "I am asleep" is not necessary. For the reply just outlined to the *reductio* argument presupposes that there is a criterion for the use of "I am sitting perfectly still." The two sentences "I am asleep" and "I am sitting perfectly still" are alike in that there is no possibility of someone's verifying that another person is using either sentence to make a judgment. If they are also alike in that there is no criterion by which a person discovers that he is using either of the sentences to say something true, then on Malcolm's argument we must conclude (falsely) that of neither sentence can we say that another person knows how to use it.

Here it will be useful to modify our example. Instead of the sentence "I am sitting perfectly still," consider "I am sitting perfectly still with my eyes closed." This latter sentence, like the former, is obviously meaningful and well understood by almost everyone who understands English; moreover, we can verify that someone knows how to use it. For surely it would count as evidence in favor of the hypothesis that someone knows how to use it if he were to say, "I would say to myself, 'I am sitting perfectly still with my eyes closed' if none of the voluntarily controllable muscles of my body were moving and if my eyes were in fact closed."

The question now is whether there is some criterion which Smith would use in order to ascertain that the state he is in is one truly described by the sentence in question. There plainly is none. Smith does not have to find out that he is sitting perfectly still and that his eyes are closed; nor does he have to make a check of any set of data in order to know that he is in this state. He need not apply to himself any of the criteria he might use to tell if some other person is sitting perfectly still with his eyes closed. In fact he applies to himself no intersubjectively applicable criterion. Nor does he examine his own mental state or bodily feelings in order to judge truly of himself that he is sitting still with his eyes closed.[9] It seems clear, then, that no criterion is needed for Smith to be able to tell that he is sitting perfectly still with his eyes closed. And, as we have noted for the case of the sentence "I am sitting perfectly still," there is no way for Jones to verify, while Smith is sitting perfectly still with his eyes closed, that Smith is saying to himself or making the judgment "I am sitting perfectly still with my eyes closed."

Thus again, on Malcolm's argument, it is true that just as Jones cannot verify in any way that Smith understands the sentence "I am asleep" so it is also true that he cannot verify that Smith understands the sentence "I am sitting perfectly still with my eyes closed." But the latter sentence is meaningful and verifiable. Therefore some of the arguments used by Malcolm in the first part of his argument must be revised. It is difficult to see, however, how Malcolm could weaken his argument at all and still show that "I am asleep" is meaningless.

As for the second part of Malcolm's argument, it relies on the fact that there could be no criterion by the use of which Smith could truly say of himself "I am asleep." We have already seen that Malcolm has not shown the necessity of such a criterion, and that, indeed, it seems unwise to demand one, since such a demand results in at least one strongly counterintuitive consequence.

9. The sentence in question is like the sentence "I have a headache," in that no criterion is used by the person who says this sentence of himself. There is, to be sure, the difference that Jones can verify that Smith uses the sentence "I have a headache" correctly, by observing that Smith holds his head and grimaces when he says it. But no one can ever say aloud the sentence of our example. That is, no one can assert it, just as one cannot assert "I am asleep"; nor can Jones ever verify directly that Smith uses the sentence correctly.

7

ROBERT L. CALDWELL

Malcolm and the Criterion of Sleep

A number of Malcolm's conclusions in his book on dreaming as well as some of the arguments he uses to reach them seem to be incompatible not only with our ordinary conception of dreaming and with commonly accepted facts, but with other statements in his own theory as well. He says, for example, ". . . that we have no way of determining *when* a dream occurred or *how long* it lasted"¹ and ". . . there is no sense in the question 'When, while he slept, did he dream?' "² These remarks are part of an argument intended to show that a dream has no genuine (experiential) content or duration and therefore that thoughts, impressions, sensations, or feelings cannot occur either in dreams or in sleep in the same sense in which they occur ordinarily. A person who dreams he is climbing a hill is not really doing so; similarly a person who dreams he is angry is not really angry, or if he gives some behavioral evidence of being angry then in that respect he is not really asleep.

It is impossible, in other words, to have experiences of any sort while asleep (except dreaming, of course) because these

---

Reprinted from the *Australasian Journal of Philosophy*, 43 (1965), 339–352, by permission of the author and the Editor of the *Australasian Journal of Philosophy*.

1. This quotation and the next are not obtained from *Dreaming* but from an article entitled "Dreaming and Scepticism" [Chapter 4 above—Ed.] The views expressed in the book and the article, however, are similar. I use this quotation because it concisely summarizes Malcolm's view.

2. *Ibid.*, p. 118.

states or activities are incompatible with the primary criterion of sleep. The frequent appeals to vivid dreams and the supposed continuity between them and waking life as evidence for the alternative view, therefore, are simply misguided. If something occurs in a dream it must be understood in a special way, even though the language used to describe it is the ordinary kind. To argue from the similarity of language to the similarity of experience is simply to overlook or ignore the distinction between the dream-telling and the historical uses of language. On the other hand, if the experience *is* the same, then the person is not really asleep.

No doubt there is something paradoxical about this view, for we normally do think that dream experiences are real in some sense or other, and although seeing or hearing may not actually occur in them, still *something* does which is rightfully described by the historical use of language. Why, then, should Malcolm fly so egregiously in the face of custom and habit by denying what most of us spontaneously affirm? His reason is that the alternative seems not to be a genuine possibility at all. In his essay entitled "Dreaming and Scepticism", Malcolm makes this quite clear. To deny his position that there are criteria for mental occurrences and states of consciousness ". . . leads one to the view that each person *teaches himself* what fright, doubt, thinking, and all other mental phenomena are, by noting his own fright, doubt, etc.: each person 'knows from his own case' what these things are." [3] Since *this* view is generally and rightfully thought to be impossible, there is nothing more to be said on the question if the disjunction is thought to be genuine. Once this is admitted, Malcolm's argument falls more or less into place, and though there may be a number of peripheral difficulties, the main question seems to be fairly, if not conclusively, resolved. But why should we accept this disjunction? So far as I can see, no proof has been offered for supposing the alternatives *are* exhaustive; the statement seems rather to be simply an assumption, apparently so obviously true that no argument is needed to justify the asserting of it. But the general unsatisfactory nature of Malcolm's argument suggests

3. *Ibid.*, p. 112.

to me, at least, that something is fundamentally wrong with the premise on which it seems to be based. Not only are there errors in reasoning, but some of the conclusions which he draws strike me as being simply wrong. Furthermore, I seriously doubt if criteria exist in at least two of the three senses in which Malcolm uses the word. Consequently, supposing these charges can be made good, there must be another alternative to those he mentions, and as a result the thesis of *Dreaming* if not shown to be false at least looks to be highly questionable.

In what follows, therefore, I shall begin by discussing what I take to be inconsistencies and errors in Malcolm's own argument, and then try to make some sense of fixing a dream in time and giving it a real content. The major portion of the paper, however, will be concerned with the question of criteria. Here I shall argue that Malcolm is mistaken in holding that behavior is the criterion of sleep, the point of this being not to show that we learn what sleep is by introspection, of course, but that we learn it in a way which is somewhat different from either of the two possibilities already mentioned. This argument will also tend to substantiate my view about the contents of dreams, and that in turn will suggest something about the meaningful uses of language.

Consider first this rather curious argument about the impossibility of anyone making judgments during sleep. Malcolm says: "If a sleeping person could note that it is raining or judge that his wife is jealous, then why could he not judge that he is asleep? The absurdity of the latter proves the absurdity of the former." [4] But arguing by analogy, if a waking person could judge that it is raining or that his wife is jealous, then surely he ought to be able to judge that he is awake. But since nothing counts for the truth of "I am awake", according to Malcolm himself, then we cannot assert it, presumably, and therefore the statement that it is raining is also absurd.

An equally curious remark which Malcolm makes in regard to the supposed continuity between dreaming and waking seems to be a clear repudiation of his repeated assertion that

4. Norman Malcolm, *Dreaming* (London: Routledge and Kegan Paul, 1959), p. 36.

testimony is the sole criterion of dreaming. Suppose a person does awaken in the middle of a dream and by testimony and behavior makes it evident that he is still in an emotional state which he claims is identical with his dream state. Ordinarily we would believe him without hesitation or question. His present state is taken as indicating the character of the contents of his dream, just as an exhilarated manner at the end of an activity is some evidence for the character of that activity. It isn't essential, however, that a particular kind of behavior be manifested; if the speaker were perfectly calm we might be a little suspicious of the claim that he is now in an agitated state which is continuous with the dream, but we would not question his dream report merely on the basis that his present behavior doesn't correspond with it. This would be to deny that testimony is the criterion for dreams and the contents of dreams. But Malcolm's comment, "How could someone show us that a dream of his was unpleasant other than by his having an *unpleasant impression* of it on awakening? . . . If he said 'It was horrible' but showed no genuine impression of horror, we should think the dream was not so bad" [5] seems to be just such a denial. Apparently testimony is not really sufficient to inform someone of the dream contents after all; one does not understand the concept of an unpleasant dream unless the teller behaves in a certain way, and if his behavior is not of the required sort, we are free, presumably, to discount his testimony. In other words, a person who tells a dream might be mistaken about it.

Finally, Malcolm says that since there is no way of verifying whether someone is both asleep and judging, the supposition that this might be so is senseless: nothing can count in favor either of its truth or falsity. This is the case even though someone might establish a relationship between the making of a judgment and electrical changes in the brain, for the induction thus formulated cannot be extended to a person who is sleeping, since it is established only with people who are awake. Presumably there is a way of verifying behaviorally whether someone is awake and judging or willing, then, inasmuch as the

5. *Ibid.*, p. 92.

behavior of a sleeping person is inconsistent with that of a person actually doing these things. But what the behavior of a person having images, for example, would be is left unsaid. Apparently it is assumed as a matter of course that some behavior would occur on the basis of which one could verify that images were being experienced. But what sort of behavior would this be? Until this is made clear and until we know what to look for, the claim that there is no way of verifying the occurrence of images in sleep is really empty. There seems to be no way of verifying them in any case unless the testimony of the person is considered to be verification—and Malcolm won't allow this by itself except in the case of dreams. I am not arguing, of course, that as a matter of fact no way exists of verifying that images are occurring to someone; there might be a way, but unless it is shown, the argument which is based on the supposition that it has already been done begs the question. An objection to everything is not also another objection to something. And is it true even in the cases of judging or willing for which verification might make sense, that these actions are always accompanied by some characteristic behavior? If there are instances in which this is not so (and surely there are such), then the argument against the possibility of judging in sleep also appears somewhat weak.

Turning now to the question of a dream's content and its temporal location, we see that Malcolm's position is influenced mainly by two considerations: that behavior is the principal criterion of sleep and that the having of images and feelings is inconsistent with that criterion. One cannot be fully asleep and give evidence of undergoing any real experience, for such evidence would indicate that the person was not fully asleep at all. One may report feelings of suffocation occurring in a dream, of course, but this is quite a different thing from reporting a genuine feeling of suffocation. One is the dream-telling use of language and the other the historical use. If an attempt were made to use these feelings as a way of locating a dream in time or giving it a real content, the effort would be bound to fail. In order to *be* suffering the victim would have to behave in the appropriate way, but then, of course, he would not be dreaming. Malcolm's view, in short, is that dreams yield no determination

in physical time nor can they contain or be identical with judging, reasoning, feeling, imagery, and so on.[6]

But consider two fairly common events which sometimes
occur in dreams—the nocturnal emission, defined in *Webster's
Third New International Dictionary* as an "involuntary discharge
of semen during sleep often accompanied by an erotic dream",
and enuresis. If testimony is the criterion for the contents of
dreams, as Malcolm argues it is, then there *are* events happening simultaneously in dreams and in actuality, and there are
dream desires and sensations which at least resemble the ordinary kind inasmuch as they culminate in the same activity.

Malcolm's rejection of similar arguments on the ground that
any activity during sleep is evidence that the person is really
partially awake doesn't seem particularly effective here. In the
first place, even if his criterion of sleep were entirely correct,
these cases would still have to be considered on other grounds.
The difference between them and those which might be elimi-
nated is that the criteria of sleeping and of dreaming could
both be satisfied and yet the activity still occur, whereas in the
case of suffocating, for example, the criterion of sleep might
not be fully satisfied. Perhaps Malcolm would say it would not
be fully satisfied in the other instance either, but surely this
would weaken rather than strengthen his argument, for then
he would be committed to saying that we cannot really tell
when a baby is fully asleep unless we observe it *au naturel*.

The experiences occurring in these dreams may not be judgments or reasoning, but they do seem to consist of genuine
feelings and desires and apparently give some sense to the notion of fixing a dream in time. Suppose a man having an erotic
dream awakens in the middle of it and discovers that he is simply not dreaming after all: the events which occurred in his

6. This is not quite right, for he does admit that testimony sometimes determines when a dream occurred. One is awakened suddenly, for example, and
claims to have been dreaming just before. Unfortunately, however, we don't
know what "just before" would amount to on the clock, Malcolm says, for it is
not that sort of determination. We are simply inclined to use this expression on
awakening. *Why* we are all so inclined Malcolm doesn't say, nor does he explain
in what sense testimony *does* determine when a dream occurred, but this is not
particularly surprising in view of his thesis that dreams do not occur in physical
time at all.

dream are happening in the real world as well. Wouldn't this circumstance be sufficient for giving the dream a temporal location? If the awakening is gradual the sleeper could even pass from the dream to the waking state without breaking the continuity, so to speak, from one to the other. As the experience builds up to a climax in the dream, so does the excitement build up in the dreamer. If this is sufficiently strong he awakens and the dream ends, but the experience continues on. In so doing, however, it does not jump an unbridgeable chasm from the dream to the waking state. One merges into the other around the core of a common event. Thus a fairly precise sense can be given to the expression "just before" inasmuch as experiences of this kind are easily timed in their ordinary manifestations and need simply be transposed to the dream.

So far this is all rather peripheral to the main argument of the paper, and is intended to show only that Malcolm's view isn't completely satisfactory, though on the surface it is clearly more plausible than the other which he rejects. I do not think that patchwork repairs can be effectively made, however, which will leave the main structure of his argument intact, for it is precisely this structure, as I've already mentioned, which I think is at fault. By this I do not mean that the argument is faulty, for the unacceptable conclusions do follow from the premises, but rather that the premises—or better, the premise—is wrong. Once doubt is cast on this, therefore, the whole edifice is in danger of crumbling; hence, instead of concentrating on the conclusions in a piecemeal way, I shall argue that Malcolm is mistaken in maintaining that behavior is the criterion of sleep.

Malcolm, of course, says that behavior is only one criterion of sleep; testimony is the other, but it has less weight. By testimony, Malcolm apparently does not mean the sleeper's claim that he was asleep but rather his ability (or inability) to give an account of the events which occurred around him during the time he supposedly was asleep. Whether he was asleep or not is therefore determined not by the person himself but by someone else. He cannot observe his behavior while he is asleep, nor would it be right to take his word that he was, since this is not the kind of testimony which Malcolm has in mind. This point is sufficiently important to warrant a fuller discussion later on, and I shall therefore let it go for the time being. The puzzling thing now, however, is the existence of two criteria and the contradiction to which Malcolm seems committed by holding them. If a criterion is something which settles the question with certainty as to whether or not a person has a sore foot or a dream, for instance, then one is asleep if the criterion of sleep is manifested. But if a conflict between criteria is possible, as Malcolm admits it is, then either one or the other cannot be a criterion at all. Surely it is contradictory to say that the criterion might be satisfied and yet the person still be awake. Malcolm's own example is relevant here and makes the point quite clearly.[7] Suppose we judge that a person is asleep by virtue of his behavior, and yet he is able to relate what had been said and done in his presence without being informed of it. Should we conclude that he was not asleep after all—that he was just pretending? Such a suggestion is incomprehensible to Malcolm: he *must* have been asleep or he would not have permitted his valuables to be destroyed. But couldn't one argue just as cogently for the other side: he must have been awake since he can relate in detail what went on when he was supposedly asleep? The criterion of testimony is clearly satisfied here, and if it is not to be accepted, then testimony is simply not a criterion for sleep though it might be something else. Assuming this is the case, I shall therefore concentrate on behavior and not consider testimony as a serious candidate for the post to which Malcolm assigns it.

Before going on to argue that behavior can't be the criterion of sleep, it would be well to get clear about what a criterion is. In addition to being something which settles the question with certainty as to whether someone has a pain, for example, a criterion is also a device for teaching the proper use of a word. The quotation cited on page 158 [above, Ed.] suggests this, at any rate, for if criteria did not exist then one would have to teach himself what mental phenomena are by introspection.

---

7. *Dreaming*, p. 26. Note in this example, incidentally, that when Malcolm says that someone must have been asleep or he would not have allowed his valuables to be destroyed, he is making an inference and hence behavior is not a criterion but evidence.

This same view is also advocated in *Dreaming:* "But it is obvious that no one would *teach* the word 'asleep' ostensibly by using examples of people who are shouting or walking. These cases would be at a considerable distance from the paradigm." [8] In another essay, however, Malcolm seems to express still another view. A criterion does not function primarily as a teaching device but as a way of determining whether someone else's claim to be frightened, in doubt, or in pain is correct: ". . . that his knowledge came about by way of the normal process of teaching is not necessary. What is necessary is that there should be something on the basis of which we may *judge* whether he *has* that knowledge." [9] Since these views do not seem to be synonymous (and perhaps are not even consistent), I shall consider them each in turn. The first and third senses of the word have to be kept separated, of course, inasmuch as we can say that a baby is asleep even though the baby itself is not capable of showing us that *he* knows what sleep is.

Is it possible, then, that behavior is a criterion of sleep in the sense that it permits us to say with certainty that someone is asleep? To deny it is apparently to admit as true the absurdity that Malcolm cites of never knowing when a baby or a dog is asleep. And since in these cases the criterion of sleep *is* behavior, according to him, one is almost bound to say it continues to be so after the development of speech. Undoubtedly if we were required to find out whether someone was asleep we would look for a certain kind of behavior, a fact which lends some plausibility to the position, but to maintain that this is what makes it certain that the person is asleep is clearly to place a greater reliance on behavior than it seems to warrant. Since feigning is possible, behavior will indicate or be a criterion of sleep only under some circumstances. But what circumstances? What makes it certain that one is not feigning? Presumably there is a criterion for the use of the sentence "He is feigning sleep" as well as for the sentence "He is asleep", and inasmuch as successful feigning requires behavior which is indistinguishable from the behavior of a person genuinely asleep, the

8. *Ibid.*, pp. 27–28.
9. Malcolm, *Knowledge and Certainty: Essays and Lectures* (Englewood Cliffs: Prentice-Hall, Inc., 1963), p. 112.

criteria for the two seem to be identical. But if this were the case there would be no difference between being asleep and pretending to be asleep, a view which is patently absurd. There is a difference, of course, but it cannot lie in behavior, apparently, if pretence is possible. The possible rebuttal that *subsequent* behavior permits us to distinguish between genuine and feigned sleep is, of course, tacitly to admit that successful feigning *is* indistinguishable from sleeping, and hence is no rebuttal at all.

The following impasse thus seems to be engendered: if behavior *is* the criterion of sleep it can function only when the possibility of feigning is ruled out. But successful feigning cannot be ruled out and still be successful. Therefore, either behavior, *per se,* is not the criterion of sleep or else so many restrictions must be placed on the affirmative statement that it becomes a mere tautology. That is to say, it must be rendered in some such fashion as this: behavior is the criterion of sleep when the person involved is not pretending to be asleep, is not unconscious, etc. In other words, behavior is the criterion for sleep when the person is genuinely asleep. Unfortunately for this criterion, however, when he is asleep seems not to be known with certainty from his behavior.

What, then, becomes of Malcolm's contention that it would be too absurd to say that we never know if a baby or a dog is asleep? Well, is the criterion for sleep here simply behavior? Haven't we ruled out the possibility of feigning in these cases, a ruling without which behavior apparently cannot function as a criterion at all? Admittedly, when we look to see whether a baby is asleep we are not generally aware of the implicit rider accompanying our inquiry, but if we were challenged to defend our judgment that the baby was asleep and not pretending, surely it would be relevant to point out the impossibility of pretence. A baby has to sleep before it can pretend, and hence up to a certain level of development, behavior functions as an indication of sleep because pretence is too sophisticated a performance for a baby to undertake. "Lying is a language-game that needs to be learned like any other." (P.I. 249) If this were not the case we would be in the same difficulty with infants as we are with adults in determining whether or not they are asleep. What I am saying, in other words, is that behavior seems to be the way we determine whether a baby is asleep only when we know in particular instances (and this is usually the case) that it cannot pretend. The adult, on the other hand, can do so, and therefore that which makes it possible to judge with certainty that a baby is asleep does not apply in his case. The difference is not so much in the criterion, however (for one can truthfully say in both cases that the criterion is behavior plus the knowledge that no pretence is occurring, though this is far from satisfactory), but in trying to find out *when* it can apply. But this, of course, is to destroy one of the functions a criterion is supposed to perform.

In addition to this difficulty, we are also faced with the problem which I alluded to earlier. If behavior were the criterion of sleep in *this* sense of the word, and if there is no other way by which it can be ascertained whether or not one *is* asleep, then it follows that someone else is always a better judge of whether I was asleep than I am. If my behavior conflicts with my belief that I *was* asleep, then my testimony is always rightfully impugned. Perhaps this doesn't seem particularly objectionable, but put in another way what it comes to is that everybody might be mistaken in his use of the sentence "I was asleep". Since we can never observe our own behavior while asleep, we can never know whether we were asleep and hence whether our present use of the sentence is correct. Someone else might know this by observing our behavior during the time we allegedly were asleep, but it is his corroboration of our claim and not the claim itself which decides the question. But this is simply to say that we really don't know how to use the sentence "I was asleep"; at best we guess that we are using it correctly, though we can, of course, verify the correctness of our guess by reference to someone else's testimony. We cannot know independently of this testimony, however, whether we were asleep; as a matter of fact, we cannot even improve our skill at guessing since the criterion by which our performance is judged is always unavailable to us. Perhaps we could still come to learn the use of the sentence "I was asleep" by being told when awake that it applies to a state just terminated, but we would never be able to tell without help that it is used correctly.

There is an incidental curiosity associated with this point which deserves passing mention, and that is Malcolm's claim that "A man's own statement is decisive for the determination by others of whether he has a sound sleep." [10] Suppose his claim to have a sound sleep is inconsistent with his behavior at that time. On the basis of behavior we judge that he is not really asleep at all; yet he says that he slept soundly. Which of these two claims shall we honor? If it is the former, then a man's own statement is not decisive about the character of his sleep; and if the latter, then behavior is not the criterion of sleep.

The second of the three senses of "criterion" which Malcolm suggests is that of teaching the proper use of a word. I suppose this one is not really thought to be independent of the other, since we could not learn what sleep is, apparently, unless a certain kind of behavior did make its presence certain. But teaching the word is clearly different from determining whether it applies when one already knows it, and this is the function with which I am now concerned. The only possibility of using a criterion as a teaching device is in respect to others, of course, and the view here is that one can come to understand the word "sleep" by observing people who are asleep. As I said earlier, this view is not one which Malcolm ever really argues for; apparently he is content to assume it is true without bothering to give it a defence. But even if there were a criterion for sleep in the first sense of the word, and this would seem to make the teaching considerably easier, would it follow that one knows what it is a criterion for? It doesn't automatically follow that one will learn what sleep is by observing the behavior which another person uses to judge that someone is asleep. A passage of some kind still has to be effected from the criterion to its concept, and since one is not logically deducible from the other, the presence of the first doesn't imply an understanding of the second. Being able to say with certainty that someone is asleep on the basis of behavior, therefore, is not equivalent to

10. *Dreaming*, p. 33.

saying that one could learn what sleep is by appealing to that criterion.

But let us take a specific instance in which the concept might be taught and try to determine whether it is really very likely to happen under the conditions visualized by Malcolm. We would need an instructor, a student, and a sleeping person, the instructor knowing already what sleep is and able to determine when the subject is really asleep. Now the question is *how* does he know? Perhaps in the excitement of the experiment the subject was unable to sleep and feigned it instead. Could one be distinguished from the other, and would it really make any difference to the teaching if it couldn't? Wouldn't the first be as effective—or ineffective—as the second? And even if the instructor could be certain that his subject was sleeping, still this gives no warrant for supposing the student understands what he is driving at. The problem is not a matter of learning an English word for a foreign equivalent or being perfectly familiar with sleep but for some reason never learning the word for it. Sleep is not like a color which can be seen unequivocally but is hidden by the veil of a criterion. Only when we have penetrated the criterion do we know it is a veil, and know that it can reveal as well as conceal. Constant staring at the veil, however, will reveal nothing. And this difficulty is not lessened by the fact that the person who is supposed to be asleep knows what sleep is only by reference to the behavior of others. From what he can observe, sleeping is simply lying down and closing the eyes.

Suppose there were a group of people who for some reason have a particular experience which we do not have. This experience is manifested behaviorally by a rapid hopping accompanied by low moans, though not of pain. We can observe this behavior and learn to talk about it, but would we know what the character of the experience is by observation? We might duplicate their behavior in an attempt to visualize what sort of experience they are having, but this would be simply a guess, and Malcolm would not permit the making of such an inference anyway: it is too close to the argument from analogy, among other things.

This example may seem a little far-fetched, but consider another which isn't. If I can believe the report of a popular magazine whose name now escapes me, there are people who have never felt pain. They can talk about it well enough, and they might go through all the recognized procedures of alleviating pain in others, but they don't know what it is. The proper way to educate another person in these circumstances would be to stick him with a pin or burn his fingers, but this won't work here for obvious reasons. Now if it wouldn't succeed in teaching him what pain is, how could the inspection of behavior ever hope to do so? But this is the position that all of us are in: we are supposed to be capable of knowing what mental phenomena are merely by scrutinizing behavior. But if this could be done at all, why couldn't it be done by anyone? There is no stipulation made that teaching by reference to a criterion works only for a person who is capable of feeling or doing and who makes the appropriate connection between his feeling states and these items of behavior. A criterion in the sense of being a teaching device therefore seems not only to be a pedagogical failure but question-begging as well. How could anyone ever know that one kind of behavior rather than another *is* the criterion of pain unless he had known both pain and its usual accompanying behavior?

The last of Malcolm's three senses of "criterion" is the one which permits us to judge on the basis of behavior that someone knows what sleep is. It is appropriate, of course, to ask that a knowledge claim be justified, even though the claim is made on behalf of someone else, but is there only one sort of thing that will qualify as a justification? Ordinarily the question about one's knowledge of sleep arises only in the case of a very small child; but even here there is probably no specific point at which one can sensibly say "Now he knows" whereas a moment ago he did not know what sleep is. A child is taught in a gradual and informal way; he is urged to sleep, praised for doing it well, asked when he awakens if he had a good sleep, etc., all of which he slowly assimilates and eventually shows that he has done so even before he can talk with any facility. He does not learn it by observing anyone's behavior nor by introspection, but by doing it in an environment of this kind. And he shows that he has learned it by behaving in a number of different ways which might range anywhere from crying to untying his shoes. Not everyone is equally good at judging whether the child has learned his lesson, therefore, for the circumstances in which the learning takes place might differ from one case to the next. What seems to be a random response in one instance may be of considerable significance to the mother who is responsible for the child's training. But this training is hardly ever a formal undertaking, and it is not unlikely that a mother would know that her child grasped the teaching without being able to specify or bring to mind exactly what it is that shows that he does. It might not *be* any one thing.

Now, admitting that some kind of behavior is requisite in order to determine whether or not someone knows the meaning of a word, how does this help to establish Malcolm's thesis that a dream cannot have a genuine content or duration? If there is only as much precision in the concept of sleep as there is in the criterion, and the criterion can be a number of different things, apparently, then the concept itself isn't especially precise. It seems doubtful in any event that the behavior of a sleeping person has to conform to such rigid limits that any deviation from them marks him as not being really asleep. Perhaps we are more justified in saying a child is asleep when he is lying quietly rather than moving, but this doesn't entail that we are not justified in the other cases as well. Malcolm, of course, doesn't deny that a person can be asleep when the normal criteria of sleep are not completely satisfied, but he feels that any sort of movement takes something away from the assertion. Hence a person who is fully asleep cannot be experiencing imagery, for example, because such an experience cannot occur without some kind of movement or facial expression. But isn't this simply a desire to have things both ways? Ordinarily we think the soundest sleep occurs to a person when he rolls over a number of times or at least moves in some way during the night. Are we to say he is not asleep then? If so, in what sense is his sleep sound? And if not, why couldn't one verify that the sleeper was experiencing imagery? Surely if a sleeper can move, his expression can also change.

But is it really necessary that a verification take place, even supposing we know what one is in this case? We certainly don't think so in the majority of normal cases, for testimony ordinarily rules here unless we have good reason to think otherwise. The same, of course, holds true for sleeping. We don't tell anyone that he slept well; we ask him because we think he is usually in the best position to know.

What seems to be underlying Malcolm's position and is responsible for most of his errors, I think, is the untenable view that the only alternative to the "one's own case" philosophy is the criteriological view. Couple this with the other assumption that we can teach someone what sleep is by reference to behavior and we have the foundation of Malcolm's argument. From this it follows that the criterion of sleep is the kind of behavior we ourselves engage in when we prepare for it. We know what sleep is, after all, and since it is not possible to learn it by introspection, we *must* have acquired it by employing a criterion. And because it is held that teaching the concept is next to impossible if we use the example of a person walking in his sleep, the real criterion must not be the fairly wide range of activity we actually observe in a sleeping person but a segment of it which supposedly will allow for easy teaching.

There is another view in addition to this which is implicit in Malcolm's thought, and the two in conjunction give some insight into Malcolm's motivation for arguing as he does, I think. This comes out more clearly, perhaps, in an essay entitled "Knowledge of Other Minds" than in *Dreaming,* and it is a variation of what Ryle calls the category mistake. In this essay Malcolm states that ". . . first-person sentences are to be thought of as similar to the natural, nonverbal, behavioral expressions of psychological states. 'My leg hurts', for example, is to be assimilated to crying, limping, holding one's leg." [11] What Malcolm seems to mean here is that these sentences have no other use than that of replacing natural pain behavior. They are learned in a certain context, play a specific part in that context, and are not permitted to deviate from it or play a different part at any later date. But to sanction the view that dreams can contain thoughts, impressions, sensations, or feelings is to violate this canon of meaningful use. Hence, since these concepts

11. Reprinted in *Knowledge and Certainty: Essays and Lectures,* p. 140.

weren't taught or learned in a dream they cannot legitimately be used in one.

These two views neatly complement one another, on one level at least, for if the criterion of sleep (in any sense of the word) is what Malcolm supposes it is, and if it be allowed that this criterion rules out the possibility of verifying the existence of mental phenomena occurring to a sleeper, then no such phenomena can occur and the restriction of the use of words to the contexts in which they are learned is preserved. If, on the other hand, Malcolm's argument that behavior is the criterion of sleep is faulty, then the concepts which we ordinarily use in respect to dreams are not to be distinguished from the so-called historical use of language in the rigid way that Malcolm suggests.

It seems to me that the fundamental question underlying the whole discussion has to do with this point and is the goal which Malcolm hopes to reach. But the trouble lies in his apparent assumption that the very points which are relevant and essential for the determination of a proper answer have already been resolved. What is needed is a defence of the view that only one alternative exists to the "one's own case" philosophy, and to present the disjunction as if it exhausted every possibility is clearly to overlook a vital point. If my argument is sound, this is precisely what cannot be done, and therefore it is still an open question as to what the proper limits are to the meaningful uses of language. Perhaps it is wildly wrong to use language in contexts in which it cannot be taught and learned, but I don't see that Malcolm has succeeded in showing that this is the case.

8

CHARLES S. CHIHARA and JERRY A. FODOR

Operationalism and Ordinary Language: A Critique of Wittgenstein

Introduction

This paper explores some lines of argument in Wittgenstein's post-*Tractatus* writings in order to indicate the relations between Wittgenstein's philosophical psychology on the one hand and his philosophy of language, his epistemology, and his doctrines about the nature of philosophical analysis on the other. We shall hold that the later writings of Wittgenstein express a coherent doctrine in which an operationalistic analysis of confirmation and language supports a philosophical psychology of a type we shall call "logical behaviorism." [1]

We shall also maintain that there are good grounds for rejecting the philosophical theory implicit in Wittgenstein's other works. In particular we shall first argue that Wittgenstein's position leads to some implausible conclusions concerning the nature of language and psychology; second, we shall maintain that the arguments Wittgenstein provides are inconclusive; and

Reprinted from the *American Philosophical Quarterly*, 2 (1965), 281–295, by permission of the authors and the *American Philosophical Quarterly*.

1. This work was supported in part by the U.S. Army, Navy, and Air Force under Contract DA 36-039-AMC-03200(E); in part by the National Science Foundation (Grant GP-2495), the National Institutes of Health (Grant MH-04737-04), the National Aeronautics and Space Administration (Ns G-496), the U.S. Air Force (ESD Contract AF 19 (628)-2487), the National Institute of Mental Health (Grant MPM 17, 760); and, in addition, by a University of California Faculty Fellowship.

third, we shall try to sketch an alternative position which avoids many of the difficulties implicit in Wittgenstein's philosophy. In exposing and rejecting the operationalism which forms the framework of Wittgenstein's later writings, we do not, however, suppose that we have detracted in any way from the importance of the particular analyses of particular philosophical problems which form their primary content.[2]

I

Among the philosophical problems Wittgenstein attempted to dissolve is the "problem of other minds." One aspect of this hoary problem is the question: What justification, if any, can be given for the claim that one can tell, on the basis of someone's behavior, that he is in a certain mental state? To this question, the sceptic answers: No good justification at all. Among the major motivations of the later Wittgenstein's treatment of philosophical psychology is that of showing that this answer rests on a misconception and is *logically* incoherent.

Characteristically, philosophic sceptics have argued in the following way. It is assumed as a premiss that there are no logical or conceptual relations between propositions about mental states and propositions about behavior in virtue of which propositions asserting that a person behaves in a certain way provide support, grounds, or justification for ascribing the mental states to that person. From this, the sceptic deduces that he has no compelling reason for supposing that any person other than himself is ever truly said to feel pains, draw inferences, have motives, etc. For, while his first-hand knowledge of the occurrence of such mental events is of necessity limited to his own case, it is entailed by the premiss just cited that application of mental predicates to others must depend upon logically fallible inferences. Furthermore, attempts to base such inferences on analogies and correlations fall short of convincing justifications.

2. In making references to Part I of Ludwig Wittgenstein's *Philosophical Investigations* (New York, 1953), cited here as PI, we shall give section numbers, e.g. (PI, §13); to Part II, we shall give page numbers, e.g. (PI, p. 220). In referring to his *The Blue and Brown Books* (New York, 1958), cited here as BB, we give page numbers. References to his *Remarks on the Foundations of Mathematics* (New York, 1956), cited here as RFM, will include both part and section numbers, e.g. (RFM, II, §26).

Various replies have been made to this argument which do not directly depend upon contesting the truth of the premiss. For example, it is sometimes claimed that, at least in some cases, no *inference* from behavior to mental states is at issue in psychological ascriptions. Thus, we sometimes *see* that someone is in pain, and in these cases, we cannot be properly said to *infer* that he is in pain. However, the sceptic might maintain against this argument that it begs the question. For the essential issue is whether anyone is *justified* in claiming to see that another is in pain. Now a physicist, looking at cloud-chamber tracks, may be justified in claiming to see that a charged particle has passed through the chamber. That is because in this case there is justification for the claim that certain sorts of tracks show the presence and motion of particles. The physicist can explain not only how he is able to detect particles, but also why the methods he uses are methods of detecting *particles*. Correspondingly, the sceptic can argue that what is required in the case of another's pain is some justification for the claim that, by observing a person's behavior, one can *see* that he is in *pain*.

Wittgenstein's way of dealing with the sceptic is to attack his premiss by trying to show that there do exist conceptual relations between statements about behavior and statements about mental events, processes, and states. Hence, Wittgenstein argues that in many cases our knowledge of the mental states of some person rests upon something other than an observed empirical correlation or an analogical argument, viz. a conceptual or linguistic connection.

To hold that the sceptical premiss is false is *ipso facto* to commit oneself to some version of *logical behaviorism* where by "logical behaviorism" we mean the doctrine that there are logical or conceptual relations of the sort denied by the sceptical premiss.[3] Which form of logical behaviorism one holds depends on

3. Philosophers of Wittgensteinian persuasion have sometimes heatedly denied that the term "behaviorism" is correctly applied to the view that logical connections of the above sort exist. We do not feel that very much hangs on using the term "behaviorism" as we do, but we are prepared to give some justification for our terminology. "Behaviorism" is, in the first instance, a term applied to a school of psychologists whose interest was in placing constraints upon the conceptual equipment that might be employed in putative psychological explanations, but who were *not* particularly interested in the analysis of the

the nature of the logical connection one claims obtains. The strongest form maintains that statements about mental states are translatable into statements about behavior. Wittgenstein, we shall argue, adopts a weaker version.

II

It is well known that Wittgenstein thought that philosophical problems generally arise out of misrepresentations and misinterpretations of ordinary language (PI, §109, §122, §194). "Philosophy," he tells us, "is a fight against the fascination which forms of expression exert upon us" (BB, p. 27). Thus, Wittgenstein repeatedly warns us against being misled by superficial similarities between certain forms of expression (BB, p. 16) and tells us that, to avoid philosophical confusions, we must distinguish the "surface grammar" of sentences from their "depth grammar" (PI, §11, §664). For example, though the grammar of the sentence "*A* has a gold tooth" seems to differ in no essential respect from that of "*A* has a sore tooth," the apparent similarity masks important conceptual differences (BB, pp. 49, 53; PI, §288–293). Overlooking these differences leads philosophers to suppose that there is a problem about our knowledge of other minds. It is the task of the Wittgensteinian philosopher to dissolve the problem by obtaining a clear view of the workings of pain language in this and other cases.

The Wittgensteinian method of philosophical therapy involves taking a certain view of language and of meaning. Throughout the *Investigations*, Wittgenstein emphasizes that "the speaking of language is part of an activity" (PI §23) and

---

mental vocabulary of ordinary language. The application of this label to a philosopher bent upon this latter task must therefore be, to some extent, analogical. Granted that there has been some tendency for the term "behaviorism" to be preempted, even in psychology, for the position held by such *radical* behaviorists as Watson and Skinner, who require that all psychological generalizations be defined over observables, insofar as C. L. Hull can be classified as a behaviorist, there does seem to be grounds for our classification. Hull's view, as we understand it, is that mental predicates are in no sense "eliminable" in favor of behavioral predicates, but that it is a condition upon their coherent employment that they be severally related to behavioral predicates and that some of these relations be logical rather than empirical—a view that is strikingly similar to the one we attribute to Wittgenstein. Cf. C. L. Hull, *Principles of Behavior* (New York, 1943).

that if we are to see the radically different roles superficially similar expressions play, we must keep in mind the countless kinds of language-using activities or "language-games" in which we participate (BB, pp. 67–68).

It is clear that Wittgenstein thought that analyzing the meaning of a word involves exhibiting the role or use of the word in the various language-games in which it occurs. He even suggests that we "think of words as instruments characterized by their use . . ." (BB, p. 67).

This notion of analysis leads rather naturally to an operationalistic view of the meaning of certain sorts of predicates. For, in those cases where it makes sense to say of a predicate that one has determined that it applies, one of the central language-games that the fluent speaker has learned to play is that of making and reporting such determinations. Consider, for example, one of the language-games that imparts meaning to such words as "length," i.e., that of reporting the dimensions of physical objects. To describe this game, one would have to include an account of the procedures involved in measuring lengths; indeed, mastering (at least some of) those procedures would be an essential part of learning this game. "The meaning of the word 'length' is learnt among other things, by learning what it is to determine length" (PI, p. 225). As Wittgenstein comments about an analogous case, "Here the teaching of language is not explanation, but training" (PI, §5). For Wittgenstein, "To understand a sentence means to understand a language." "To understand a language means to be master of a technique" (PI, §199).

In short, part of being competent in the language-game played with "length" consists in the ability to arrive at the truth of such statements as "x is three feet long" by performing relevant operations with, e.g., rulers, range-finders, etc. A philosophic analysis of "length," insofar as it seeks to articulate the language-game played with that word, must thus refer to the operations which determine the applicability of length predicates. Finally, insofar as the meaning of the word is itself determined by the rules governing the language-games in which it occurs, a reference to these operations will be essential in characterizing the meaning of such predicates as "three feet long."

It is in this manner that we are led to the view that the relevant operations for determining the applicability of a predicate are conceptually connected with the predicate.[4]

By parity of reasoning, we can see that to analyze such words as "pain," "motive," "dream," etc., will *inter alia* involve articulating the operations or observations in terms of which we determine that someone is in pain, or that he has such and such a motive, or that he has dreamed, etc. (PI, p. 224). But clearly, such determinations are ultimately made on the basis of the behavior of the individual to whom the predicates are applied (taking behavior in the broad sense in which it includes verbal reports). Hence, for Wittgenstein, reference to the characteristic features of pain behavior on the basis of which we determine that someone is in pain is essential to the philosophical analysis of the word "pain" just as reference to the operations by which we determine the applicability of such predicates as "three feet long" is essential to the philosophical analysis of the word "length." In both cases, the relations are conceptual and the rule of language which articulates them is in that sense a rule of logic.

III

But what, specifically, is this logical connection which, according to Wittgenstein, is supposed to obtain between pain behavior and pain? Obviously, the connection is not that of simple entailment. It is evident that Wittgenstein did not think that some proposition to the effect that a person is screaming, wincing, groaning, or moaning could entail the proposition that the person is in pain. We know that Wittgenstein used the term "criterion" to mark this special connection, but we are in need of an explanation of this term.

We have already remarked that one of the central ideas in Wittgenstein's philosophy is that of a "language-game." Ap-

4. Cf. "Let us consider what we call an 'exact' explanation in contrast with this one. Perhaps something like drawing a chalk line round an area? Here it strikes us at once that the line has breadth. So a color-edge would be more exact. But has this exactness still got a function here: isn't the engine idling? And remember too that we have not yet defined what is to count as overstepping this exact boundary; *how, with what instruments, it is to be established*" (PI, §88, italics ours). Cf., also RFM, I. §5.

parently Wittgenstein was passing a field on which a football game was being played when the idéa occurred to him that "in language we play *games* with *words*." [5] Since this analogy dominated so much of the later Wittgenstein's philosophical thinking, perhaps it would be well to begin the intricate task of explicating Wittgenstein's notion of criterion by considering some specific game.

Take basketball as an example. Since the object of the game is to score more points than one's opponents, there must be some way of telling if and when a team scores. Now there are various ways of telling that, say, a field goal has been scored. One might simply keep one's eyes on the scoreboard and wait for two points to be registered. Sometimes one realizes that a field goal has been scored on the basis of the reactions of the crowd. But these are, at best, indirect ways of telling, for if we use them we are relying on someone else: the score-keeper or other spectators. Obviously, not every way of telling is, in that sense, indirect; and anyone who is at all familiar with the game knows that, generally, one *sees* that a field goal has been scored in seeing the ball shot or tipped through the hoop. And if a philosopher asks, "Why does the fact that the ball went through the basket show that a field goal has been scored?" a natural reply would be, "That is what the rules of the game say; that is the way the game is played." The ball going through the basket satisfies a *criterion* for scoring a field goal.

Notice that though the relation between a criterion and that of which it is a criterion is a logical or conceptual one, the fact that the ball goes through the hoop does not entail that a field goal has been scored. First, the ball must be "in play" for it to be possible to score a field goal by tossing the ball through the basket. Second, even if the ball drops through the hoop when "in play," it need not follow that a field goal has been scored, for the rules of basketball do not cover all imaginable situations. Suppose, for example, that a player takes a long two-handed shot and that the ball suddenly reverses its direction, and after soaring and dipping through the air like a swallow in flight, gracefully drops through the player's own basket only to

5. Norman Malcolm, *Ludwig Wittgenstein: A Memoir* (Oxford, 1958), p. 65.

change into a bat, which immediately entangles itself in the net. What do the rules say about that?

An analogous situation would arise, in the case of a "language-game," if what seemed to be a chair suddenly disappeared, reappeared, and, in general, behaved in a fantastic manner. Wittgenstein's comment on this type of situation is:

Have you rules ready for such cases—rules saying whether one may use the word "chair" to include this kind of thing? But do we miss them when we use the word "chair"; and are we to say that we do not really attach any meaning to this word, because we are not equipped with rules for every possible application of it? [PI §80]

For Wittgenstein, a sign "is in order—if, under normal circumstances it fulfils its purpose" (PI, §87).

It is only in normal cases that the use of a word is clearly prescribed; we know, are in no doubt, what to say in this or that case. The more abnormal the case, the more doubtful it becomes what we are to say. [PI, §142]

Let us now try to make out Wittgenstein's distinction between *criterion* and *symptom*, again utilizing the example of basketball. Suppose that, while a game is in progress, a spectator leaves his seat. Though he is unable to see the playing court, he might realize that the home team had scored a field goal on the basis of a symptom—say, the distinctive roar of the crowd—which he had observed to be correlated with home-team field goals. This correlation, according to Wittgenstein, would have to be established *via* criteria, say, by noting the sound of the cheering when the home team shot the ball through the basket. Thus, a symptom is "a phenomenon of which experience has taught us that it coincided, in some way or other, with the phenomenon which is our defining criterion" (BB, p. 25). Though both symptoms and criteria are cited in answer to the question, "How do you know that so-and-so is the case?" (BB, p. 24), symptoms, unlike criteria, are discovered through experience or observation: that something is a symptom is not given by the rules of the "language-game" (not deducible from the rules alone). However, to say of a statement that it expresses a symptom is to say something about the relation between the statement and the rules, viz., that it is not derivable from them. Hence, Wittgenstein once claimed that "whereas 'When it rains the pavement gets wet' is not a grammatical statement at all, if we say 'The fact that the pavement is wet is a *symptom* that it has been raining' this statement is 'a matter of grammar'." [6] Furthermore, giving the criterion for (e.g.) another's having a toothache "is to give a grammatical explanation about the word 'toothache' and, in this sense, an explanation concerning the meaning of the word 'toothache'" (BB, p. 24). However, given that there is this important difference between criteria and symptoms, the fact remains that Wittgenstein considered both symptoms and criteria as "evidences" (BB, p. 51).

Other salient features of criteria can be illuminated by exploiting our illustrative example. Consider Wittgenstein's claim that "in different circumstances we apply different criteria for a person's reading" (PI, §164). It is clear that in different circumstances we apply different criteria for a person's scoring a field goal. For example, the question whether a player scored a field goal may arise even though the ball went nowhere near the basket: in a "goal-tending" situation, the question will have to be decided on the basis of whether the ball had started its descent before the defensive player had deflected it. According to the rules it would be a decisive reason for not awarding a field goal that the ball had not reached its apogee when it was blocked.

One can now see that to claim that X is a criterion of Y is not to claim that the presence, occurrence, existence, etc., of X is a necessary condition of the applicability of 'Y', and it is not to claim that the presence, occurrence, existence, etc., of X is a sufficient condition of Y, although if X is a criterion of Y, it may be the case that X is a necessary or a sufficient condition of Y.

Again, consider the tendency of Wittgenstein, noted by Albritton,[7] to write as if X (a criterion of Y) just *is* Y or is what is called 'Y' in certain circumstances. We can understand a philosopher's wanting to say that shooting the ball through the basket

6. G. E. Moore, "Wittgenstein's Lectures in 1930–33," *Philosophical Papers* (London, 1959), pp. 266–267.

7. Rogers Albritton, "On Wittgenstein's Use of the Term 'Criterion'," *Journal of Philosophy*, 56 (1959), 851–854.

in the appropriate situation just *is* scoring a field goal or is what we call "scoring a field goal."

Consider now the following passage from the *Investigations* (§376) which suggests a kind of test for "non-criterionhood":

> When I say the ABC to myself, what is the criterion of my doing the same as someone else who silently repeats it to himself? It might be found that the same thing took place in my larynx and in his. (And similarly when we both think of the same thing, wish the same, and so on.) But then did we learn the use of the words: "to say such-and-such to oneself" by someone's pointing to a process in the larynx or the brain?

Obviously not. Hence, Wittgenstein suggests, something taking place in the larynx cannot be the criterion. The rationale behind this "test" seems to be this: For the teaching of a particular predicate 'Y' to be successful, the pupil must learn the rules for the use of 'Y' and hence must learn the criteria for 'Y' if there are such criteria. Thus, if the teaching could be entirely successful without one learning that X is something on the basis of which one tells that 'Y' applies, X cannot be a criterion of Y. For example, since a person could be taught what "field goal" means without learning that one can generally tell that the home team has scored a field goal by noting the roar of the home crowd, the roar of the home crowd cannot be a criterion of field goals.

Finally, let us examine the principle, which Wittgenstein appears to maintain, that any change of criteria of X involves changing the concept of X. In the *Investigations*, Wittgenstein makes the puzzling claim:

> There is *one* thing of which one can say neither that it is one metre long, nor that it is not one metre long, and that is the standard metre in Paris.—But this is, of course, not to ascribe any extraordinary property to it, but only to mark its peculiar role in the language-game of measuring with a metre-rule.—Let us imagine samples of colour being preserved in Paris like the standard metre. We define: "Sepia" means the colour of the standard sepia which is there kept hermetically sealed. Then it will make no sense to say of this sample either that it is of this colour or that it is not. [PI, §50]

Wittgenstein evidently is maintaining not only that the senses of the predicates "x is one meter long" and "x is sepia" are given by the operations which determine the applicability of the respective predicates (the operations of comparing objects in certain ways with the respective standards),[8] but also that these operations cannot be performed on the standards themselves and hence neither standard can be said to be an instance of either the *predicate* for which it is a standard or of its negation. (Cf., "A thing cannot be at the same time the measure and the thing measured" [RFM, I, §40, notes].)

Wittgenstein would undoubtedly allow that we might introduce a new language-game in which "meter" is defined in terms of the wave length of the spectral line of the element krypton of atomic weight 86.[9] In this language-game, where such highly accurate and complex measuring devices as the interferometer are required, the standard meter does not have any privileged position: it, too, can be measured and "represented." In this language-game, the standard meter is or is not a meter. But here, Wittgenstein would evidently distinguish two senses of the term "meter." Obviously what is a meter in one language-game need not be a meter in the other. Thus, Wittgenstein's view seems to be that by introducing a new criterion for something's being a meter long, we have introduced a new language-game, a new sense of the term "meter," and a new concept of meter. Such a position is indicated by Wittgenstein's comment:

We can speak of measurements of time in which there is a different, and as we should say a greater, exactness than in the measurement of time by a pocket-watch; in which the words "to set the clock to the exact time" have a different, though related meaning. . . . [PI, §88]

Returning to our basketball analogy, suppose that the National Collegiate Athletic Association ruled that, henceforth, a player can score a field goal by pushing the ball *upward* through

8. Note Wittgenstein's suggestion that we can "give the phrase 'unconscious pain' sense by fixing experiential criteria for the case in which a man has pain and doesn't know it" (BB, p. 55). Cf., also: "If however we do use the expression 'the thought takes place in the head,' we have given this expression its meaning by describing the experience which would justify the *hypothesis* that the thought takes place in our heads, by describing the experience which we wish to call observing thought in our brain" (BB, p. 8).

9. Adopted by the eleventh General International Conference on Weights and Measures in the fall of 1960.

the basket. Obviously, this would involve changing the rules of basketball. And to some extent, by introducing this new criterion, the rules governing the use or "grammar" of the term "field goal" would be altered. To put it somewhat dramatically (in the Wittgensteinian style), a new *essence* of field goal would be created. (Cf. "The mathematician creates *essence*" [RFM, I, §32].) For Wittgenstein, not only is it the case that the criteria we use "give our words their common meanings" (BB, p. 57) and that to explain the criteria we use is to explain the meanings of words (BB, p. 24), but also it is the case that to introduce a new criterion of *Y* is to define a new concept of *Y*.[10]

In summary, we can roughly and schematically characterize Wittgenstein's notion of criterion in the following way: *X* is a criterion of *Y* in situations of type *S* if the very meaning or definition of '*Y*' (or, as Wittgenstein might have put it, if the "grammatical" rules for the use of '*Y*')[11] justify the claim that one can recognize, see, detect, or determine the applicability of '*Y*' on the basis of *X* in *normal* situations of type *S*. Hence, if the above relation obtains between *X* and *Y*, and if someone admits that *X* but denies *Y*, the burden of proof is upon him to show that something is abnormal in the situation. In a normal situation, the problem of gathering evidence which justifies concluding *Y* from *X* simply does not arise.

IV

The following passage occurs in the *Blue Book* (p. 24):

When we learnt the use of the phrase "so-and-so has toothache" we were pointed out certain kinds of behavior of those who were said to have toothache. As an instance of these kinds of behavior let us take holding your cheek. Suppose that by observation I found that in certain cases whenever these first criteria told me a person had toothache, a red patch appeared on the person's cheek. Supposing I now said to someone "I see *A* has toothache, he's got a red patch on his cheek." He may ask me "How do you know *A* has toothache when you see a red patch?" I would then point out that certain phenomena had always coincided with the appearance of the red patch.

10. RFM, II, §24; III, §29; and I, Appendix I, §15–16. See also C. S. Chihara "Mathematical Discovery and Concept Formation," *The Philosophical Review*, 72 (1963), 17–34.

11. Cf., "The person of whom we say 'he has pain' is, *by the rules of the game*, the person who cries, contorts his face, etc." (BB, p. 68, italics ours).

Now one may go on and ask: "How do you know that he has got toothache when he holds his cheek?" The answer to this might be, "I say, *he* has toothache when he holds his cheek because I hold my cheek when I have toothache." But what if we went on asking:—"And why do you suppose that toothache corresponds to his holding his cheek just because your toothache corresponds to your holding your cheek?" You will be at a loss to answer this question, and find that here we strike rock bottom, that is we have come down to conventions.

It would seem that, on Wittgenstein's view, empirical justification of the claim to see, recognize, or know that such and such is the case *on the basis of some observable feature or state of affairs,* would have to rest upon inductions from observed correlations, so that, if a person claims that Y is the case on the grounds that X is the case, in answer to the question "Why does the fact that X show that Y?" he would have to cite either conventions or observed correlations linking X and Y. Thus, Wittgenstein appears to be arguing that the possibility of ever inferring a person's toothache from his behavior requires the existence of a criterion of toothache that can sometimes be observed to obtain. A generalized form of this argument leads to the conclusion that "an 'inner process' stands in need of outward criteria" (PI, §580).

As an illustration of Wittgenstein's reasoning, consider the following example: It appears to be the case that the measurement of the alcohol content of the blood affords a reasonably reliable index of intoxication. On the basis of this empirical information, we may sometimes justify the claim that X is intoxicated by showing that the alcohol content of his blood is higher than some specified percentage. But now consider the justification of the claim that blood-alcohol is in fact an index of intoxication. On Wittgenstein's view, the justification of *this* claim must rest ultimately upon correlating cases of intoxication with determinations of high blood-alcohol content. But, the observations required for this correlation could be made only if there exist independent techniques for identifying each of the correlated items. In any particular case, these independent techniques may themselves be based upon further empirical correlations; we might justify the claim that the blood-alcohol content is high by appealing to some previously established correlation between the presence of blood-alcohol and some test result. But ultimately according to Wittgenstein, we must come upon identifying techniques based not upon further empirical correlations, but rather upon definitions or conventions which determine criteria for applying the relevant predicates. This is why Wittgenstein can say that a symptom is "a phenomenon of which experience has taught us that it coincided, in some way or other with the phenomenon which is our defining criterion" (BB, p. 25).

A similar argument has recently been given by Sydney Shoemaker who writes:

If we know psychological facts about other persons at all, we know them on the basis of their behavior (including, of course, their verbal behavior). Sometimes we make psychological statements about other persons on the basis of bodily or behavioral facts that are only contingently related to the psychological facts for which we accept them as evidence. But we do this only because we have discovered, or think we have discovered, empirical correlations between physical (bodily and behavioral) facts of a certain kind and psychological facts of a certain kind. And if *all* relations between physical and psychological facts were contingent, it would be impossible for us to discover such correlations. . . . Unless some relationships between physical and psychological states are not contingent, and can be known prior to the discovery of empirical correlations, we cannot have even indirect inductive evidence for the truth of psychological statements about other persons, and cannot know such statements to be true or even probably true.[12]

Malcolm argues in a similar manner in *Dreaming.*[13]

Of course, Wittgenstein did not claim that all predicates presuppose criteria of applicability. For example, Wittgenstein probably did not think that we, in general, see, tell, determine, or know that something is red on the basis of either a criterion or a symptom. The relevant difference between ascriptions of "red" and third-person ascriptions of "pain" is that we generally see, recognize, determine, or know that another is in pain on the basis of something which is not the pain itself (as for example, behavior and circumstances) whereas, if it made any sense at all to say we generally see, recognize, etc., that an ob-

12. Sydney Shoemaker, *Self-knowledge and Self-identity* (Ithaca, 1963), pp. 167–168.

13. Norman Malcolm, *Dreaming* (London, 1959), pp. 60–61.

ject is red on the basis of something, what could this something be other than just the object's redness? But Wittgenstein's use of the term "criterion" seems to preclude redness being a criterion of redness. If someone asks "How do you know or tell that an object is red?" it would not, in general, do to answer "By its redness." (Cf. Wittgenstein's comment "How do I know that this color is red?—It would be an answer to say: 'I have learnt English' " [PI, §381].) Evidently, some color predicates and, more generally, what are sometimes called "sense datum" predicates (those that can be known to apply—as some philosophers put it—*immediately*), do not fall within the domain of arguments of the above type. But the predicates with which we assign "inner states" to another person are not of this sort. One recognizes that another is in a certain mental state, Y, on the basis of something, say, X. Now it is assumed that X must be either a criterion or symptom of Y. If X is a symptom, X must be known to be correlated with Y, and we may then inquire into the way in which this correlation was established. Again, X must have been observed to be correlated with a criterion of Y or with a symptom, X_1, of Y. On the second alternative, we may inquire into the basis for holding that X_1 is a symptom of Y. . . . Such a chain may go on for any distance you like, but it cannot go on indefinitely. That is, at some point, we must come to a criterion of Y. But once this conclusion has been accepted, there appears to be no reasonable non-sceptical alternative to Wittgenstein's logical behaviorism, for if "inner" states require "outward" criteria, behavioral criteria are the only plausible candidates.

V

As a refutation of scepticism, the above argument certainly will not do; for, at best, it supports Wittgenstein's position only on the assumption that the sceptic is not right. That is, it demonstrates that there must be criteria for psychological predicates by assuming that such predicates are sometimes applied justifiably. A sceptic who accepts the argument of Section IV could maintain his position only by allowing that no one could have any idea of what would show or even indicate that another is in pain, having a dream, thinking, etc. In this section we shall show how Wittgenstein argues that that move would lead the sceptic to the absurd conclusion that it must be impossible to teach the meaning of these psychological predicates.

"What would it be like if human beings showed no outward signs of pain (did not groan, grimace, etc.)? Then it would be impossible to teach a child the use of the word 'toothache' " (PI, §257). For just imagine trying to teach a child the meaning of the term "toothache," say, on the supposition that there is absolutely no way of telling whether the child—or anyone else for that matter—is actually in pain. How would one go about it, if one had no reason for believing that gross damage to the body causes pain or that crying out, wincing, and the like indicate pain? ("How could I even have come by the idea of another's experience if there is no possibility of any evidence for it?" [BB, p. 46; cf. also BB, p. 48].)

Again, what would show us that the child had grasped the teaching? If anything would, the argument of Section IV requires that there be a criterion of having succeeded in teaching the child. (As Wittgenstein says of an analogous case, "If I speak of communicating a feeling to someone else, mustn't I in order to understand what I say know what I shall call the criterion of having succeeded in communicating?" (BB, p. 185).) But the only plausible criterion of this would be that the child applies the psychological predicates correctly (cf. PI, §146); and since the sceptical position implies that there is no way of knowing if the child correctly applies such predicates, it would seem to follow that nothing could show or indicate that the child had learned what these terms mean.

We now have a basis for explicating the sense of "logical" which is involved in the claim that scepticism is a logically incoherent doctrine. What Wittgenstein holds is not that "*P* and not-*P*" are strictly deducible from the sceptic's position, but rather that the sceptic's view presupposes a deviation from the rules for the use of key terms. In particular, Wittgenstein holds that if the sceptic were right, the preconditions for teaching the meaning of the mental predicates of our ordinary language could not be satisfied.[14]

14. Cf., " 'Before I judge that two images which I have are the same, I must recognize them as the same.' . . . Only if I can express my recognition in some

We now see too the point to the insistence that the sceptic's position must incorporate an extraordinary and misleading use of mental predicates. The sceptic's view is logically incompatible with the operation of the ordinary language rules for the application of these terms, and these rules determine their meanings. (Cf. "What *we* do is to bring words back from their metaphysical to their everyday usage" [PI, §116].) As Wittgenstein diagnoses the sceptic's view, the sceptic does not have in mind any criteria of third person ascriptions when he denies that he can know if anyone else has pains (cf. PI, §272). The sceptic tempts us to picture the situation as involving "a barrier which doesn't allow one person to come closer to another's experience than to the point of observing his behavior"; but, according to Wittgenstein, "on looking closer we find that we can't apply the picture" (BB, p. 56); no clear meaning can be attached to the sceptic's claim: no sense can even be given the hypothesis that other people feel "pains," as the sceptic uses the term "pain." ("For how can I even make the hypothesis if it transcends all possible experience?" [BB, p. 48].) And if the sceptic says, "But if I suppose that someone has a pain, then I am simply supposing that he has just the same as I have so often had." Wittgenstein can reply:

That gets us no further. It is as if I were to say: "You surely know what 'It is 5 o'clock here' means; so you also know what 'It's 5 o'clock on the sun' means. It means simply that it is just the same time there as it is here when it is 5 o'clock."—The explanation by means of *identity* does not work here. For I know well enough that one can call 5 o'clock here and 5 o'clock there "the same time," but what I do not know is in what cases one is to speak of its being the same time here and there. [PI, §350]

Thus, we can see how Wittgenstein supports his logical behaviorism: the argument in Section IV purports to show that the only plausible alternative to Wittgenstein's philosophical psychology is radical scepticism; and the argument in the present section rules out this alternative. For Wittgenstein, then, "the person of whom we say 'he has pains' is, by the rules of the game, the person who cries, contorts his face, etc.," (BB, p. 68).

---

other way, and if it is possible for someone else to teach me that 'same' is the correct word here" (PI, §378).

Undoubtedly, there is much that philosophers find comforting and attractive in Wittgenstein's philosophical psychology, but there are also difficulties in the doctrine which mar its attractiveness. To some of these difficulties, we shall now turn.

VI

In this section, we shall consider some consequences of applying the views just discussed to the analysis of dreaming, and we shall attempt to show that the conclusions to which these views lead are counter-intuitive.

According to Wittgenstein, we are to understand the concept of dreaming in terms of the language-game(s) in which "dream" plays a role and, in particular, in terms of the language-game of dream telling. For, to master the use of the word "dream" is precisely to learn what it is to find out that someone has dreamed, to tell what someone has dreamed, to report one's own dreams, and so on. Passages in the *Investigations* (e.g., PI, pp. 184, 222–223) indicate that, for Wittgenstein, a criterion of someone's having dreamed is the dream report. On this analysis, sceptical doubts about dreams arise when we fail to appreciate the logical bond between statements about dreams and statements about dream reports. The sceptic treats the dream report as, at best, an empirical correlate of the occurrence of a dream: a symptom that is, at any event, no more reliable than the memory of the subject who reports the dream. But, according to Wittgenstein, once we have understood the criterial relation between dream reporting and dreaming, we see that "the question whether the dreamer's memory deceives him when he reports the dream after waking cannot arise . . ." (PI, p. 222). (Compare: "Once we understand the rules for playing chess, the question whether a player has won when he has achieved check-mate cannot arise.")

The rules articulating the criteria for applying the word "dream" determine a logical relation between dreaming and reporting dreams. Moreover, the set of such rules fixes the language-game in which "dream" has its role and hence determines the meaning of the word.

It is important to notice that there are a number of *prima facie* objections to this analysis which, though perhaps not conclusive, supply grounds for questioning the doctrines which lead to it. Though we could perhaps learn to live with these objections were no other analyses available, when seen from the vantage point of an alternative theory they indicate deep troubles with Wittgenstein's views.

(1) Given that there exist no criteria for first person applications of many psychological predicates ("pain," "wish," or the like) it is unclear how the first person aspects of the game played with these predicates are to be described. Wittgenstein does not appear to present a coherent account of the behavior of predicates whose applicability is not determined by criteria. On the other hand, the attempt to characterize "I dreamt" as criterion-governed leads immediately to absurdities. Thus, in Malcolm's *Dreaming* it is suggested that:

> If a man wakes up with the impression of having seen and done various things, and if it is known that he did not see and do those things, then it is known that he dreamt them. . . . When he says "I dreamt so and so" he implies, first, that it seemed to him on waking up as if the so and so had occurred and second, that the so and so did not occur. [p. 66]

That this is an incredibly counter-intuitive analysis of our concept of dreaming hardly needs mentioning. We ask the reader to consider the following example: A person, from time to time, gets the strange feeling that, shortly before, he had seen and heard his father commanding him to come home. One morning he wakes with this feeling, knowing full well that his father is dead. Now we are asked by Malcolm to believe that the person *must have dreamt* that he saw and heard his father: supposedly, it would be logically absurd for the person to claim to have this feeling and deny that he had dreamt it!

(2) Wittgenstein's view appears to entail that no sense can be made of such statements as "Jones totally forgot the dream he had last night," since we seem to have no criteria for determining the truth of such a statement. (We have in mind the case in which Jones is totally unable to remember having dreamed and no behavioral manifestations of dreaming were exhibited.) It is sometimes denied that observations of what people ordinarily say are relevant to a description of ordinary language. But, in-

sofar as statements about what we would say are susceptible to empirical disconfirmation, the claim that we would feel hesitation about saying that someone completely forgot his dream appears to be just false.[15]

(3) The Wittgensteinian method of counting concepts is certainly not an intuitive one. Consider Malcolm's analysis of dreaming again. Malcolm realizes that sometimes, on the basis of a person's behavior during sleep, we say that he had a dream, even though he is unable to recall a dream upon awaking. But, in such cases, Malcolm claims, "our words . . . have no clear sense" (*Dreaming*, p. 62). On the other hand, Malcolm admits that there is a *sense* of the term "nightmare" where behavior during sleep is the criterion. However, a different concept of dreaming is supposedly involved in this case. An analogous situation is treated in the *Blue Book* (p. 63), where Wittgenstein writes:

If a man tries to obey the order "Point to your eye," he may do many different things, and there are many different criteria which he will accept for having pointed to his eye. If these criteria, as they usually do, coincide, I may use them alternately and in different combinations to show me that I have touched my eye. If they don't coincide, I shall have to distinguish between different senses of the phrase "I touch my eye" or "I move my finger towards my eye."

Following this suggestion of Wittgenstein, Malcolm distinguishes not only different senses of the term "dream," but also different concepts of sleep—one based upon report, one based upon nonverbal behavior. But surely, this is an unnatural way of counting concepts. Compare Malcolm's two concepts of sleep with a case where it really does seem natural to say that a special concept of sleep has been employed, viz., where we say of a hibernating bear that it sleeps through the winter.

(4) As Malcolm points out, the language-game *now* played with "dream" seems to exhibit no criteria which would enable

15. Thus consider the following: "Up until the night I opened the door, I remembered my dreams. Soon after, I ceased to recall them. I still dreamed, but my waking consciousness concealed from itself what sleep revealed. If the recurrent nightmare of the iron fence awoke me, I recognized it. But if any other nightmare broke my sleep, I forgot what it was about by morning. And of all the other dreams I had during the night I remembered nothing" (Windham, D., "Myopia," *The New Yorker,* July 13, 1963).

one to determine the precise duration of dreams. Hence, it would seem to follow (as Malcolm has noticed) that scientists who have attempted to answer such questions as, "How long do dreams last?" are involved in conceptual confusions rather than empirical determinations. For such questions cannot be answered without adopting criteria for ascribing the relevant properties to dreams. But since, on Wittgenstein's view, to adopt such new criteria for the use of a word is, to that extent, to change its meaning, it follows that the concept of "dream" that such researchers employ is not the ordinary concept and hence that the measurements they effect are not, strictly speaking, measurements of *dreams*.[16] The notion that adopting any test for dreaming which arrives at features of dreams not determinable from the dream report thereby alters the concept of a dream seems to run counter to our intuitions about the goals of psychological research. It is not immediately obvious that the psychologist who says he has found a method of measuring the duration of dreams *ipso facto* commits the fallacy of ambiguity.[17]

(5) Consider the fact that such measures as EEG, eye-movements and "dream-behavior" (murmuring, tossing, etc., during sleep) correlate reasonably reliably with one another and dream reports. The relation between, say, EEG and dream reports is clearly not criterial; no one holds that EEG is a criterion of dream reports. It would seem then that, on Wittgenstein's view, EEG provides us with, at best, a symptom of positive dream reports; and symptoms are supposedly discovered

16. In *Dreaming,* Malcolm gives a number of arguments, not to be found in Wittgenstein's published writings, for the position that psychologists attempting to discover methods of measuring the duration of dreams must be using the term "dream" in a misleading and extraordinary way. For a reply to these arguments, see C. S. Chihara "What Dreams Are Made On" forthcoming in *Theoria* [Chapter 11 below]. See also H. Putnam's criticism of Malcolm, "Dreaming and 'Depth Grammar'," *Analytical Philosophy,* ed. R. J. Butler (Oxford, 1962), pp. 211–235.

17. The implausibility of this view is even more striking when Wittgenstein applies it in his philosophy of mathematics to arrive at the conclusion that every new theorem about a concept alters the concept or introduces a new concept. When the notion of conceptual change is allowed to degenerate this far, it is not easy to see that anything rides on the claim that a conceptual change has taken place. Cf. C. S. Chihara, "Mathematical Discovery and Concept Formation," the *Philosophical Review,* 72 (1963), 17–34.

by observing co-occurrences. The difficulty, however, is that this makes it unclear how the expectation that such a correlation must obtain could have been a rational expectation even *before* the correlation was experimentally confirmed. One cannot have an inductive generalization over no observations; nor, in this case, was any higher level "covering law" used to infer the probability of a correlation between EEG and dream reports. Given Wittgenstein's analysis of the concept of dreaming, not only do the researches of psychologists into the nature of dreams appear mysterious, but even the expectations, based upon these researches, seem somewhat irrational.

The difficulties we have mentioned are not peculiar to the Wittgensteinian analysis of dreams. Most of them have counterparts in the analyses of sensation, perception, intention, etc. Whether or not these difficulties can be obviated, in some way, noticing them provides a motive for re-examining the deeper doctrines upon which Wittgensteinian analyses of psychological terms are based.

VII

The Wittgensteinian argument of Section IV rests on the premiss that if we are justified in claiming that one can tell, recognize, see, or determine that 'Y' applies on the basis of the presence of X, then either X is a criterion of Y or observations have shown that X is correlated with Y. Wittgenstein does not present any justification for this premiss in his published writings. Evidently, some philosophers find it self-evident and hence in need of no justification. We, on the other hand, far from finding this premiss self-evident, believe it to be false. Consider: one standard instrument used in the detection of high-speed, charged particles is the Wilson cloud-chamber. According to present scientific theories, the formation of tiny, thin bands of fog on the glass surface of the instrument indicates the passage of charge particles through the chamber. It is obvious that the formation of these streaks is not a Wittgensteinian criterion of the presence and motion of these particles in the apparatus. That one can detect these charged particles and determine their paths by means of such devices is surely not, by any stretch of the imagination, a *conceptual* truth.

C. T. R. Wilson did not learn what "path of a charged particle" means by having the cloud-chamber explained to him: he *discovered* the method, and the discovery was contingent upon recognizing the empirical fact that ions could act as centers of condensation in a supersaturated vapor. Hence, applying Wittgenstein's own test for non-criterionhood (see above), the formation of a cloud-chamber track cannot be a criterion of the presence and motion of charged particles.

It is equally clear that the basis for taking these streaks as indicators of the paths of the particles is not observed *correlations* between streaks and some criterion of motion of charged particles. (What criterion for determining the path of an electron could Wilson have used to establish such correlations?) Rather, scientists were able to give compelling explanations of the formation of the streaks on the hypothesis that high-velocity, charged particles were passing through the chamber; on this hypothesis, further predictions were made, tested, and confirmed; no other equally plausible explanation is available; and so forth.

Such cases suggest that Wittgenstein failed to consider all the possible types of answers to the question, "What is the justification for the claim that one can tell, recognize, or determine that Y applies on the basis of the presence of X?" For, where Y is the predicate "is the path of a high-velocity particle," X need not have the form of either a criterion or a correlate.

Wittgensteinians may be tempted to argue that cloud-chamber tracks really are criteria, or symptoms observed to be correlated with criteria, of the paths of charged particles. To obviate this type of counter, we wish to stress that the example just given is by no means idiosyncratic. The reader who is not satisfied with it will easily construct others from the history of science. What is at issue is the possibility of a type of justification which consists in neither the appeal to criteria nor the appeal to observed correlations. If the Wittgensteinian argument we have been considering is to be compelling, some grounds must be given for the exhaustiveness of these types of justification. This, it would seem, Wittgenstein has failed to do.

It is worth noticing that a plausible solution to the problem raised in VI (5) can be given if we consider experiments with dreams and EEG to be analogous to the cloud-chamber case. That is, we can see how it could be the case that the correlation of EEG with dream reports was anticipated prior to observation. The dream report was taken by the experiments to be an indicator of a psychological event occurring prior to it. Given considerations about the relation of cortical to psychological events, and given also the theory of EEG, it was predicted that the EEG should provide an index of the occurrence of dreams. From the hypothesis that dream reports and EEG readings are both indices of the same psychological events, it could be deduced that they ought to be reliably correlated with one another, and this deduction in fact proved to be correct.

This situation is not at all unusual in the case of explanations based upon theoretical inferences to events underlying observable syndromes. As Meehl and Cronbach have pointed out, in such cases the validity of the "criterion" is often nearly as much at issue as the validity of the indices to be correlated with it.[18] The successful prediction of the correlation on the basis of the postulation of a common etiology is taken both as evidence for the existence of the cause and as indicating the validity of each of the correlates as an index of its presence.

In this kind of case, the justification of existential statements is thus identical neither with an appeal to criteria nor with an appeal to symptoms. Such justifications depend rather on appeals to the simplicity, plausibility, and predictive adequacy of an explanatory system as a whole, so that it is incorrect to say that relations between statements which are mediated by such explanations are either logical in Wittgenstein's sense or contingent in the sense in which this term suggests simple correlation.

It cannot be stressed too often that there exist patterns of justificatory argument which are not happily identified either with appeals to symptoms or with appeals to criteria, and which do not in any obvious way rest upon such appeals. In these

18. P. M. Meehl and H. J. Cronbach, "Construct Validity in Psychological Tests," *Minnesota Studies in the Philosophy of Science*, vol. I, ed. H. Feigl and M. Scriven (Minneapolis, 1956), pp. 174–204. We have followed Meehl and Cronbach's usage of the terms "reliability" and "validity" so that *reliability* is a measure of the correlation between criteria while *validity* is a measure of the correlation between a criterion and the construct whose presence it is supposed to indicate.

arguments, existential claims about states, events, and processes, which are *not* directly observable are susceptible of justification despite the fact that no *logical* relation obtains between the predicates ascribing such states and predicates whose applicability *can* be directly observed. There is a temptation to hold that in such cases there *must* be a criterion, that there must be some set of possible observations which would settle *for sure* whether the theoretical predicate applies. But we succumb to this temptation at the price of postulating stipulative definitions and conceptual alterations which fail to correspond to anything we can discover in the course of empirical arguments. The counter-intuitive features of philosophic analyses based on the assumption that there must be criteria are thus not the consequences of a profound methodological insight, but rather a projection of an inadequate philosophical theory of justification.

VIII

It might be replied that the above examples do not constitute counter-instances to Wittgenstein's criterion-correlation premise since Wittgenstein may have intended his principle to be applicable only in the case of ordinary language terms which, so it might seem, do not function within the framework of a theory. It is perhaps possible to have indicators that are neither criteria nor symptoms of such highly theoretical entities as electrons and positrons, but the terms used by ordinary people in everyday life are obviously (?) in a different category. (Notice that Wittgenstein considers "making scientific hypotheses and theories" a different "game" from such "language-games" as "describing an event" and "describing an immediate experience" [BB, pp. 67–68; Cf. PI,§23].) Hence, Wittgenstein might argue, it is only in the case of ordinary language terms that the demand for criteria is necessary.

Once one perceives the presuppositions of Wittgenstein's demand for criteria, however, it becomes evident that alternatives to Wittgenstein's analyses of ordinary language mental terms should at least be explored. Perhaps, what we all learn in learning what such terms as "pain" and "dream" mean are not criterial connections which map these terms severally onto characteristic patterns of behavior. We may instead form complex conceptual connections which interrelate a wide variety of mental states. It is to such a conceptual system that we appeal when we attempt to explain someone's behavior by reference to his motives, intentions, beliefs, desires, or sensations. In other words, in learning the language, we develop a number of intricately interrelated "mental concepts" which we use in dealing with, coming to terms with, understanding, explaining, interpreting, etc., the behavior of other human beings (as well as our own). In the course of acquiring these mental concepts we develop a variety of beliefs involving them. Such beliefs result in a wide range of expectations about how people are likely to behave. Since only a portion of these beliefs are confirmed in the normal course, these beliefs and the conceptual systems which they articulate are both subject to correction and alteration as the consequence of our constant interaction with other people.

On this view, our success in accounting for the behavior on the basis of which mental predicates are applied might properly be thought of as supplying *evidence* for the existence of the mental processes we postulate. It does so by attesting to the adequacy of the conceptual system in terms of which the processes are understood. The behavior would be, in that sense, analogous to the cloud-chamber track on the basis of which we detect the presence and motion of charged particles. Correspondingly, the conceptual system is analogous to the physical *theory* in which the properties of these particles are formulated.

If something like this should be correct, it would be possible, at least in theory, to reconstruct and describe the conceptual system involved and then to obtain some confirmation that the putative system is in fact employed by English speakers. For example, confirmation might come *via* the usual methods of "reading off" the conceptual relation in the putative system and *matching them* against the linguistic intuitions of native speakers. Thus, given that a particular conceptual system is being employed, certain statements should strike native speakers as nonsensical, others should seem necessarily true, others should seem ambiguous, others empirically false, and so on, all of which would be testable.

To maintain that there are no criterial connections between pains and behavior does not commit us to holding that the fact that people often feel *pains* when they cry out is *just* a contingent fact (in the sense in which it is just a contingent fact that most of the books in my library are unread). The belief that other people feel pains is not gratuitous even on the view that there are no criteria of pains. On the contrary, it provides the only plausible explanation of the facts I know about the way that they behave in and *vis à vis* the sorts of situations I find painful. These facts are, of course, enormously complex. The "pain syndrome" includes not only correlations between varieties of overt behaviors but also more subtle relations between pain and motivations, utilities, desires, and so on. Moreover, I confidently expect that there must exist reliable members of this syndrome other than the ones with which I am currently familiar. I am in need of an explanation of the reliability and fruitfulness of this syndrome, an explanation which reference to the occurrence of pains supplies. Here, as elsewhere, an "outer" syndrome stands in need of an inner process.

Thus, it is at least conceivable that a non-Wittgensteinian account ought to be given of the way children learn the mental predicates. (It is, at any event, sufficient to notice that such an account *could* be given, that there exist alternatives to Wittgenstein's doctrine.) For example, if the concept of dreaming is *inter alia* that of an inner event which takes place during a definite stretch of "real" time, which causes such involuntary behavior as moaning and murmuring in one's sleep, tossing about, etc., and which is remembered when one correctly reports a dream, then there are a number of ways in which a child might be supposed to "get" this concept other than by learning criteria for the application of the word "dream." Perhaps it is true of many children that they learn what a dream is by being told that what they have just experienced was a dream. Perhaps it was also true of many children that, having grasped the notions of *imagining* and *sleep*, they learn what a dream is when they are told that dreaming is something like imagining in your sleep.

But does this imply that children learn what a dream is "from their own case?" If this is a logical rather than psychological question, the answer is "Not necessarily": a child who never dreamed, but who was very clever, might arrive at an understanding of what dreams are just on the basis of the sort of theoretical inference we have described above. For our notion of a dream is that of a mental event having various properties that are required in order to explain the characteristic features of the dream-behavior syndrome. For example, dreams occur during sleep, have duration, sometimes cause people who are sleeping to murmur or to toss, can be described in visual, auditory, or tactile terms, are sometimes remembered and sometimes not, are sometimes reported and sometimes not, sometimes prove frightening, sometimes are interrupted before they are finished, etc. But if these are the sorts of facts that characterize our concept of dream, then there seems to be nothing which would, in principle, prevent a child who never dreamed from arriving at this notion.

A similar story might be told about how such sensation terms as "pain" are learned and about the learning of such quasi-dispositionals as "having a motive." In each case, since the features that we in fact attribute to these states, processes, or dispositions are just those features we know they must have if they are to fulfill their role in explanations of behavior, etiology, personality, etc., it would seem that there is nothing about them the child could not in principle learn by employing the pattern of inference we have described above, and hence nothing that he could in principle learn *only* by an analogy to his own case.

Now it might be argued that the alternative to Wittgenstein's position we have been sketching is highly implausible. For, if children do have to acquire the complicated conceptual system our theory requires to understand and use mental predicates, surely they would have to be taught this system. And the teaching would surely have to be terribly involved and complex. But as a matter of fact, children do not require any such teaching at all, and hence we should conclude that our alternative to Wittgenstein's criterion view is untenable.

The force of this argument, however, can to some extent be dispelled if we consider the child's acquisition of, e.g., the grammar of a natural language. It is clear that, by some process we are only now beginning to understand, a child, on the basis of a relatively short "exposure" to utterances in his language, develops capacities for producing and understanding "novel" sentences (sentences which he has never previously heard or seen). The exercise of these capacities, so far as we can tell, "involve" the use of an intricate system of linguistic rules of very considerable generality and complexity.[19] That the child is not taught (in any ordinary sense) any such system of rules is undeniable. These capacities seem to develop naturally in the child in response to little more than contact with a relatively small number of sentences uttered in ordinary contexts in everyday life.[20] Granting for the moment that the apparent complexity of such systems of rules is not somehow an artifact of an unsatisfactory theory of language, the fact that the child develops these linguistic capacities shows that a corresponding "natural" development of a system of mental concepts may not, as a matter of brute fact, require the sort of explicit teaching a person needs to master, say, calculus or quantum physics.

IX

It is easily seen that this unabashedly non-behavioristic view avoids each of the difficulties we raised regarding Wittgenstein's analyses of mental predicates. Thus, the asymmetry between first and third person uses of "dream" discussed in Section VI need not arise since there need be no criteria for "X dreamed," *whatever* value X takes: we do not have the special problem of characterizing the meaning of "I dreamed" since "dream" in this context means just what it means in third person contexts, viz., "a series of thoughts, images, or emotions occurring during sleep." Again, it is now clear why people find such remarks as "Jones totally forgot what and that he dreamed last night" perfectly sensible. It is even clear how such assertions might be confirmed. Suppose, for example, that there exists a neurological state α such that there is a very high

19. This point is susceptible of direct empirical ratification, for it can be demonstrated that in perceptual analysis, speech is analyzed into segments which correspond precisely to the segmentation assigned by a grammar.

20. Cf. N. Chomsky's "A Review of Skinner's *Verbal Behavior*," reprinted in J. Fodor and J. Katz, *The Structure of Language* (Englewood Cliffs, 1964).

correlation between the presence of α and such dream behavior as tossing in one's sleep, crying out in one's sleep, reporting dreams, and so on. Suppose, too that there exists some neurological state β such that whenever β occurs, experiences that the subject has had just prior to β are forgotten. Suppose, finally, that sometimes we observe sequences, α, β, and that such sequences are not followed by dream reports though the occurrences of α are accompanied by other characteristic dream behaviors. It seems clear that the reasonable thing to say in such a case is that the subject has dreamed and forgotten his dream. And since we have postulated no criterion for dreaming, but only a syndrome of dream behaviors each related to some inner psychological event, we need have no fear that, in saying what it is reasonable to say, we have changed the meaning of "dream." We leave it to the reader to verify that the other objections we raised against the Wittgensteinian analysis of "dream" also fail to apply to the present doctrine.

Thus, once we have abandoned the arguments for a criterial connection between statements about behavior and statements about psychological states, the question remains open whether applications of ordinary language psychological terms on the basis of observations of behavior ought not themselves be treated as theoretical inferences to underlying mental occurrences. The question whether such statements as "He moaned because he was in pain" function to explain behavior by relating it to an assumed mental event cannot be settled simply by reference to ordinary linguistic usage. Answering this question requires broadly empirical investigations into the nature of thought and concept formation in normal human beings. What is at issue is the question of the role of theory construction and theoretical inference in thought and argument outside pure science. Psychological investigations indicate that much everyday conceptualization depends on the exploitation of theories and explanatory models in terms of which experience is integrated and understood.[21] Such pre-scientific theories, far

21. Among the many psychological studies relevant to this point, the following are of special importance: F. Bartlett, *Remembering, A Study in Experimental and Social Psychology* (Cambridge, 1932); J. Piaget, *The Child's Conception of the World* (London, 1928); J. Brunner, "On Perceptual Readiness," reprinted in

from being mere functionless "pictures," play an essential role in determining the sorts of perceptual and inductive expectations we form and the kind of arguments and explanations we accept. It thus seems *possible* that the correct view of the functioning of ordinary language mental predicates would assimilate applying them to the sorts of processes of theoretical inference operative in scientific psychological explanation. If this is correct, the primary difference between ordinary and scientific uses of psychological predicates would be just that the processes of inference which are made explicit in the latter case remain implicit in the former.

We can now see what should be said in reply to Wittgenstein's argument that the possibility of teaching a language rests upon the existence of criteria. Perhaps teaching a word would be impossible if it could not sometimes be determined that the student has mastered the use of the word. But this does not entail that there need be *criteria* for "X learned the word *w*." All that is required is that we must sometimes have good reasons for saying that the word has been mastered; and this condition is satisfied when, for example, the simplest and most plausible explanation available of the verbal behavior of the student is that he has learned the use of the word.

Readings in Perception, ed. M. Wertheimer and D. Beardsley (Princeton, 1958), pp. 686–729.

9

DAVID F. PEARS

Dreaming

The thesis of this monograph [*Dreaming*, by Norman Mal-
colm] is that dreams are not identical with, or composed of
thoughts, impressions, feelings, images or any other mental
phenomena occurring during sleep (pp. 4, 45, 51). This does
not mean that dreams do not occur during sleep, nor that they
cannot be classified as mental phenomena (52). The point is
that, if they are so classified, they are a unique and peculiar exception. They are unique, because they are the only mental
phenomena that do occur during sleep (50). They are peculiar,
because the criterion of the truth of the statement that a person
has had a certain dream is, essentially, his saying so (49).

The last contention is qualified in three ways. First, it is applied only to the primary concept of dreaming (62, 63, 70). Secondly, the person's report might be untruthful (55). And
thirdly, there is one way in which his report might be mistaken:
what he reported might in fact be part of his waking life. This
does not mean that, when he says that it was a dream, he has
made an inference, but only that he might have defended what
he said by pointing out that it was not part of his waking life
(65). It is important that he could not make any other kind of
mistake (66). For no sense can be made of the suggestion that
his impression of memory might fail to correspond to his

Reprinted from *Mind*, 70 (1961), 145–163, by permission of the author and
the publisher (Basil Blackwell, Oxford); originally titled "Professor Norman
Malcolm: Dreaming."

dream (56). If his report of his dream is false, and if this is not because it corresponds to something in his waking life, then the only possible explanation is that he is being untruthful. For, given that there is no correspondence with waking life, a truthful report of a dream simply is the criterion of the occurrence of that dream.

It would be too much to expect that this closely packed monograph should contain a full investigation of the concept of truthfulness. But there are certain difficulties in it. Of course, the person who reports the dream does not use his own report as the criterion of its occurrence: only his audience do that (63). But does he, therefore, as Professor Malcolm maintains, use no criterion? Suppose that it takes him some time to achieve a narrative that he really accepts. Perhaps he even experiments with slightly varying versions until he arrives at one which feels exactly right. Might he not then be said to be using a criterion? Maybe not. But the word "criterion" needs to have its own criterion fixed. Certainly the dreamer corrects himself in such cases, and he would not explain the rejected version by saying that it was the result of untruthfulness. Or, if he did say this, he would have to point out that his truthfulness sometimes cost him an effort, not because he knew what he ought to say but could not bring himself to say it, but because he had to work his way through various versions until he reached an acceptable one. Not that this process is typical. But it does occur sometimes, and its occurrence is important. For it suggests that there might sometimes be an alternative to the account according to which the dreamer simply wakes up with an impression of memory, and the only mistake that he might make is saying that it is a dream when in fact it is a piece of real life (57). Malcolm mentions these untypical cases but sees no need to modify his account in the light of them. This is probably because he is preoccupied with his main point, that no sense can be attached to the suggestion that the report might be mistaken because it did not correspond to the dream. For this point certainly makes the investigation of the exact process leading up to the report of the dream look rather small, since, if there is no question of correspondence between the report and the dream, the dreamer is the final arbiter, and his penultimate arbitrations do not seem to be very important. And, in any case, even if their importance is admitted, it may be that the concept of truthfulness can be made to cover this area. But with what modifications?

Another difficulty, of an entirely different kind, is that Malcolm's criterion of the truth of the statement that a person has had a certain dream does not seem to fit our concept of dreaming. It is, of course, not easy to decide whether it does or does not fit our concept, or, if it does not, how far it diverges. For the implications of his criterion are not quite clear, and it is a difficult matter to determine exactly what our concept is. In general, it is well known that supporters of this kind of reductive theory often attribute double vision to their critics, only to be met with the counter-charge of blindness either to the implications of the reduction or to certain aspects of the material. However, one thing is clear; we ordinarily think that a waking experience can be recapitulated in a subsequent dream. But the suggested criterion does not seem to allow for this possibility, since Malcolm appears to say that, given the impression of memory, absence of correspondence with anything in the person's waking life is not only a sufficient condition of his having dreamt it, but also a necessary condition (51, 68, 80, 97). If he says this, it is probably a slip. But how should the criterion be amended? Is the occurrence of a recapitulating dream always to be left an open and undecidable possibility every time anyone remembers anything from his waking life? Certainly we do not ordinarily think that there is such a large area of undecidability here. But perhaps our ordinary thoughts on this matter are confused? Or is Malcolm's account of remembering too thin and Humean?

We might also raise the converse objection, that we ordinarily think that a sincere memory-claim might fail to correspond with anything, either in the person's waking life or in his dreams. For we do not think that all the sincere memory-claims of a person who had never slept in his life would be true. So it is unrealistic to suggest that, whenever a sleeper makes a sincere memory claim that does not correspond with anything in his waking life, it should be treated as the criterion that he has dreamt it. But Malcolm has a stronger defence against this objection. For he would argue that, since we could never establish that he has not dreamt it, the idea that this is an open possibility really is confused.

Problems of the same kind, but more complicated ones, are raised by the question whether dreams can be timed. What do we ordinarily think? And what does Malcolm's criterion allow? First, we certainly think that dreams can only occur during sleep; and he makes this a matter of definition (49, 83, 98). Secondly, we almost certainly think that dreams occur at particular times during periods of sleep; but he refuses to allow that any sense can be attached to this belief. Indeed, he even denies that dreams occur in physical time (43, 70). This denial appears to be incompatible with his concession that we do dream during sleep. But he claims that the appearance of incompatibility ought to vanish as soon as we whole-heartedly accept his criterion for the truth of the statement that a dream occurred during a period of sleep (77). If it lingers, spatial imagery must be exercising an undue influence.

This part of his thesis is not easy to understand. He is almost certainly offering a reductive analysis of the statement that dreams occur during periods of sleep, and so he is not rejecting this part of what we ordinarily think about the timing of dreams. But why, in that case, does he say that dreams do not occur in physical time? This is a very puzzling remark. Dr. Johnson would have tried to refute it by going off and having a dream. But, of course, it ought to mean that they do not occur in physical time in a sense that is governed by other criteria than Malcolm's. But, why, then, does he reject the second thing that we ordinarily think? That is, why does he refuse to allow that any sense can be attached to the belief that dreams occur at particular times during periods of sleep? The reason he gives is that, though indications of specific times are sometimes given in dreamers' reports, they are never precise enough to satisfy physical science (75, 76). But this does not seem to be a sufficient reason. These imprecise indications place dreams imprecisely in physical time. Moreover, it ought to make sense to say that, if the sleeper had awoken ten minutes earlier, he would not have had the dream, even if we cannot know whether this is so. For, if this did not make sense, why should it make sense to say that, if he had not slept at all that night, he would not have had the dream?

It looks as if Malcolm is offering a reductive analysis of part of what we ordinarily think, and rejecting the other part of what we ordinarily think. In general, this is a possible programme. But in this particular case, when one part is the thought that dreams occur during periods of sleep, and the other part is the thought that they occur at particular times during periods of sleep, it is hard to see how it could be carried out. If he really intended his thesis to be taken in this way, the explanation may be that he believed that, if he allowed that dreams occurred at particular times during periods of sleep, his reductive analysis would be unable to cover this possibility. But why should the exact timing of dreams escape his analysis if the inexact timing of them does not? Because exact timing would imply that what was timed was concrete and historical? But this suggestion, even if it were intelligible, would be irrelevant to the question of analysis. Then is the reason that counterfactual conditionals, like the one beginning "If he had awoken ten minutes earlier . . .", are unverifiable? But there could be indirect evidence for them.

However, suppose that he were to insist that sense should be given not only to the statement that a dream occurred at a particular time during sleep, but also to the further statement that it was composed of, say, images, on the ground that the first statement would have very little content unless the second statement, or something like it, were added. If he insisted on this, he could argue that, if the statement that dreams occur at particular times during periods of sleep is to have a substantial content, it cannot be analysed reductively in the way that he favours. For there would be nothing in the dreamer's subsequent report which could possibly give sense to the statement that a particular dream was composed of images rather than, say, unspoken words, and so the use of physiological evidence would seem to be unavoidable. But this would be contemporary. Therefore it would be impossible to carry out a reductive analysis that appealed to no contemporary facts except the bare fact that the dreamer slept.

This would provide him with a reason for thinking that at

least such statements as "The dream was composed of images" cannot be given a reductive analysis of the kind that he favours, and therefore must be rejected by him. But it does not seem to have been his reason. For he never considers the possible difference in sense between the statement that a particular dream was composed of images, and the statement that it was composed of something else. He simply takes the statement that dreams, in general, are composed of images, thoughts, feelings, etc., and argues, in general, that the only sense that it could possibly have is that people dream that they have images, thoughts, feelings, etc.; and, if there are occasions when people would not actually call the thing a dream, this can only be because it is too brief; and this is unimportant, since it will still have the same logical status as a dream—i.e. the criterion of its occurrence will be, essentially, his subsequent report (42, 47, 84, 85). In any case, even if he had followed this line of thought, it would not have diminished the difficulty that has already been mentioned: *viz.* it is difficult to accept and reduce the statement that dreams occur during periods of sleep without giving the same treatment to the statement that dreams occur at particular times during periods of sleep. For the argument which shows that the reductive analysis would deprive the second statement of substantial content would also show that the reductive analysis deprives the first statement of substantial content.

Alternatively, it may be that he simply did not think of the possibility that the statement, that a particular dream was composed of, say, images, might be given a reductive analysis of the kind that he favours.

Finally, it is just possible that he is not offering a reductive analysis even of the statement that dreams occur during periods of sleep. For his puzzling remark, that dreams do not occur in physical time, may be intended quite generally. If so, his concept of dreaming really does diverge considerably from ours. But again what he rejects, if he is rejecting it, may seem to him to be confused.

It is important to try to determine the exact meaning of Malcolm's thesis, and its relation to our concept of dreaming. For, if it is felt to be paradoxical, it is necessary to decide whether this is because it rejects part of our concept, or because it accepts it all, but gives a new and strange reductive analysis of it. Now it is doubtful how the questions of detail that have just been raised ought to be answered. But there is no doubt that, in the main, he accepts and reduces. Nor is there much doubt that most people will find his reduction paradoxical. But some of the arguments for it are very strong. However, when a conclusion is felt to be paradoxical, and perhaps even fantastic, the very strength of the arguments is a source of irritation which could cause them to be neglected. This would be regrettable, since, even if they are not conclusive, they are important challenges. And even those of his arguments that are less strong are of great interest. For he raises difficult questions, which were almost totally neglected by philosophers until Wittgenstein wrote about dreams, and he pursues them with pertinacity.

His main argument is that there could be no criterion for the truth of the statement that a person had an image, thought, feeling, etc., in his sleep, unless it merely meant that he dreamed that he had one (10, 16, 35). For anything that tended to show that he was at that moment having one would necessarily show that he was at that moment not asleep, and it is no good appealing to his subsequent memory claims if there are no possible criteria for establishing the truth of their contents (11, 40). Our only resource is to interpret them as reports of dreams, and then, subject to the qualifications already given, they are the criteria of their own truth.

Unfortunately this argument does not always succeed in disentangling itself from a subsidiary argument, which looks like it, but is in fact different from it (7, 18). The subsidiary argument simply says that the hypothesis that a person might have an image, thought, feeling, etc. in his sleep is contradictory: for all these things entail that he was aware at the time, and awareness is incompatible with sleep. The difference between the two arguments is that, according to the subsidiary one, the hypothesis is contradictory; whereas, according to the main one what is contradictory is the hypothesis that we might verify the hypothesis.[1] The subsidiary argument, of course, invites the retort that there might be another kind of awareness, and then the main argument would have to be invoked.

One reason why the main argument does not always succeed in disentangling itself from the subsidiary argument is that Malcolm's investigation of alleged mental phenomena during sleep develops out of a discussion of the statement "I am asleep". For it is very easy to assimilate this statement to the statements "I am dead", and "I do not exist", and in fact he makes both these assimilations. When he makes the first, he says that the assertion of both "I am asleep" and "I am dead" is incompatible with their truth (7). And this is clearly the subsidiary argument. When he makes the second assimilation, he says that I cannot wonder whether I am asleep any more than I can wonder whether I exist (18). And this too ought to be the subsidiary argument, since it seems to be too strong a statement for the main argument: but in fact it comes immediately after the first exposition of the main argument. The trouble is that the statement "I am asleep" looks very like a member of a class of statements that are perfect targets for the subsidiary argument, and so a general investigation, which happens to begin with it, but really relies on the main argument, naturally tends to neglect the distinction between the two arguments.

There are traces of the subsidiary argument at other points in the monograph. For example, Malcolm argues that my dreaming that I had thoughts and feelings does not establish that I had them while asleep any more than my dreaming that I climbed a mountain establishes that I climbed it while asleep (51, 52. Cf. pp. 65, 95). Certainly. But I might retort that I could have a very quiet thought in my sleep, whereas even a small mountain would wake me up; so that, even if neither of these two things would be established, one of them could be true. And here again the main argument would have to be invoked.

This discussion of the difference between the two arguments might provoke the reply that it really does not matter. For if we find it contradictory to suppose that we could verify a hypothe-

1. This distinction is clearly drawn on page 36.

sis, this is just as bad as finding that the hypothesis itself is contradictory: in neither case does the hypothesis express a possibility. It is not certain that Malcolm would make this reply (37).
It raises a profound question about sense. This question, and
the problem of interpreting his views on this point may be postponed for the moment, until the main argument has been examined.

The main argument is directed against the very natural belief that, at the times during sleep when we dream, we enjoy
another mode of consciousness. It is not clear exactly what this
mode of consciousness is supposed to be, but at least it is not
supposed to be the same as waking consciousness, so that the
belief is immune to the subsidiary argument. Presumably it
would be some trance-like state, like that of a person who has
been drugged, or even of someone who is totally absorbed in a
work of art. If people were asked to say more exactly what the
stuff of dreams is, they would probably suggest images, and
some kind of narrative or unspoken words. Against this belief
the main argument simply says that it is contradictory to suppose that it might be verified. And, as has already been pointed
out, the possibility that it might have a purely subsequent verification is not considered, perhaps for good reasons: the verification which is considered and rejected as impossible includes
at least some contemporary things, and may even be purely
contemporary.

Various doubts might be raised about the main argument.
First, must every type of memory-claim be verified sometimes,
or at least confirmed sometimes? If so, what counts as a type?
And, if memory-claims that purport to transcend a plane of
consciousness count as a type for this purpose, may they not be
confirmed in cases where the sleeper exhibits some behaviour,
or is subjected to some stimulus? And, if so, might not this type
of confirmation be used to give sense to what appears to be our
ordinary belief about dreams in the other cases where it is not
available? Particularly if in all cases there is, or could be physiological confirmation as well?

It would be a lengthy matter to discuss these doubts properly, and to show how Malcolm tries to preserve the main argument against them. He has a strong position, built on three

lines of defence. First, in his description of cases he tends to deny, but does not actually deny outright that there are grounds for saying that, when the sleeper exhibits behaviour or is subjected to a stimulus, he is aware in any special sense. Secondly, he denies that these cases are central cases of sleep, and implies that any attempt to extrapolate from them to the central cases would be illicit. His third, and most important line of defence is to maintain, at least about the physiological phenomena in central cases, and probably also about stimulus and behaviour in borderline cases, that we cannot give any separate sense to the hypothesis that these evidences are alleged to confirm, so that they are either irrelevant to dreaming, or else must be treated as a new criterion of dreaming, different from ours.

Let us begin with his first line of defence. Now the debate in the monograph starts from an examination of the statement "I am asleep", and some kind of behaviour on the sleeper's part might naturally be used as a ground for the belief that he made this statement; and later it passes on to a general discussion of all alleged mental phenomena during sleep, including things which would not be classified as activities, and for which, therefore, some kind of stimulus might be taken to be a plausible ground. So let us first concentrate on activities.

Now the making of statements is only one activity among many, but it is very important for this investigation, because it is closely related to one of the things which might be held to be the stuff of dreams—unspoken narration, so that its relevance is not restricted to the dreams inside which the dreamer makes a statement. This tends to be obscured in the monograph where it is assumed that the particular dreamer dreams that he makes a statement. Moreover, the statement which he dreams that he makes, "I am asleep", is a peculiar one. For, if he did make this statement in his sleep, it would be a reflection on the plane of consciousness on which it itself existed; or, on Malcolm's view, a reflection on the status of the memory-claim in which it was reported.

Suppose that this dreamer talked in his sleep, and "made" this peculiar statement. Then, as Malcolm observes, outside his dream he would not be making a claim, asserting or communicating, since all these performances require that the words should be deliberately addressed or at least sent off, and the dreamer does not, and perhaps could not even know that they are going out into the world (8). Nevertheless might they not be taken as providing ground for thinking that he is at that moment making this judgement during a dream? (9, 10). "Only if he is aware at that moment." But if a special kind of awareness is envisaged—as it must be, if this problem is going to be investigated—are his words not sufficient ground for thinking that he is aware at that moment, at least in those cases where he subsequently reports that he dreamt that he made the judgement? Malcolm considers talking in one's sleep, but, when he considers it, he does not ask himself this question (10, 62). So it is not quite certain how he would have answered it if he had asked it. In similar, but more extreme cases—e.g. where the person's behaviour shows that he is having a nightmare—he tends to say that he is not fully asleep (28, 100). Perhaps this means that he would allow that there is some ground for thinking, at least in extreme cases, that he is aware. If he did allow this, he would, of course, mean ordinary awareness. But, if it is admitted that there is ground for thinking that there is any sort of awareness in such cases, would it not be more plausible to say that it is the sort of awareness that most people believe themselves to have when they are dreaming? For a person in the throes of a nightmare is not like a person just waking up: perhaps neither is fully asleep, but the person in the throes of a nightmare is not faintly aware that he is doing things in the real world. However, in his description of this case, Malcolm does not concede this point. But he does concede more when he raises the question whether there are any grounds for thinking that things in which the mind is passive—e.g. images—occur during sleep.

If we now took up this question, the debate would follow a roughly parallel course. For suppose that the hypothesis were that dreams are composed partly of images. Then it would be important that these images would be thought to occur not only at those moments when the sleeper was dreaming that he was having an image (93). So, if he were subjected to a stimulus—e.g. if there were a loud noise in his vicinity—the idea would be that this noise might be woven into the images that composed his dream. And the same view would be taken of proprioceptive sensations. Now, if this hypothesis had a sense, it would not imply that the sleeper heard the noise in the full way: for he would not refer it to the world outside his dream, or, perhaps even think of that world. (This is parallel to the fact, already noted, that the person who talks in his sleep does not communicate, etc.) Malcolm suggests that, in order to make this clear, the sleeper should say, after waking up, "I *must* have heard the noise" (98, 99, cf. p. 32). This he might well do. But Malcolm then interprets this remark as a causal hypothesis, and not as a report of an actual experience. Obviously his theory necessitates this interpretation of the remark, but it is an unnatural one. And even he finds himself unable to extend this kind of treatment to the asthmatic sleeper, who both is, and dreams that he is suffocating (99). This man's feeling of suffocation is, he concedes, partly dreamt, and the context makes it fairly clear that he means that it is dreamt at the moment when he is actually suffocating. So this is a very important concession; it comes very close indeed to the admission that at that moment the sleeper is aware in a special sense. He seeks to neutralize it by observing that he is not fully asleep and that, since his suffering and behaviour yield a criterion of the occurrence of his dream, it is not a dream in the primary sense—i.e. the sense that is governed by the recommended criterion. But, even if this were correct, it would still leave us with a borderline case where there is some contemporary ground for thinking that there is a special kind of awareness.

At several points in his discussion of things in which the mind is passive Malcolm is influenced by an argument which is connected with a point already made here, the point that his criterion of dreaming appears to rule out, probably by an oversight, dreams that recapitulate a past experience in waking life. According to this argument the following restriction must be put on the ways in which a dream can be true of the real world: if a person dreams that he saw something happen, or heard it, etc., then the content of his dream cannot correspond to the real world in his immediate vicinity at the time when the dream would ordinarily be taken to have occurred.[2] (There is, as has been noted, some doubt whether he would extend this restriction to earlier times too, and thus rule out recapitulating dreams.) But why is contemporary correspondence impossible? Certainly the view that it did correspond would not normally be held by the person himself, either later, or in the dream (however that is to be analysed): nor, of course, would his statement that he dreamed that he had the experience imply that view. Nevertheless the view might be correct: the content of the dream might correspond to the contemporary events in his room; and, if it did, there would probably be a causal explanation of the correspondence. So any support that this argument might give to Malcolm's case must be subtracted.

There is also anothe point at which his first line of defence might be attacked. The phenomenology of going to sleep and waking up might be cited against it. For at those moments we sometimes find that dreaming and waking experience overlap. Admittedly, these are cases where the person is not fully asleep, so that we could not argue that, if he is aware at all, his awareness must be the special kind of awareness. But this does not matter, since this time he himself could testify that he was conscious on two different planes, or at least that he experienced the transition from one plane to the other.

If the attack on Malcolm's first line of defence had any effect he might make a stand on the second line that he has prepared, and say that we cannot understand awareness in deep sleep by extrapolating from cases of disturbed sleep (99, 100). But this would be a more difficult position to defend. For, once it is clearly understood that the kind of awareness that is meant is not ordinary awareness, it is hard to maintain the dilemma, that either reports of dreams in undisturbed sleep have a completely different sense, or else they are unintelligible. Must all extrapolation be disallowed? Must every type of statement get its sense entirely directly? If so, what counts as a type?

But his third line of defence is the most important one. For so far we have used the unanalysed notion of "a ground". But

2. Pages 68, 98. Cf. p. 8 footnote.

he would say that we must always ask whether a ground provides confirmation or verification: if it provides the latter, it is a
criterion; while, if it provides the former, something else will
have to provide the criterion of what is being confirmed, if it is
going to have a definite sense (44). He would probably apply
this dilemma to stimulus and behaviour, in order to defend his
descriptions of cases which have just been challenged. But he
certainly applies it to physiological phenomena (43, 76, 77, 81,
82). So let us first examine its application there.

Now it is very important that his thesis is reductive only in
the sense that his criterion of the truth of the statement that a
dream occurred is parsimonious. He carefully guards himself
against the interpretation that would credit him with the unintelligible view that the dream is to be identified with his criterion of its occurrence (59, 60, 61). So, when he suggests the
possibility that in central cases of sleep physiological phenomena, like rapid eye movements, might be taken as a new criterion of dreaming, he is not suggesting an absurd identification.
But what is the justification of his dilemma, that such phenomena are either irrelevant to dreaming or else must be taken as a
new criterion of dreaming, i.e. as a criterion of dreaming in a
secondary sense? It is clear that, if the hypothesis, that in the
central cases the sleeper is aware in a special way, could get its
sense by extrapolation from the borderline cases, the dilemma
would not be valid in the central cases. So let us go back to the
borderline cases, and see how he applies the dilemma to them.

But the trouble is that it is not certain that he does apply the
dilemma to borderline cases, where there is stimulus and
behaviour. If he did apply it to borderline cases, he would not
have the same reason for saying that the criterion would necessarily be a new one that he has for saying this in central cases.
For if physiological phenomena were used as a criterion of
dreaming, this would necessarily be a new criterion, since the
phenomena have only been discovered recently and are not
generally known. But this is not true of stimulus and behaviour
in borderline cases.

Moreover, if he did apply the dilemma to borderline cases,
he might find that it could be turned against himself. For, if he
said that the physical state and behaviour of the asthmatic

sleeper could provide only confirmation for the hypothesis that he had some special kind of awareness, on the ground that this awareness must amount to more than the observable phenomena, then the ordinary awareness of people who are awake will often be no more than confirmed. If, on the other hand, he says that it would provide verification, he will have to go on to establish that, if it is accepted as verification, a new criterion will, in fact, have been introduced. And this is never established in the monograph. It might look as if it is established, because he says that his criterion is the one that we use, and that it fixes the primary concept of dreaming (74, 79, 80, 81, 82). But the case for doubting whether it is the one that we use has already been sketched, and he never justifies his assertion that it fixes the primary concept, and not just part of the concept of dreaming.

There is, underlying this state of his main argument, the idea that every kind of statement must have a definite criterion whose fulfilment conclusively verifies it, and whose non-fulfilment conclusively falsifies it. Guided by this idea he goes to human behaviour in order to find out what the criterion for reports of dreams is. But perhaps the search is misguided. If dreaming really does involve a special kind of awareness at the time, why should we not think that we have two independent indications of this awareness, and therefore of dreams—subsequent memory-claims and contemporary behaviour? Given certain conditions, each could be taken as sufficient ground for saying that a dream occurred; and the absence of one of them would not be taken as sufficient ground for saying that a dream did not occur, so that, e.g. the fact that the dreamer had not behaved appropriately in his sleep would not show that his subsequent memory-claim was mistaken. And, if he objects that, in that case, we should never have anything more than contemporary confirmation for the hypothesis that a sleeper was aware in the special way and therefore dreaming, how could he avoid extending this objection to the hypothesis that people who are awake are aware in the ordinary way? Whatever the result of this debate, it ought to take place before the word "criterion" is used.

The main argument has been examined at length because

the whole subject is difficult and uncertain, and because our ordinary beliefs in the matter are apt to exercise an undue influence, before their content has been exactly determined and before they have been shown to involve more than Malcolm's criterion allows in a reductive way. There is also a small group of auxiliary arguments which do not need much comment. According to one of these arguments, if the statement "I am asleep" came from the mouth of a sleeper, it could not be taken as reliable testimony (5). According to another, I could not verify the judgement "I am asleep": for I could not observe the state of my body, and I could not tell by noticing that I was having a certain experience, since there is no experience that is necessarily connected with sleep (12); and, if it were suggested that there was a contingent connection between being asleep and having a certain experience, how could this be verified? (40) Both these arguments would presumably be applied to the statement "I am dreaming", which entails the statement "I am asleep".

Now these arguments are directed against the man who refuses to accept a reductive analysis of the statement "I have visited the world of my dreams". They reply, in effect, that, if *per impossible*, he were right, there would be no way in which he could then establish whether he was asleep and dreaming. But the reply is not convincing. For, whatever the correct analysis of the statement "I dreamed that I was having a dream", and whatever the status of the verdict that it reports, there is no doubt that both are often true. Now it is a very mysterious fact that the verdict is often true: for at least often I am totally unable to say what the basis of my verdict was. But this mysterious fact cannot be used as an objection against the man who rejects the reductive analysis. For any theory, including the reductive one, has to admit that it is a fact, and a mysterious one. So these arguments do not advance Malcolm's case beyond the point where the main argument left it. His contention, that the statement "I dreamed that I was having a dream" must be analysed reductively, may be right; and, if it is right, the verdict can be verified, but *not by my waiting to see*. But the contention gains no support from these arguments, and must, therefore, rest on the main argument.

Imagine a world in which things were made easier for the main argument, because in it there was no correlation between dreaming and stimulus, behaviour or physiological phenomena, and no overlapping of the two planes of consciousness. What exactly ought the conclusion to be? Ought it to be that, in this world, the hypothesis that the dreamer was aware in a special way during sleep had no sense, or that it did not have a sense that we could understand? The profound question that was postponed earlier was the question whether there is any difference between these two theses. Now to say that it would have no sense is ambiguous. It might mean that it was contradictory, so that what it expressed was not a possibility. But, as has been shown, one argument for this view, the subsidiary argument, is invalid. Nor is there any plausibility in arguing for it in the way in which some people have argued that the survival of death is contradictory: for there is no reason to think that all kinds of awareness are incompatible with sleep. Suppose, on the other hand, that the ambiguous thesis were taken to mean that it had not been given a sense, and so did not express an identifiable possibility. This, of course, might be for the uninteresting reason that nobody had tried to give it a sense. Alternatively, it might be because our best efforts to give it the sense that it seemed that it ought to have had always failed, so that the words were never connected with an identifiable possibility. This second alternative could be expressed by saying that the words did not have a sense that we could understand, and this, of course, is the second thesis. But, if the first thesis is interpreted in the first way, it differs from the second thesis.

Would either of them be a correct conclusion in the imagined world? Certainly it looks as if, even in the imagined world, we should have no reason to say that what was expressed by the hypothesis that the dreamer is aware in a special way during sleep was not a possibility. But would we have any reason to say that we could not connect it with an identifiable possibility? This is a more difficult question. First, suppose that we concede that reports of dreams are a type of memory-claim that needs to be verified, or at least confirmed sometimes, in order to avoid being treated as self-supporting in the way that

Malcolm recommends. The reason for conceding this would be that, if the report of a dream were alleged to mean anything more than he allows, then in the imagined world nothing in waking life could count either in favour of or against the surplus possibility. Nevertheless it might still be a possibility, and, if it were, it is arguable that we could verify it while dreaming. For would we not then know that this was it, and do we not now understand what it would be like to know that then?

So we might argue. But would we be right? For verification involves the fitting together of a situation and a statement. And how could we understand now what it would be like to know then that we had remembered the right statement? How could we even understand now what it would be like for us to remember, at the moment in a dream when we judge that we are dreaming, that our judgment bears its usual sense? How could constancy of meaning be known to have been preserved across an impervious gap between two planes of consciousness? (54) This is rather an abstruse question. If it is unanswerable, then in the imagined world the hypothesis that the dreamer is aware in a special way during sleep would not be connected with an identifiable possibility. However, it would not follow that this result applied to our world, in which dreaming is sometimes connected with stimulus, behaviour and physiological phenomena, and the two planes of consciousness do sometimes overlap. And, even if it did apply to our world, it would not follow that what the hypothesis expressed would not be a possibility.

The invalidity of this second step is extremely important, but it is not absolutely certain that it is recognized in the monograph. Two things suggest that it might not be recognized. Both happen because Malcolm approaches the problem by way of an examination of the statements "I am asleep", and "I am dreaming". The first thing, which has already been noted, is this: if it is possible for a sleeper to make either of these two judgements, it must be possible for him to be aware at the time; and, though the main argument shows, if it is successful, only that we cannot connect the hypothesis, that he is aware at the time, with an identifiable possibility, the subsidiary argument insinuates that what it is connected with is not a possibility. He probably did not intend this to happen. The second thing is that he argues that, because neither of the two statements has a correct use, neither of them expresses a possibility. At least these are the words that he sometimes employs (18). But he also sometimes phrases his conclusion in a different way, and says that neither of the two statements expresses a possibility that we can think (18, 118). Now this second version must be the one that he intends. For, while it is obvious that neither of the two statements can have a correct use in the way in which the statement "I am now approaching the target area" has a correct use, this shows, at the most, that the connection of each statement with a possibility is not that it expresses it, and not that what each is connected with is not a possibility. The second version, however, is still ambiguous. For when can I not think the possibilities? He makes it clear that he does not mean that I cannot think them in the past tense when awake; which would obviously be false. So he must mean that I cannot think them in the present tense when asleep. But what is the case for saying that I cannot think them when asleep? This time he seems to have avoided one categorical assertion of impossibility only by making another, which, like the first, gets no support from the main argument, and can only be treated as the untenable conclusion of the subsidiary argument.

This analysis of his remarks about possibility shows that it is not absolutely certain that he would disallow the inference from the premiss that the hypothesis cannot be connected with an identifiable possibility to the conclusion that what it is connected with is not a possibility. Yet he seems to disallow it in several passages, and, in the course of his discussion of the question [3] whether, perhaps, I might now be asleep and dreaming, he makes it very clear that he is not denying that this is a possibility. If we are going to understand that discussion it is of the utmost importance that we should understand what he really thinks about possibility.

What he says about the possibility that I might now be asleep and dreaming is succinct. First, he says that the classical way of answering the question by appealing to the coherence of my experiences is useless since I might only be dreaming that they

3. Pages 117–118. This passage is an answer to an objection raised by Mr. G. J. Warnock. It looks like a later addition to the original theory.

cohered (108). Secondly he says that in any case the question is not about a possibility that I can think (18, 109, 110, 118). But though this is succinct, it is not simple.

First, inside a dream—or perhaps we should say, alongside a dream—one seldom takes the dream for reality, if only because one seldom raises this question. This is a fact, and, of course, it remains a fact even when it is analysed in his reductive way. But now suppose that I say to myself that at this moment I might be dreaming. Does he think that if I immediately told myself that what my words were connected with was not a possibility, I would be right? No. For in the passage mentioned just now he explicitly says that a determined sceptic would realize that he might be dreaming that he was wondering whether he was dreaming (117, 118). And from this it follows that he thinks that what my original words were connected with was a possibility, since they might have been inside, or alongside a dream.

Now this passage confirms the interpretation of his views about possibility that was suggested above. But it also does much more than this. For, since his determined sceptic, or at least he himself is supposed to be awake, it implies that even for a man who is awake the possibility is identifiable: i.e. it implies that a man who is awake understands now what it would be like to verify the possibility then. But this is incompatible with the reductive analysis of reports of dreams. For, according to that analysis, the statement that a person is dreaming means, essentially, that, if he wakes up, he will say that he has dreamt, and means no more than this. Consequently, if anyone who accepted this analysis suggested, when he was awake, that he might at that moment be dreaming, and therefore only dreaming that he was suggesting it, he ought to be suggesting no more than that, at that moment, a certain future conditional statement might be true. But how could he avoid adding to what he meant the fact that he was doing something which, if he were right, would be dreaming that he was suggesting it? It would be relevant.

This objection does not owe its force to the assumption that the sceptic is in fact awake. It makes the general point that, if a philosopher maintains that the barrier between any two planes of consciousness is so impervious that on either of the two planes statements about the other must be analysed reductively, then he cannot consistently allow that a sceptic could understand the possibility that he might be on a different plane from the one on which he is in fact. Of course, the sceptic himself would specify the possibility that he believed himself to understand: just as a person who says "I thought your yacht was bigger than it is" has a specific size in mind. But the point made against the philosopher who maintains that the barrier is impervious is entirely general. It could also be made against a philosopher who maintained that inside a dream the meaning of the statement that an event occurred in waking life should be reduced, essentially, to the report of it in the dream. Now it so happens that Malcolm specifies the possibility that his determined sceptic wants to understand, and maintains that the plane of waking consciousness, on which the sceptic is, is the only one that really is a plane of consciousness. And against this position the objection too can be made specific; if the sceptic is awake, and if the barrier is so impervious that statements about dreams must be analysed reductively, tnen the sceptic cannot understand the possibility that he might at that moment be dreaming. Therefore, when Malcolm admits that he cannot refute the sceptic because the sceptic might suggest that he was at that moment dreaming that he was suggesting that he might be dreaming, he is abandoning his reductive analysis.

Malcolm, of course, never claimed to be able to refute the sceptic, but only to show that the possibility that he suggests is not a possibility that he can think. But this is still an exaggerated claim. For he specifies the possibility, which, according to him, the sceptic cannot think. But even if the sceptic had been convinced by the monograph that he could not understand the possibility that he might be on the other plane of consciousness, he would still be unable to specify what he did not understand, since he would not know which plane of consciousness he was, in fact, on.

If, in our world, the sceptic's question has a sense that he can understand, can he answer it? Malcolm says that he could not use coherence in order to establish his state, unless he already knew that he was not dreaming that he was establishing it in

226 David F. Pears

this way: and presumably he would say the same about the phenomenology of his experiences. But why should the nature of his experiences not tell him whether he was establishing it or dreaming that he was establishing it? Perhaps there is only the illusion of a circle here. But might the method not be unreliable? Certainly it might fail, and on rare occasions it does fail. But, if it were to become generally unreliable, dreams would have to become far less recessive in our lives, and this would involve radical changes. For example, when we entered the dream-world, it would always have to be at the place where we left it, unless someone had moved our dream-bodies while we were awake: after an absence from the dream-world we would find, on our return, that other people had kept their identities: logic would be generally respected: one thing would perplex us—the strange actions that we seemed to remember having performed in the waking life, and perhaps we should regard them as the expressions of wishes that we suppressed in dream life, etc.

Philosophers have always been fascinated by dreams, and rightly so. But they have not always seen the full range of problems that they raise. Many of these problems are profound, and many of them have analogues in other philosophical topics. Malcolm identifies and explores some of the neglected ones, and those who are not convinced by his solutions will find it easier to be under the impression that they have refuted his main argument than to refute it.

10

DANIEL C. DENNETT

Are Dreams Experiences?

The "received view" of dreams is that they are *experiences that occur during sleep,* experiences which we can often recall upon waking. Enlarged, the received view is that dreams consist of sensations, thoughts, impressions, and so forth, usually composed into coherent narratives or adventures, occurring somehow in awareness or consciousness, though in some other sense or way the dreamer is *un*conscious during the episode.[1] *Received* it certainly is; as Norman Malcolm pointed out in his book, *Dreaming,* not only has it been virtually unchallenged, it has been explicitly endorsed by Aristotle, Descartes, Kant, Russell, Moore, and Freud.[2] That was in 1959, and I think it is fair to say that in spite of Malcolm's arguments against the received view, it is still the received view. I want to reopen the case, and though my aims and presuppositions are quite antagonistic to Malcolm's, those familiar with his attack will see many points at which my discussion agrees with and gains insight and direction from his. I will not, though, go into a detailed extraction and defense of what I find valuable in Malcolm's book. My immediate purpose in what follows is to undermine the authority

Reprinted from the *Philosophical Review,* 85 (1976), 151–171, by permission of the author and the *Philosophical Review.*
1. Cf. Hilary Putnam's version of "a natural lexical definition": "a series of impressions (visual, etc.) occurring during sleep; usually appearing to the subject to be of people, objects, etc.; frequently remembered upon awakening" ("Dreaming and 'Depth Grammar'," in R. J. Butler, ed., *Analytical Philosophy,* Oxford, 1962, p. 224).
2. Norman Malcolm, *Dreaming* (London, 1959), p. 4.

of the received view of dreams. My larger purpose is to introduce a view about the relationship between experience and memory that I plan to incorporate into a physicalistic theory of consciousness, a theory considerably different from the theory I have hitherto defended.[3]

The most scandalous conclusion that Malcolm attempted to draw from his analysis of the concept of dreaming was to the effect that contemporary dream research by psychologists and other scientists was conceptually confused, misguided, ultimately simply *irrelevant* to dreaming.[4] This conclusion strikes many as bizarre and impertinent. If scientists can study waking experience, waking sensation, thought, imagination, consciousness, they can surely study the varieties of these phenomena that occur during sleep, in dreaming. This riposte is not, of course, a consideration that would impress Malcolm, for it is simply an announcement of faith in the received view, the view that dreams do consist of sensations, thoughts, and so forth occurring during sleep, and Malcolm already knows that the view he is attacking inspires such faith. In any event, as everyone expected, Malcolm's words have had little or no discouraging effect on dream researchers. Their work continues apace to this day, apparently with a degree of fruition that makes a mockery of Malcolm's view. So let us suppose, *contra* Malcolm, that the researchers are neither the perpetrators nor the victims of a conceptual crime, and see where it leads us. Let us suppose that the dream researcher's concept of dreaming is not only received, but the true and unconfused concept of dreaming. What are the prospects, then, for the scientific elaboration of the received view?

It is well known that periods of rapid eye movements (REMs) occur during sleep, and correlate well with subsequent reports of having dreamed. There are also characteristic EEG patterns usually concurrent with the REM episodes, and other physiological correlates that go to suggest that dreams do indeed occur during sleep, and can now be timed, confirmed to occur, and measured in all manner of ways. One tantalizing finding

3. In *Content and Consciousness* (London, 1969), and more recently in "On the Absence of Phenomenology" (unpublished).
4. *Dreaming*, p. 82.

has been the apparent occasional content-relativity of the REMs. A person whose REMs are predominantly horizontal is awakened and reports a dream in which he watched two people throwing tomatoes at each other. A predominantly vertical pattern in REMs is correlated with a dream report of picking basketballs off the floor and throwing them up at the basket.[5] A neurophysiological model [6] of dreaming would plausibly construe these REMs as relatively gross and peripheral effects of a more determinate content-relative process deeper in the brain, which we might hope some day to *translate,* in this sense: we might be able to *predict* from certain physiological events observed during sleep that the subsequent dream report would allude to, for example, fear, falling from a height, eating something cold, even (in the Golden Age of neurocryptography) buying a train ticket to New Haven for $12.65 and then forgetting which pocket it was in. The prospect of a *generalized* capacity to predict dream narratives in such detail would be vanishingly small in the absence of a highly systematic and well-entrenched theory of representation in the brain, but let us suppose for the nonce that such a theory is not only in principle possible, but the natural culmination of the research strategies that are already achieving modest success in "translating" relatively gross and peripheral nervous-system activity.[7]

Now some people claim never to dream, and many people waken to report that they have dreamed but cannot recall any details. The latter usually have a strong conviction that the dream *did* have details, though they cannot recall them, and even when we can recall our dreams, the memories fade very fast, and the mere act of expressing them seems to interfere, to

5. David Foulkes, *The Psychology of Sleep* (New York, 1966).
6. Putnam (*op. cit.*) points out that a crucial lacuna in Malcolm's verificationist arguments against REMs as evidence confirming the received view is his failure to consider the confirmation relations arising from the use of developed theories and models (p. 226). At a number of points this paper attempts to fill that gap.
7. I have in mind such work as Hubel and Wiesel's "translation" of optic nerve signals in the cat. I argue against optimism regarding the prospects for a generalized neural theory of representation in "Brain Writing and Mind Reading," in Keith Gunderson, ed., *Language, Mind, and Knowledge, Minn. Studies in Philosophy of Science* VII (1975), but nothing in what follows relies on the considerations I raise there.

speed up the memory loss. Here the impression of details *there then* but *now lost* is very strong indeed. REM researchers now confidently state that their research shows that *everybody* has dreams (and every night); some of us just seldom—or never—recall them. It must be unsettling to be assured that one has dreamed when one is positive one has not; Malcolm could be expected to diagnose one's reaction to such an assurance as the shudder of conceptual violation,[8] but that would be an over-statement. The data of common experience strongly suggest a gradation in people's capacities to recall (both dreams and other items) and it should be nothing worse than an odd but obvious implication of the received view that one could *dream* without recalling just as one can promise without recalling or be raucously drunk without recalling.

Guided by common experience and the received view, then, we can imagine our scientists of the future isolating the memory mechanisms responsible for dream recall, and finding ways of chemically facilitating or inhibiting them. This is surely plausible; research into the chemistry of memory already suggests which chemicals might have these powers. We would expect that the scientists' claims to a theory of the dream-recall mechanism would be buttressed by systematic ties to a theory of memory mechanisms in general and by results, such as, perhaps, their ability to cure the dream-amnesiac.

So we imagine future dream theory to posit two largely separable processes: first, there are neural events during sleep (more specifically during REM periods having certain characteristic EEG correlates) that systematically represent (are systematically correlatable with) the "events occurring in the dream," and during this process there is a second, memory-loading process so that these events can be recalled on waking (when the memory process works). Dreams are *presented,* and simultaneously *recorded* in memory, and we might be able to interfere with or prevent the recording without disturbing the presentation.

This posited process of memory-loading and playback must be saved from simplistic interpretation if we are to maintain

8. See Norman Malcolm, "Dreaming and Skepticism" [Chapter 4 above], esp. sec. VIII.

any vestige of realism for our fantasy. It is rarely if ever the case that a dreamer awakens and proceeds to recite with vacant stare a fixed narrative. Dream recall is like recall generally. We interpret, extrapolate, revise; it sometimes seems that we "relive" the incidents and *draw conclusions* from this reliving—conclusions that are then expressed in what we actually *compose* then and there as our recollections. It is not easy to analyze what must be going on when this happens. What is the *raw material*, the evidence, the basis for these reconstructions we call recollections?

Consider a fictional example. John Dean, a recently acclaimed virtuoso of recollection, is asked about a certain meeting in the Oval Office. Was Haldeman present? Consider some possible replies.

(1) "No."
(2) "I can't (or don't) recall his being there."
(3) "I distinctly recall that he was not there."
(4) "I remember noticing (remarking) at the time that he was not there."

If Dean says (1) we will suspect that he is saying less than he *can* say, even if what he says is sincere and even true. At the other extreme, (4) seems to be a nearly *complete* report of the relevant part of Dean's memory. Answer (2), unlike all the others, reports an inability, a blank. Under the right circumstances, though, it carries about as strong a pragmatic implication of Haldeman's absence as any of the others (we ask: could Dean conceivably fail to recall Haldeman's presence if Haldeman had been there?). The stronger these pragmatic implications, the more disingenuous an answer like (2) will seem. Consider: "Was Dan Rather at that meeting in the Oval Office?" "I can't *recall* his being there." The answer is seen to be disingenuous because we know Dean knows, and we know, the additional supporting premises which, in conjunction with (2), imply something like (1), and we expect Dean to be reasonable and draw this conclusion for—and with—us. Then what should Dean say, if asked the question about Dan Rather? Certainly not (4), unless the paranoia in the White House in those days knew no bounds, but (3) can be heard to carry a similar, if weaker, implication. We would not expect Dean to say this because it suggests (presumably misleadingly) that his answer is closer to being *given* in his recollection, less a conclusion quickly drawn. (1) is clearly the best answer on the list under these circumstances. It *looks* like a conclusion he reaches on the basis of things he remembers. He remembers Nixon and Ehrlichman talking with him, forming a sort of triangle in the room, and on the basis of *this* he concludes that Haldeman, and Rather, were absent, though he took no notice of the fact at the time, or if he did he has forgotten it. Now suppose Dean says (1). Perhaps when he does this he recalls in his mind this triangle, but does not bother to tell us that—he does not close his eyes on the witness stand and do a little phenomenology for us; he simply offers up his conclusion as a dictate of memory. But he need not have gone through this conscious process of reliving and reasoning at all. He may say, directly, "No," and if he is pressed to be more forthcoming, any reasoning he offers based on other things he recalls will not be expressing any reasoning he knows he went through before his initial negative reply. He may not even be able to explain why or how his memory dictates this answer to the question, and yet be sure, and deservedly sure, that his reply is a sincere and reliable dictate of memory.

To summarize: sometimes we can sincerely answer a question of recollection with an answer like (4), but often we cannot, and sometimes we draw a blank, but in *all* these cases there are conclusions we can draw based on what in some sense we directly remember in conjunction with common and proprietary knowledge, and these conclusions need not be drawn in a process of *conscious* reasoning. Whatever it is that is directly remembered can play its evidentiary role in prompting an answer of recollection without coming into consciousness. This suggests that when we remember some event, there is some limited amount of information that is *there,* not necessarily in consciousness but available in one way or another for utilization in composing our recollections and answering questions we or others raise. Perhaps what occupies this functional position is an immensely detailed recording of our experience to which our later access is normally imperfect and partial (although under hypnosis it may improve). Perhaps there is enough information in this position to reconstitute completely our past experience and present us, under special circumstances, with a vivid hallucination of reliving the event.[9] However much is in this position in Dean, however, it is not possible that Dan Rather's absence is there except by implication, for his absence was not experienced by Dean at the time, any more than up to this moment you have been experiencing Rather's absence from this room. What the posited memory-loading process records, then, is whatever occupies this functional position at a later time. The "playback" of dream recollections, like other recollections, is presumably seldom if ever complete or uninterpreted, and often bits of information are utilized in making memory claims without being played back in consciousness at all.

In dreaming there is also a third process that is distinguished both in the layman's version of the received view and in fancier theories, and that is the *composition* of what is presented and recorded. In various ways this process exhibits intelligence: dream stories are usually coherent and realistic (even surrealism has a realistic background), and are often gripping, complex, and of course loaded with symbolism. Dream composition utilizes the dreamer's general and particular knowledge, her recent and distant experience, and is guided in familiar ways by her fears and desires, covert and overt.

Studying these three processes will require tampering with them, and we can imagine that the researchers will acquire the technological virtuosity to be able to influence, direct, or alter the composition process, to stop, restart, or even transpose the presentation process as it occurs, to prevent or distort the recording process. We can even imagine that they will be able to obliterate the "veridical" dream memory and substitute for it an undreamed narrative. This eventuality would produce a strange result indeed. Our dreamer would wake up and report her dream, only to be assured by the researcher that she never dreamed *that* dream, but rather another, which they proceed to relate to her. Malcolm sees that the scientific elaboration of the received view countenances such a possibility-in-principle and

9. Cf. Wilder Penfield's descriptions of electrode-induced memory hallucinations, in *The Excitable Cortex in Conscious Man* (Springfield, Ill., 1958).

for him this amounts to a *reductio ad absurdum* of the received view,[10] but again, this is an overreaction to an admittedly strange circumstance. Given the state of the art of dream research today, were someone to contradict my clear recollection of what I had just dreamed, my utter skepticism would be warranted, but the science-fictional situation envisaged would be quite different. Not only would the researchers have proved their powers by correctly predicting dream recollections on numerous occasions, but they would have a theory that explained their successes. And we need not suppose the dream they related to the dreamer would be entirely *alien* to her ears, even though she had no recollection of it (and in fact a competing recollection). Suppose it recounted an adventure with some secretly loved acquaintance of hers, a person unknown to the researchers. The stone wall of skepticism would begin to crumble.

The story told so far does not, I take it, exhibit the conceptual chaos Malcolm imagines; strange as it is, I do not think it would evoke in the layman, our custodian of ordinary concepts, the nausea of incomprehension. As a premise for a science-fiction novel it would be almost pedestrian in its lack of conceptual horizon-bending.

But perhaps this is not at all the way the theory of dreaming will develop. Malcolm notes in passing that it has been suggested by some researchers that dreams may occur during the moments of waking, not during the prior REM periods. Why would anyone conjecture this? Perhaps you have had a dream leading logically and coherently up to a climax in which you are shot, whereupon you wake up and are told that a truck has just backfired outside your open window. Or you are fleeing someone in a building, you climb out a window, walk along the ledge, then fall—and wake up on the floor having fallen out of bed. In a recent dream of mine I searched long and far for a neighbor's goat; when at last I found her she bleated *baa-a-a*—and I awoke to find her bleat merging perfectly with the buzz of an electric alarm clock I had not used or heard for months. Many people, I find, have anecdotes like this to relate, but the

10. "Dreaming and Skepticism," sec. VIII, esp. p. 119.

scientific literature disparages them, and I can find only one remotely well-documented case from an experiment: different stimuli were being used to waken dreamers, and one subject was wakened by dripping cold water on his back. He related a dream in which he was singing in an opera. Suddenly he *heard and saw* that the soprano had been struck by water falling from above; he ran to her and as he bent over her, felt water dripping on his back.[11]

What are we to make of these reports? The elaboration of the received view we have just sketched can deal with them, but at a high cost: precognition. If the terminal events in these dreams are strongly *prepared for* by the narrative, if they do not consist of radically juxtaposed turns in the narrative (for example, the goat turns into a telephone and starts ringing), then the composition process must have been directed by something having "knowledge" of the future. That is too high a price for most of us to pay, no doubt. Perhaps all these anecdotes succumb to a mixture of reasonable skepticism, statistics (coincidences do happen, and are to be "expected" once in a blue moon), the discovery of subtle influences from the environment, and various other deflating redescriptions. But if all else failed we could devise any number of variant dream theories that accommodated these "miracles" in less than miraculous ways. Perhaps, to echo the earlier conjecture, dreams are composed and presented *very fast* in the interval between bang, bump, or buzz and full consciousness, with some short delay system postponing the full "perception" of the noise in the dream until the presentation of the narrative is ready for it. Or perhaps in that short interval dreams are composed, presented, and recorded *backwards* and then remembered front to back. Or perhaps there is a "library" in the brain of undreamed dreams with various indexed endings, and the bang or bump or buzz has the effect of retrieving an appropriate dream and inserting it, cassette-like, in the memory mechanism.

None of these theories can be viewed as a mere variation or rival elaboration of the received view. If one of them is true,

11. William Dement and E. A. Wolpert, "The Relation of Eye Movements, Bodily Motility and External Stimuli to Dream Content," *Journal of Experimental Psychology,* 55 (1958), 543–553.

236 Daniel C. Dennett

then the received view is false. And since these rival theories, including the theory inspired by the received view, are all empirical, subject to confirmation and refutation, and since the rival theories even have some (admittedly anecdotal) evidence in their favor, we are constrained to admit that the received view might simply turn out to be false: dreams, it might turn out, are not what we took them to be—or perhaps we would say that it turns out that there are not dreams after all, only dream "recollections" produced in the manner described in our confirmed theory, whichever it is. Malcolm sees that all this is implied by the received view and takes it to be yet another *reductio ad absurdum* of it: any view that could permit the discovery that "we are always only under the *illusion* of having had a dream" is "senseless." [12] But again, Malcolm's response to this implication is too drastic. The claim that we had been fooled for millennia into believing in dreams would be hard to swallow, but then we would not have to swallow it unless it had the backing of a strongly confirmed scientific theory, and then this claim would put no greater strain on our credulity than we have already endured from the claims of Copernicus, Einstein, and others. It would be rather like learning that dream-recall was like *déjà vu*—it only *seemed* that you had experienced it before—and once you believed *that,* it would no longer even seem (as strongly) that you were recalling. The experience of "dream recall" would change for us. [13]

My attack on the received view is not, however, a straightforward empirical attack. I do not wish to aver that anecdotal evidence about dream anticipation disproves the received view, but I do want to consider in more detail what the issues would be were a rival to the received view to gain support. I hope to show that the received view is more vulnerable to empirical disconfirmation than its status as the received view would lead us to expect. Of the rival theories, the cassette-library theory runs most strongly against our pretheoretical convictions, for on the

12. "Dreaming and Skepticism," p. 121.
13. Cf. Putnam, *op. cit.*, p. 227. The naive subject of *déjà vu* says, "I vaguely remember experiencing all this before"; the sophisticated subject is not even tempted to say this, but says, perhaps, "Hm, I'm having a *déjà vu* experience right now." The experience has changed.

other two there still is some vestige of the presumed presentation process: it is just much faster than we had expected, or happens backwards. On the cassette view, our "precognitive" dreams are never dreamed at all, but just spuriously "recalled" on waking. If our memory mechanisms were empty until the moment of waking, and then received a whole precomposed dream narrative in one lump, the idea that precognitive dreams are *experienced episodes* during sleep would have to go by the board.

Suppose we generalize the cassette theory to cover all dreams: all dream narratives are composed directly into memory banks; which, if any, of these is available to waking recollection depends on various factors—precedence of composition, topicality of waking stimulus, degree of "repression," and so forth. On this view, the process of presentation has vanished, and although the dream cassettes would have to be filled at some time by a composition process, that process might well occur during our waking hours, and spread over months (it takes a long time to write a good story). The composition might even occur aeons before our birth; we might have an *innate* library of undreamed dream cassettes ready for appropriate insertion in the playback mechanism. Stranger things have been claimed. Even on the received view the composition process is an unconscious or subconscious process, of which we normally have no more *experience* than of the processes regulating our metabolism; otherwise dreams could not be suspenseful. (I say "normally" for there does seem to be the phenomenon of self-conscious dreaming, where we tinker with a dream, run it by several times, attempt to resume it where it left off. Here the theatrical metaphor that enlivens the received view seems particularly apt. After tinkering like the playwright, we must sit back, get ourselves back into the audience mood, suspend disbelief, and re-enter the play. Some researchers call these occasions *lucid dreams*. But usually we are not privy to the composition process at all, and so have no inkling about when it might occur.) Research might give us good grounds for believing that dream narratives that were composed onto cassettes in the morning decayed faster than cassettes composed in the afternoon, or during meals.

A more likely finding of the cassette-theorist would be that the composition process occurs during sleep, and more particularly, during periods of rapid eye movements, with characteristic EEG patterns. One might even be able to "translate" the composition process—that is, predict dream recollections from data about the composition process. This theory looks suspiciously like the elaboration of the received theory, except for lacking the presentation process. Cassette narratives, we are told, are composed in narrative order, and long narratives take longer to compose, and the decay time for cassettes in storage is usually quite short; normally the dream one "recalls" on waking was composed just minutes earlier, a fact attested to by the occasional cases of content-relativity in one of the by-products of cassette composition: rapid eye movements. On this theory dream memories are produced just the way the received theory says they are, except for one crucial thing: the process of dream-memory production is entirely unconscious, involves no awareness or experiencing at all. Even "lucid dreams" can be accommodated easily on this hypothesis, as follows: although the composition and recording processes are entirely unconscious, on occasion the composition process inserts traces of itself into the recording via the literary conceit of a dream within a dream.

Now we have a challenge to the received view worth reckoning with. It apparently accounts for all the data of the REM researchers as well as the received view does, so there is no reason for sober investigators not to adopt the cassette theory forthwith if it has any advantages over the received view. And it seems that it does: it has a simple explanation of precognitive dreams (if there are any) and it posits one less process by eliminating a presentation process whose point begins to be lost.

But what greater point could a process have? In its presence we have experience; in its absence we have none. As Thomas Nagel would put it, the central issue between these two theories appears to be whether or not it is like anything to dream.[14] On

14. Thomas Nagel, "What Is It Like to Be a Bat?" *Philosophical Review*, 83 (1974), 435–450.

the cassette theory it is not like anything to dream, although it is like something *to have dreamed*. On the cassette theory, dreams are not experiences we have during sleep; where we had thought there were dreams, there is only an unconscious composition process and an equally unconscious memory-loading process.

A few years ago there was a flurry of experimentation in learning-while-you-sleep. Tape recordings of textbooks were played in the sleeper's room, and tests were run to see if there were any subsequent signs of learning. As I recall, the results were negative, but some people thought the results were positive. If you had asked one of them *what it was like* to learn in one's sleep, the reply would presumably have been: "It was not like anything at all—I was sound asleep at the time. I went to sleep not knowing any geography and woke up knowing quite a bit, but don't ask me what it was like. It wasn't like anything." If the cassette theory of dreams is true, dream-recollection production is a similarly unexperienced process. If asked what it is like to dream one *ought* to say (because it would be the truth): "It is not like anything. I go to sleep and when I wake up I find I have a tale to tell, a 'recollection' as it were." It is Malcolm's view that this is what we ought to say, but Malcolm is not an explicit champion of the cassette theory or any other empirical theory of dreaming. His reasons, as we shall see, are derived from "conceptual analysis." But whatever the reasons are, the conclusion seems outrageous. *We all know better,* we think. But do we? We are faced with two strikingly different positions about what happens when we dream, and one of these, the received view, we are not just loath to give up; we find it virtually unintelligible that we could be wrong about it. And yet the point of difference between it (as elaborated into a theory by scientists) and its rival, the cassette theory, is apparently a technical, theoretical matter about which the layman's biases, his everyday experience, and even his personal recollections of dreams are without authority or even weight. What should we do? Sit back and wait for the experts to tell us, hoping against hope that dreams will turn out to be, after all, experiences? That seems ridiculous.

If that seems ridiculous, perhaps it is ridiculous. Can some way be found to protect the received view from the possibility of losing this contest? If we do not for a minute believe it could lose, we must suppose there is some principled explanation of this. One might set out in a verificationist manner.[15] What could possibly settle the issue between the received view and the cassette theory if subjects' recollections were deemed neutral? The conclusion of one view is that dreams are experiences, and of the other that they are not, but if subjects' recollections were not held to be *criterial,* nothing else could count as evidence for or against the rival theories, at least with regard to this disputed conclusion. Therefore the claimed difference between the two theories is illusory, or perhaps we should say they are both pseudo-theories. This will not do. We can easily imagine the two theories to share a concept of experience, and even to agree on which data would go to show that dreams were, in this shared technical sense, experiences. Nor would this technical concept of experience have to look all that unordinary. We have many common ways of distinguishing which among the events that impinge on us are experienced and which are not, and we can imagine these theories to build from these ordinary distinctions a powerful shared set of well-confirmed empirically necessary and sufficient conditions for events to be experienced. If, for instance, some part of the brain is invariably active in some characteristic way when some event in waking life is, as we ordinarily say, experienced, and if moreover we have a theory that says why this should be so, the absence of such brain activity during REM periods would look bad for the received view and good for the cassette view.

But if that is what we should look for, the received view is in trouble, for one routinely recognized condition for having an experience is that one be conscious, or awake, and dreamers are not. A well-confirmed physiological condition for this is that one's reticular activating system be "on," which it is not during sleep. The fact that one is in a sound sleep goes a long way to confirming that one is *not* having experiences, as *ordinarily* understood. Malcolm would make this criterial, but that is

15. This argument is inspired by the verificationist arguments of Malcolm and its rebuttal is inspired by Putnam's objections, but Malcolm does not commit himself to this argument.

one more overstatement. Lack of reticular system activity strongly suggests that nothing is being experienced during REMs, but the defender of the received view can plausibly reply that reticular activation is only a condition of *normal* experience, and can point to the frequent occurrence during REM periods of the normal physiological accompaniments of fear, anxiety, delight, and arousal as considerations in favor of an extended concept of experience. How could one exhibit an emotional reaction to something not even experienced? The debate would not stop there, but we need not follow it further now. The fact remains that the physiological data would be clearly relevant evidence in the dispute between the theories, and not all the evidence is on the side of the received view.

Still, one might say, the very relevance of physiological evidence shows the dispute not to involve our ordinary concept of experience at all, but only a technical substitute. For suppose we were told without further elaboration that the theory inspired by the received view had won the debate, had proved to be the better theory. We would not know what, if anything, had been confirmed by this finding. Which of our hunches and biases would be thereby vindicated, and are any of them truly in jeopardy?

This plausible rhetorical question suggests that none of our precious preconceptions about dreaming *could* be in jeopardy, a conclusion that "conceptual analysis" might discover for us. How might this be done? Let us return to the comparison between the cassette view of dreams and the speculation that one might learn in one's sleep. I suggested that subjects in either circumstance should, on waking, deny that it was like anything to have undergone the phenomenon. But there would be a crucial difference in their waking states, presumably. For the dreamer, unlike the sleep-learner, would probably want to add to his disclaimer: "Of course it *seems to me* to have been like something!" The sleep learner has new knowledge, or new beliefs, but not new *memories*. This is surely an important difference, but just what difference does it make? Is it that the claim

(5) It was not like anything, but it seems to me to have been like something,

is a covert contradiction? Can one sustain the following principle?

(6) If it seems to have been like something, it was like something.

The present tense version of the principle is unassailable:

(7) If it seems to me to be like something to be x, then it is like something to me to be x.

That is what we mean when we talk of what it is like: how it seems to us.[16] When we try to make the principle extend through memory to the past, however, we run into difficulties. There is no good reason to deny that memories can be spurious, and there is plenty of confirmation that they can. This is somewhat obscured by some looseness in our understanding of the verb "remember." Sometimes we draw a distinction between remembering and seeming to remember such that remembering, like knowing, is veridical. On this reading it follows that if you remember something to have been x, it was x. If it was not x you only seem to remember that it was. But when I say, about a restaurant we are dining in, "This isn't the way I remember it," my claim is equivocal. I may not be claiming the restaurant has changed—it may be that my memory is at fault. On this reading of "remember" there is still a distinction between remembering and seeming to remember, but it is not a distinction with veridicality on one side: for example one tells a tale of one's childhood that is shown to be false and one wonders whether one has mistaken fantasizing or confabulating for (mis)remembering. On *either* reading, however, there is no claim that can be made of the form:

(8) Since I remember it to have been like something, it was like something.

On the first reading of "remember" the claim, while logically impeccable, does not work unless one claims a capacity to tell one's memories from one's seeming memories that one simply does not have. On the second reading, even if we could always tell fantasy from memory the consequent would not follow. So

16. Cf. Nagel, *op. cit.*, p. 440n. "[T]he analogical form of the English expression 'what is it *like*' is misleading. It does not mean 'what (in our experience) it resembles,' but rather 'how it is for the subject himself.' "

(5) represents a possible state of affairs. We had in fact already countenanced this state of affairs as an abnormality in supposing that the dream researchers could, by tampering, insert a spurious dream recollection. Now we are countenancing it as a possible and not even improbable account of the normal case.

Malcolm sees that nothing like (6) or (8) can be exploited in this context; we can seem to have had an experience when we have not, and for just this reason he denies that dreams are experiences! His argument is that *since* one can be under the impression that one has had an experience and yet not have had it, and since if one is under the impression that one has had a dream, one *has* had a dream,[17] having had a dream cannot be having had an experience, hence dreams are not experiences.

The "criteriological" move has a curious consequence: it "saves" the authority of the wakened dream-recaller, and this *looks like* a rescue of subjectivity from the clutches of objective science, but it "saves" dreaming only at the expense of experience. What Malcolm sees is that if we permit a distinction between remembering and seeming to remember to apply to dream recollections, the concept of dreaming is cast adrift from any criterial anchoring to first-person reports, and becomes (or is revealed to be) a theoretical concept. Once we grant that subjective, introspective or retrospective evidence does not have the authority to settle questions about the nature of dreams—for instance, whether dreams are experiences—we have to turn to the other data, the behavior and physiology of dreamers, and to the relative strengths of the theories of these, if we are to settle the question, a question which the subject is not in a privileged position to answer. Malcolm avoids this by denying that dreams are experiences, but this only concedes that one

---

17. "That he really had a dream and that he is under the impression that he had a dream: these are the same thing" ("Dreaming and Skepticism," p. 121). This is the central premise of Malcolm's work on dreaming, and one he gets from Wittgenstein: "The question whether the dreamer's memory deceives him when he reports the dream after waking cannot arise unless indeed we introduce a completely new criterion for the report's 'agreeing' with the dream, a criterion which gives us a concept of 'truth' as distinguished from 'truthfulness' here" (*Philosophical Investigations*, pp. 222–223). It is Malcolm's unswerving loyalty to this remark that forces his account into such notorious claims.

does *not* have a privileged opinion about one's own past experiences.[18] This concession is unavoidable, I think, and Malcolm's is not the only philosophic position caused embarrassment by it. A defender of the subjective realm such as Nagel must grant that in general, whether or not it was like something to be *x*, whether or not the subject *experienced* being *x*—questions that *define* the subjective realm—are questions about which the subject's subsequent subjective opinion is not authoritative. But if the subject's own convictions do not settle the matter, and if, as Nagel holds, no objective considerations are conclusive either, the subjective realm floats out of ken altogether, except, perhaps for the subject's convictions about the specious present. Dreams are particularly vulnerable in this regard only because, as Malcolm observes, sleepers do not and cannot *express* current convictions about the specious present (if they have any) while they are dreaming. Since our only expressible access to dreams is retrospective, dreams are particularly vulnerable, but they are not alone. The argument we have been considering is more general; the dispute between the rival theories of memory-loading can be extended beyond dreaming to all experience. For instance, just now, while you were reading my remarks about Nagel, were you experiencing the peripheral sights and sounds available in your environment? Of course you were, you say, and you can prove it to your own complete satisfaction by closing your eyes and recalling a variety of events or conditions that co-occurred with your reading those remarks. While not *central* in your consciousness at the time, they were certainly *there*, being *experienced*, as your recollections show. But the cassette theorist, emboldened by the success with dreams, puts forward the *subliminal peripheral recollection-production* theory, the view that the variety of peripheral details in such cases are not consciously experienced, but merely unconsciously recorded for subsequent recall. Events outside our immediate attention are not experienced at all, our theorist says, but they do have subliminal effects on short-term memory. Our capacity to recall them for a short period does not establish that they were

18. Sometimes Malcolm seems to want to "save" all "private states" in this way, thus either having to deny that experiences are private states, or having to adopt after all some principle like (8). See *Dreaming*, p. 55.

experienced, any more than our capacity to "recall" dreams shows that they were experienced. But this is nonsense, you say: *recording those peripheral items for subsequent recollection just is experiencing them.*

If only this bold claim were true! Look what it would do for us. The difference between the received view of dreams and the cassette theory would collapse; the presumably unconscious memory-loading process of the cassette theory would turn out to be the very presentation process dear to the received view. A "conceptual relationship" could be established between experience and memory that avoided the difficulties heretofore encountered in such claims, as follows. The conceptual relationship is *not* between experiencing and subsequent subjective convictions of memory (the latter are *not* criterial), but between experiencing and something perfectly objective: the laying down thereupon of a memory trace—for however short a time and regardless of subsequent success or failure at recollection.[19] The conceptual relationship would be identity. *Experire est recordare.*

Much can be said in support of this principle, but at this time I will restrict myself to a few brief persuasions. First, is remembering a *necessary* condition for experiencing? Arguably, yes, if you grant that memories may not last long. The idea of a subject, an "I," experiencing each successive state in a stream of consciousness with *no* recollection of its predecessors is a hopelessly impoverished model of experience and experiencers. The *familiarity* and *continuity* in the world of current experiences is a necessary background for recognition and discrimination and only short-term memory can provide this. Items that come and go so fast, or so inconspicuously, as to leave no reverberations behind in memory at all are plausibly viewed as simply not experienced. So if remembering is a necessary condition, is it also a *sufficient* condition for experiencing? Yost and Kalish say so, without supporting argument: "Dreaming is a

19. Not completely regardless of subsequent success or failure at recollection, for identifying some process as the laying down of a memory trace is identifying some process by its function, and nothing that did not have as its normal effect enabling the subject to report truly about the past could be picked out functionally as the memory-loading process.

real experience. And since dreams can be remembered they must be conscious experiences." [20] Martin and Deutscher, in their article, "Remembering," concur:

> So long as we hold some sort of 'storage' or 'trace' account of memory, it follows that we can remember only what we have experienced, for it is in our experience of events that they "enter" the storehouse.[21]

So remembering, in the sense of storing away in the memory for some time, is arguably a necessary and sufficient condition for experiencing. These are, I think, philosophically respectable arguments for the claimed identity, and to them can be added an ulterior consideration which will appeal to physicalists if not to others. The proposed identity of experiencing and recording promises a striking simplification for physicalist theories of mind. The problematic (largely because utterly vague) presentation process vanishes as an extra phenomenon to be accounted for, and with it goes the even more mysterious *audience* or *recipient* of those presentations. In its place is just a relatively prosaic short-term memory capacity, the sort of thing for which rudimentary but suggestive physical models already abound.

The principle as it stands, however, is too strong, on two counts. Consider again Martin and Deutscher's commentary on the "storehouse" model of memory: "It is in our experience of events that they 'enter' the storehouse." What, though, of forcible or illegal entry? We need an account of something like *normal* entry into memory so that we can rule out, as experiences, such abnormally entered items as the undreamed dream surgically inserted by the dream researchers. We want to rule out such cases, not by declaring them impossible, for they are not, but by denying that they are experiences for the subject. As we shall see in a moment, the best way of doing this may have a surprising consequence. The second failing of our principle is simply that it lacks the status we have claimed for it. It is not self-evident; its denial is not a contradiction. We must not make

20. R. M. Yost and Donald Kalish, "Miss MacDonald on Sleeping and Waking" [Chapter 3 above]. Malcolm discusses this claim in *Dreaming*.
21. C. B. Martin and Max Deutscher, "Remembering," *Philosophical Review*, 75 (1966), 189.

the mistake of asserting that this is a discovered conceptual truth about experience and memory. We must understand it as a proposal, a theoretically promising adjustment in our ordinary concepts for which we may have to sacrifice some popular preconceptions. For instance, whether animals can be held to dream, or to experience anything, is rendered an uncertainty depending on what we mean by *recall*. Can animals *recall* events? If not, they cannot have experiences. More radically, subjective authority about experience goes by the board entirely. Still, we get a lot in return, not the least of which is a way of diagnosing and dismissing the Pickwickian hypothesis of subliminal peripheral recollection-production.

We are still not out of the woods on dreaming, though, for we must define normal memory-entry in such a way as to admit ordinary experience and exclude tampering and other odd cases.

When the memory gets loaded by accident or interference we will not want this to count as experience, and yet we want to grant that there is such a thing as nonveridical experience. The memory-loading that occurs during a hallucination occurs during abnormal circumstances, but not so abnormal as to lead us to deny that hallucinations are experiences. But look at a slightly different case. (I do not know if this ever occurs, but it might.) Suppose at noon Jones, who is wide awake, suffers some event in her brain that has a delayed effect: at 12:15 she will "recall" having seen a ghost at noon. Suppose her recollection is as vivid as you like, but suppose her actual behavior at noon (and up until recollection at 12:15) showed no trace of horror, surprise, or cognizance of anything untoward. Had she shown any signs at noon of being under the impression that something bizarre was happening, we would be strongly inclined to say she had had a hallucination then, was experiencing it then, even if she could not recount it to us until fifteen minutes later. But since she did not *react* in any such telling way at noon, but proceeded about her business, we are strongly inclined to say the hallucination occurred later, at 12:15, and was a *hallucination of recollection* of something she had never experienced, even though the cause of the hallucination occurred at noon. Since the events responsible for her later capacity to recall did not contribute to her behavior-controlling state at the time, they did not enter her experience then, whatever their later repercussions. But then when we apply this distinguishing principle to dreams, we find that it is quite likely that most dreams are not experiences. Whereas nightmares accompanied by moans, cries, cowering, and sweaty palms *would* be experiences, bad dreams dreamed in repose (though remembered in agony) would not be, unless, contrary to surface appearances, their entry into memory is accomplished by engagements of the whole behavior-controlling system sufficiently normal to distinguish these cases sharply from our imaginary delayed hallucination.[22]

If it turns out that sleep, or at least that portion of sleep during which dreaming occurs, is a state of more or less peripheral paralysis or inactivity; if it turns out that most of the functional areas that are critical to the governance of our wide awake activity are in operation, then there will be good reason for drawing the lines around experience so that dreams are included. If not, there will be good reason to deny that dreams are experiences.

Some of the relevant data are already familiar. The occurrence of REMs suggests that more than a little of the visual processing system is active during dream periods, and it should be a fairly straightforward task—perhaps already accomplished—to determine just how much is. Even strongly positive results would not be overwhelming grounds for deciding that dreams are experiences, however, for in various sorts of hysteric or psychosomatic blindness there is substantial apparently normal activity in the visual processing system, and in so-called subliminal perception the same is true, and in neither case are we inclined to suppose visual experience occurs. More compelling, in many ways, is the evidence that dreams serve a purpose: they seem to be used to redress emotional imbalances caused by frustrating experiences in waking life, to rationalize cognitive dissonances, allay anxieties, and so forth. When this

---

22. Malcolm too sees an important distinction between "violent nightmares" and normal dreams dreamed in repose, a distinction that forces him to claim we have several different concepts of sleep. Only thus can he save as a *conceptual* truth the claim that we have no experiences while we sleep.

task is too difficult, it seems, the dream mechanisms often go into a looping cycle; troubled people often report recurring obsessive dreams that haunt them night after night. It is implausible that such recurrent dreams must be recomposed each night,[23] so if a recurrent physiological process can be correlated with these dreams, it will appear to be a presentation process, and the presentation process will have a point: namely, to provide the emotional and cognitive-processing functional parts with the raw material for new syntheses, new accommodations, perhaps permitting a more stable or satisfying self-image for the dreamer. But even this function could easily be seen to be accomplished entirely *unconsciously.* The self-presentation tactics and perceptual interpretation ploys posited by theorists as diverse as Freud and Erving Goffman are no less plausible for being presumed to be entirely unconscious, and they serve a similar self-protective maintenance function. As Malcolm points out, dreamers' narratives can be used by Freudians and others as a valuable source of information about the internal processes that shape us, without our having to suppose that these are recollections of experiences.[24]

It is an *open,* and *theoretical* question whether dreams fall inside or outside the boundary of experience.[25] A plausible theory of experience will be one that does justice to *three* distinguishable families of intuitions we have about experience and consciousness: those dealing with the role of experience in guiding current behavior, those dealing with our *current* procli-

23. I am indebted to Robert Nozick for raising this consideration.

24. *Dreaming,* p. 122. Malcolm quotes with approval this methodological suggestion of Freud's (from *A General Introduction to Psychoanalysis,* [Garden City, 1943], p. 76):

> Any disadvantage resulting from the uncertain recollection of dreams may be remedied by deciding that exactly what the dreamer tells is to count as the dream, and by ignoring all that he may have forgotten or altered in the process of recollection.

25. Foulkes (*op. cit.*) cites a number of telling, if inconclusive, further observations: in one study no association was found between "the excitement value of dream content and heart or respiration rate" (p. 50), a datum to be balanced by the curious fact that there are usually action-potentials discoverable in the motor neurons in the bicep of one who is asked to *imagine* bending one's arm; similar action-potentials are found in the arms of deaf mute dreamers—people who talk with their hands. There are also high levels of activity in the sensory cortex during dreaming sleep.

vities and capacities to *say* what we are experiencing, and those dealing with the *retrospective* or *recollective* capacity to say. In earlier work I have sharply distinguished the first and second of these, but underestimated the distinctness and importance of this third source of demands on a theory of consciousness. A theory that does justice to these distinct and often inharmonious demands must also do justice to a fourth: the functional saliencies that emerge from empirical investigation. In the end, the concept of experience may not prove to differentiate any one thing of sufficient theoretical interest to warrant time spent in determining its boundaries. Were this to occur, the received view of dreams, like the lay view of experience in general, would not be so much disproved as rendered obsolete. It my seem inconceivable that this could happen, but armchair conceptual analysis is powerless to establish this.

11

CHARLES S. CHIHARA

What Dreams Are Made On

In his well-known monograph on dreaming, Norman Malcolm argues that the notion of images or visions appearing to one during sleep is unintelligible [1] so that dreaming cannot consist in experiencing imagery during sleep. According to Malcolm a person simply wakes up with the impression of having seen and done various things, and if it is known that he did not see and do those things, then it is known that he dreamt them' (66). From this amazing position, Malcolm goes on to claim that scientists are simply confused in trying to find ways of determining either the precise time of occurrence or the duration of dreams, and it is this claim which is the primary target of my paper. I shall begin, however, by arguing that Malcolm has failed to give any solid grounds for accepting his strange doctrine of dreaming and that Malcolm's position is fundamentally unsound.

I

I shall consider first of all Malcolm's claim that the criterion of someone's having had a dream is that upon awaking he

Reprinted from *Theoria*, 31 (1965), 145–158, by permission of *Theoria*.
NOTE: This paper was read at the 1962 meeting of the Pacific Division of the American Philosophical Association held in Berkeley, California. I am indebted to L. Linsky and J. Fodor for helpful criticisms.
1. Norman Malcolm, *Dreaming* [London: Routledge and Kegan Paul, 1959], p. 45. Hereafter, in referring to passages in this monograph, I shall simply put its page number in parentheses.

relates a dream (49). Unfortunately, what Malcolm means by 'criterion' is not perfectly clear, but we can form some notion of the way he is using the term from what he says about dreaming. Malcolm tells us that a statement of the criterion for the use of the sentence 'He dreamt' gives 'the conditions that determine whether the statement "He dreamt" is true or false' (61). And as Wittgenstein had contrasted criterion with *symptom* in *The Blue Book*,[2] Malcolm contrasts criterion with *evidence* (60–2): when we know that the criterion of *y* is satisfied, then the question as to whether or not *y* is settled with certainty (60). It is not that we have strong evidence for *y* since that something is evidence for *y* is learned generally from experience and is a fact which is justified ultimately by an appeal to observations and experiences of some sort whereas 'that so-and-so is the criterion of *y* is a matter, not of experience, but of "definition" '.[3] Thus, since Malcolm takes the dream report as the principal criterion of dreaming, he is led to make the surprising assertion that it is 'a matter of definition that someone who told a dream had dreamt' (81).

According to Malcolm then, if a person wakes up with the impression of having seen and done various things, and if as a matter of fact he did not see and do those things, then in some sense, it follows *by definition* that he dreamt he saw and did those things, and we can tell that he had a dream on the basis of his dream report and the fact that he did not actually see and do the things related in the dream report.

Now it is clear that Malcolm takes not having seen and done the things reported as a necessary condition of having dreamt (51, 64–8, 80, 97), but this doctrine obviously needs qualification, as David Pears points out in his review of Malcolm's book,[4] since people sometimes have dreams, even recurring

2. Ludwig Wittgenstein, *The Blue and Brown Books* (Oxford: Blackwell, 1958), pp. 24–25.

3. Norman Malcolm, 'Wittgenstein's *Philosophical Investigations*', *Philosophical Review*, 63 (1954), 544. So far as I can see, Malcolm's use of the term 'criterion' in his monograph is, at least in certain respects, very similar to the use of the term described by Malcolm in the above review of the *Philosophical Investigations*.

4. David F. Pears, 'Professor Norman Malcolm: Dreaming,' [Chapter 9 above, "Dreaming"] pp. 207, 216–217.

dreams, which are repetitions of actual waking experiences which they at one time had.

More damaging to Malcolm's position, however, is the fact that he has not given sufficient conditions for having dreamt either. Surely a person might very well wake up with the mistaken impression of having seen and done various things and yet not have dreamt that he had. Suppose, for example, that a person, from time to time, is struck by the strange feeling that, shortly before, he had been talking with his wife. One morning, he awakes with this impression. Now it seems quite obvious that, although the person might realize that he could not have been talking with his wife, he need not conclude that he had dreamt it.

If a person awakes with an impression that he had done and seen certain things, Malcolm considers only two alternatives which he holds to be mutually exclusive: either the person really did see and do those things or the person dreamt it (51, 64–6). It is difficult to see why anyone would want to defend such a position. Hence, rather than continue criticizing Malcolm's reductive analysis of dreams, let us see if we can discern what underlies Malcolm's position. Deeper criticisms can then be given.

II

Malcolm begins Chapter Twelve of his monograph by asserting that we do not arrive at the concept of dreaming through introspection, and moving from this claim to the Wittgensteinian doctrine that a person's description of his 'inward state' provides a determination of what the state is, he concludes that the concept of dreaming must be derived from the familiar phenomenon of telling dreams and that we must take dream reports as the criterion of having dreamt (55). I suspect that Malcolm, accepting the above Wittgensteinian doctrine, is led to hold that, since no one can describe his own dream as it is taking place, we must use what a person says when he awakes as the criterion of the occurrence and content of his dream. Now Malcolm seems to think that it is by examining typical teaching situations that one can bring to mind criteria,[5] and

5. See Malcolm's 'Wittgenstein's *Philosophical Investigations*,' pp. 543–544.

evidently he follows Wittgenstein in taking the typical situation in which a child learns what 'I dreamt so-and-so' means to be the one in which a child wakes up with the mistaken impression that he has seen and done certain things. Perhaps in this way, Malcolm came to his positive account of dreaming. I think Malcolm can see no alternative to this view. He is committed to the position that there must be a criterion for determining that someone had a dream since he believes that otherwise, the sentence 'He had a dream' would have no use (61). And he is unable to see what the criterion could be other than the dream report (59).

Now it is difficult to evaluate the above reasoning since the crucial terms in the argument, i.e. 'criterion' and 'use,' are not precisely defined. But I think we are entitled to ask for a justification of his claim that without a criterion, the sentence 'He had a dream' would have no use. But I do not see that Malcolm has explicitly given any argument for this claim in his monograph. He does consider the position that, although we have no criterion of dreaming, we do have knowledge of various 'outer' phenomena correlated with dreams. Against this, he asserts that without a criterion of dreaming no empirical correlates could be established (60–1). Unfortunately, he fails to provide the reader with any cogent reasons for accepting this strong claim.[6]

But suppose Malcolm can justify his assertion that the dream report is the criterion of dreaming. He would still have to justify his positive account of dreaming, for even if the criterion of dreaming is the dream report, it does not follow from this, for example, that saying 'I dreamt so-and-so' implies that I woke up with the mistaken impression that so-and-so occurred. But where is Malcolm's argument which bridges that gap? If

6. Malcolm seems to have been influenced greatly by Wittgenstein's well-known private language argument. He quotes (13) with approval Wittgenstein's remarks: 'In the present case I have no criterion of correctness. One would like to say: whatever is going to seem right to me is right. And that only means that here we can't talk about "right" '. It should be kept in mind however that the E-example of Wittgenstein is a special case. The E is supposedly a 'private object', and the lack of criterion of correctness results in special difficulties because it is not clear how a connection can be established between the E and anything public.

Malcolm has provided us with such an argument, it is well hidden in his monograph.

III

I cannot see that Malcolm has justified anywhere his positive account of dreaming. Returning then to his negative thesis, why cannot a person have a dream which simply consists in various images appearing to him during sleep? Consider the following example: A person, having recently been in a terrible automobile accident in which he struck and killed a six year old girl, cannot forget the look of horror and pain in the child's face at the moment of impact. He tells us: 'I keep seeing her face! And no matter what I do, I cannot keep that image out of my mind. Even during sleep, the image appears to me.'

Of course, for Malcolm the whole notion of images appearing in a person's sleep is senseless: he feels that we can have no reason for thinking that images ever appear to anyone during sleep and he suggests that, in this regard, no reliance can be placed on what a person tells you when he awakes (37, 49).

It is difficult to see why Malcolm maintains this position, but it is connected with his conviction that if a person said that various images appeared to him while he was asleep, a legitimate and proper question which would absolutely 'cry to be asked' is: 'How do you know this occurred while you slept?' (84) and this question, Malcolm feels, is in the end unanswerable primarily because no one can be aware of the fact that he is asleep while he is asleep.

Now it certainly does not seem to me that in the above situation the question 'How do you know this occurred while you slept?' would cry to be asked. Indeed, I would not be even slightly tempted to ask such a question. But I can imagine a situation in which I might want to ask a somewhat similar question. Suppose a person claimed that an image of his dead father appeared to him during his sleep at exactly 1:45 a.m. Here, I think it would be quite natural to ask, How do you know this occurred at 1:45? since a sleeping person is generally not thought to be in a position to know the exact time of such an occurrence. But this case is quite different from the one Malcolm considers. For to know the precise time of an occurrence, one would normally need to see or hear something which would in some way 'give one the time'—obviously something a sleeping person is in no position to do. In the former case however, there is no comparable question about how he knows the image appeared during sleep. He simply remembers that the image appeared just before he awoke. He may remember getting into bed, becoming drowsy and drifting off to sleep at about 10:00 p.m. He may remember the image of the face appearing just before he woke up with a start. And he may remember looking at his alarm clock immediately after this and seeing that it was 6:15 a.m. In other words, he may remember not just that the image appeared, but also that the image appeared after drifting off to sleep and just before waking up—to remember that an image appeared to him during sleep, it is not necessary that he remember having been aware of being asleep when the image appeared. After all, one generally remembers a temporal sequence of events and to remember that an event took place in an interval of time, one need only remember that the event occurred after the beginning of the interval and before the end.

IV

I have stressed this memory element involved in our notion of dreaming since Malcolm seems to have left no real place for it in his account. He tells us that when a person says "I dreamt so and so" he implies, first, that it seemed to him on waking up as if the so and so had occurred and, second, that the so and so did not occur' (66). It is not clear to me why Malcolm insists that one must have this impression *upon waking up*. But since he states this queer time-condition in a number of places (66, 77, 49), it is hard to believe it is a mere slip. Noting Malcolm's treatment of the question, How do you know the imagery appeared during sleep? it may be that Malcolm thinks he can avoid, with this requirement, the kind of difficulty which he feels faces those who hold that dreaming consists in experiencing images and ideas in sleep. By tying the waking impression to the dream in this way, in answer to the question, How do you know the dream took place on Tuesday rather than Monday? one need only remember when one had the waking impression which, Malcolm feels, does not involve any special difficulties. Another possibility is that Malcolm, looking to typical teaching situations in order to discern the criterion of dreaming, finds this 'time-factor' present and is thus led to include it in his account.

But whatever reasons Malcolm may have had for producing this account of dreaming, his reductive analysis is surely contradicted by the common phenomenon of people waking up not remembering having dreamt at all and ony recalling a dream hours and perhaps many days later because, for example, some event triggers the recollection of the dream. Furthermore, sometimes upon waking, a person is not sure whether or not he had a dream. His uncertainty need not be (if it ever is) an uncertainty as to whether he has an impression of the sort described by Malcolm or whether the impression is false. Memory being what it is, he is simply not sure whether or not he *had* a dream.

I suggest then that Malcolm completely obscures the place memory has in our common notion of dreaming by analyzing dreaming and dream reports in terms of impressions we have upon awaking. Malcolm puts himself into the position of seeing little more than what he takes to be the criterion of dreaming, viz. the dream report. Thus, in one place he writes:

People declare on awaking that various incidents *took* place (past tense) which did not take place. We then say that these incidents were *dreamt* (past tense). This is merely how we label the above facts. . . . [77]

No wonder Malcolm can find 'no clear sense' in the 'notions of location and duration of a dream in physical time' (70)! Given this strange view of dreaming, it is not difficult to see why Malcolm would claim that 'in the familiar concept of dreaming there is no provision for the duration of dreams in physical time' (79). His defense of these extraordinary claims is based on his principle that 'there can be only as much precision in the common concept of dreaming as is provided by the common criterion of dreaming' (75).

Now I shall attempt to throw more doubt on Malcolm's position by defending philosophers, physiologists and psychologists against Malcolm's charge that they are confused in 'supposing that a dream *must* have a definite location and duration in physical time' (75).

Imagine a society of people who, not having a great deal of scientific knowledge, measure distances solely in terms of measuring rods and pieces of string. Now if these people have some concept of space, would it not make sense for them to wonder whether or not the moon is closer to the earth than the sun is, and even try to discover methods of deciding this question though it is absolutely inconceivable to them that they might be able to stretch a string to the sun and measure the string? Indeed would it not be correct for them to maintain that the sun and the moon have some determinate location in physical space relative to the earth even though, at this time, given their methods of establishing distances, there is simply no way of determining what the distances are? Certainly one must consider factors other than criteria.

We can, of course, imagine a genuine question arising as to whether the sun and the moon have determinate locations in space, since, to some members of the tribe, it might seem reasonable to suppose that these observable things are really very much like rainbows. But surely this question would not be decidable simply on grounds of ordinary usage.

In the case of dreaming, is there any reason for denying on logical grounds the possibility of constructing a scientific theory that would provide us with the theoretical framework within which methods of determining the location and duration of dreams in physical time could be developed? One would think that, with sufficiently great scientific advances, one might be able to establish precisely, on the basis of certain physiological occurrences, the duration of a person's dream. Scientists would not have to start with an isolated Humean 'idea' completely lacking in theoretical and conceptual connections: dream reports and dreams are connected by memory. And it does not seem inconceivable to me that scientists might someday discover a great deal more about memory on the one hand and physiological processes during waking experiences on the other which would provide the basis for a general theory the laws of which would relate memory and mental phenomena of various kinds and which would also encompass dreaming. Given such a theory, the physiological states of a person during a period of time might show not only that the person had a dream of a certain sort, but also that the person for example:

1. remembers the dream clearly;
2. vaguely remembers some of the dream but would be able to remember more of it if X were done to him;
3. remembers having dreamt though not the dream itself but would be able to remember the dream if Y were done to him;
4. remembers neither having dreamt nor the dream but would be able to remember the dream if Z were done to him;
5. remembers neither having dreamt nor the dream and would not be able to remember any of the dream even if X, Y, Z and W were done to him.

Obviously these implications of the theory could be tested, and confirmation of the theory by way of such tests would certainly be a start in the direction Malcolm finds impossible. In terms of the laws of the theory, scientists might then be able to explain and throw light on a variety of dream phenomena and discover new and important facts about the effect dreaming has on people. Now why could not a physiological test of the duration of dreams also be discovered?

V

From what Malcolm says in his monograph, one can gather that he would regard such scientific methods of 'determining the occurrence and duration of dreams' as essentially irrelevant to his own position regarding dreaming on the grounds that no matter what scientists discover, the use of such methods would require, in effect, a new convention, a 'stipulation' of a new criterion of dreaming (78), which would be tantamount to creating a 'new concept under an old label' (79), and indeed, one which 'only remotely resembled the old one' (81).

Now I do not find this defense at all satisfactory. Let us first consider his claim that were we to adopt such methods of testing dream reports we would have a concept so different from our present concept of dreaming that 'to use the name "dreaming" for the new concept would spring from confusion and result in confusion' (81). Now what are these 'radical conceptual changes' which Malcolm cites to support his claim? He suggests that if physiological occurrences could be used to establish the fact that a person had a dreamless sleep, then it would be conceivable that a person could wake up thinking he had dreamt when, as a matter of fact, he had not, 'even if his impression that he had seen and done various things was false' (80). And this, Malcolm thinks, is a radical conceptual change. But is it? In our present state of knowledge, we do not generally question a person's dream report or wonder whether or not the person really dreamt. After all, why should one? What would be the point? Especially since we now have no way of conclusively checking his dream report. But even now, I do not think it is inconceivable that a person might awake thinking he had dreamt he had won money at the race track when actually he had neither dreamt that night nor won any money. Malcolm also argues that if we used a criterion other than the dream report, 'people would have to be *informed* on waking up that they had dreamt or not—instead of their informing us, as it now is' (80). But how does Malcolm know this? We do not use a person's memory claim that he had been to the movies yesterday as the criterion for determining that he had been to the movies, but does it follow from this that a person who had gone to the movies would have to be informed of this fact the next day? Malcolm goes on to assert that if we adopt physiological tests of dream reports, it would be possible for there to be a tribe of people who never told dreams but dreamt every night (80)—as if this showed some radical change in our concept of dreaming! I see nothing logically absurd at all in the supposition that there might be a tribe of people who dream but never relate their dreams any more than I see any absurdity in the statement that dogs dream. Finally, there is the teaching-argument: Malcolm asks us to consider how differently a child would have to be taught—'to teach him the new concept of dreaming we should have to explain the physiological experiment that provides the new criterion' (81). But why could not the child first learn what dreams are as we now do and later learn how scientists test dream reports? Is the case we are considering so different from the case of a child acquiring the concept of distance? It is difficult to explain to a child complicated methods of measuring distances using precise optical instruments, and even more difficult to explain the methods by which scientists measure immense astronomical distances. Would Malcolm also say here that the use of the term 'distance,' where neither rod nor string is employed in measuring, 'would spring from confusion and result in confusion?'

Perhaps at this point, we should consider Malcolm's weaker claim that to bring in the notion of duration of dreams in physical time 'is to create a new concept under an old label.' So far as I can tell, in Malcolm's writings 'concept', like 'criterion', is a technical term which Malcolm evidently inherited from Wittgenstein. And for Malcolm as for Wittgenstein, criterion and concept are intimately connected notions so that any vagueness in the meaning of the term 'criterion' tends to spill over and contaminate the clarity of the term 'concept.' Now we are told by Malcolm that there are different concepts of dreaming: the primary concept, the sole criterion of which is the dream report, and a secondary one, the criterion of which is behaviour during sleep (61–3, 70). Malcolm goes so far as to claim that we even have more than one concept of *sleep* since with adults and older children we use the two criteria of testimony and behaviour wheareas with animals and infants we use only the criterion of behaviour (23). One begins to wonder where Malcolm would halt this proliferation of concepts. Wittgenstein, it should be noted, held that a proof that 200 and 200 added together yield 400 provides us with a criterion of correct addition, and thereby 'defines a new concept: "the counting of 200 and 200 objects together.' " [7] Wittgenstein was even tempted to say that 'every new proof alters the concept of proof in one way or another' (RFM, p. 126). At this point, one might want to know how it is to be determined whether any two given persons have the same concept of proof.[8] Unfortunately, nowhere in Malcolm's monograph nor in Wittgenstein's

7. Ludwig Wittgenstein, *Remarks on the Foundations of Mathematics* (Oxford: Blackwell, 1956), p. 76. Cited here as RFM.
8. See in this regard my "Mathematical Discovery and Concept Formation," *Philosophical Review*, 72 (January 1963).

published writings do I find any clear statement of how this term 'concept' is being used. Wittgenstein's explanation that a concept is 'something like a picture with which one compares objects' (RFM, p. 195) is not very enlightening, and he indicated in various places in the *Remarks on the Foundations of Mathematics* that he was not clear about the use of this term.[9] Hence I shall not quarrel with Malcolm over the charge that a new concept would have been created in the envisaged situation since, without an adequate explication of this term 'concept,' there is little solid ground for disagreement, and it may well be the case that nothing very important hangs on whether or not we would have a new concept of dreaming. All this talk of new concepts, changed concepts and the like is worth little until this blank check 'concept' is filled in. Therefore, I do not see that Malcolm's defense can rest here.

Now we have seen that Malcolm claims not only that there is no sense in the claim that dreams have duration in physical time but also that to provide us with a concept of duration of dreams, scientists would have to *stipulate* what will establish the duration of dreams. This would not be a matter of discovering something—it would simply be a case of adopting a new convention. Well, suppose a group of scientists got together and stipulated that the duration of a person's dream will henceforth be said to be equal to the length of time it takes the person to get dressed after awaking. Would this stipulation give sense to the notion of 'duration of dreams'? Would this be a case of stipulating a criterion of the length of a dream? I do not think so. I think it can be seen that not anything will count as establishing the duration of dreams. Given a scientific theory of dreaming of the sort sketched above, there may be no question as to what establishes the duration of dreams, nor any room for stipulation.

Malcolm at one point says:

If someone tells a dream or says he had one he is not making a 'subjective' report which may or may not agree with 'objective' fact. His waking impression is what establishes that he had a dream, and his account of his dream establishes what the content of his dream was. [79]

9. See pages 188, 195.

I have tried to show that these claims are neither obviously true nor justified by Malcolm in his monograph. Is it possible that Malcolm, himself, has been held captive by a picture of language? Might it not be the case that our ordinary concept of dreaming—if there is such a thing—does not have the neat and tidy character attributed to it by Malcolm? Perhaps most people have no idea of what would establish for certain that a person actually dreamt what he says he dreamt but use the term 'dream' anyhow in a way that requires dream reports to be taken as 'subjective' reports which may or may not agree with 'objective' facts. I suppose, Malcolm would say that anyone who used the term 'dream' in that way would have to be confused. But confused or not, what if most people, as a matter of fact, do use the term in that way? Has Malcolm proved this to be impossible? I do not think so. And if most people do use the term in that way, just what are we to make of Malcolm's remarkable claims concerning the *actual use* of the term 'dream' and *our* ordinary concept of dreaming?

Malcolm sees part of his task as that of getting people to regard dream reports differently: he argues from his analysis of what he calls 'our ordinary concept of dreaming' to the conclusion that our ordinary conception of dreaming is confused. Following Wittgenstein, he feels he is clearing away 'prejudices' produced by 'grammatical illusions' (75). But perhaps our common notions concerning the nature of dreams are more than 'houses of cards.' After all, what we say and how we regard what we say reflect our view of the world. Now perhaps the various beliefs about human nature, memory, and mental processes, which we share, which are reflected in our common notions concerning the nature of dreams, and in virtue of which our dream reports have the particular significance for us which they have, provide us with the framework upon which a scientific theory can be built that will enable us to measure the duration of dreams. A scientific theory that encompasses these beliefs, that preserves most of our common ideas about the nature of dreaming in a way that renders intelligible and coherent such phenomena as dream behaviour and dream utterances, and that enables us to explain and predict important things, could reasonably be said, on my view, to give us significant insights into the nature of dreams. If such a scientific theory were successfully developed, and if, on such a theory, dreams are connected with certain physiological occurrences in a way that enables scientists to measure the duration of dreams, then even if it could be said that a new concept of dreaming had been introduced I, for one, should not say that scientists had made a stipulation that such and such is what we shall henceforth call the 'duration of dreams'—I should say that a scientific method of measuring the duration of dreams had been *discovered*.

My conclusion is that even if, in the envisaged situation in which one would be able to check dream reports by means of scientific instruments, we could be said to have introduced a new concept of dreaming in some vague Wittgensteinian sense of the term 'concept,' we should not overlook the fact that there would be a core of ideas about dreaming, preserving important conceptual relations that remained invariant under this growth of scientific knowledge, which would both entitle us to use the term 'dream' in this new context and justify our saying that scientists had discovered a method of measuring the duration of dreams. Whether or not such a method will be discovered remains to be seen—in spite of Malcolm.

12

FREDERICK A. SIEGLER

Remembering Dreams [1]

There are two unusual and obvious features of the concept
of dreaming, and both are examined by Malcolm in his book
Dreaming.[2] The first is about the verb 'to dream'. There is no
first person present tense. The second is that dreams are not
public phenomena, and so in reporting a dream one is not
reporting something that can be checked by the reports of
others.

Malcolm develops some of the further features of the concept of dreaming from an analysis of the implications of these
two features. I want to examine a two-part thesis about the concept of dreaming which Malcolm seems to hold. The two parts
rest on two more general theses about the concepts of remembering and correctness. The general theses are: one cannot
remember what one could not have reported in the present
tense. One cannot learn to make memory reports if there is no
public referent. The thesis about dreaming is: since we do report our dreams, it follows that the ordinary concepts of *memory*
and *correctness* do not apply to dream reports. I think that the
two general theses are false and consequently do not support

Reprinted from the *Philosophical Quarterly,* 17 (1967), 14–24, by permission of
Dorothy Siegler and the *Philosophical Quarterly.*

1. I have had helpful discussions of this paper with Professors R. C. Coburn
and V. C. Chappell, and particularly with Mr. Andrew Naylor and Mr. D. F.
Wallace.

2. Norman Malcolm, *Dreaming* (London, 1959).

the two-part thesis about dreaming. Also I think that the two-part thesis about dreaming is false.

Malcolm may well deny that he holds the two-part thesis. He accepts Chappell's example of misremembering a dream,[3] and replies to the example, "That one cannot misremember a dream? I do not make that claim".[4] But clearly Malcolm holds the more general thesis about "remembering":

> When we think philosophically about memory the following sort of paradigm comes most naturally to our minds: I spoke certain words to you yesterday. Today I am requested to give an account of what those words were. The account I give is right or wrong. This is determined by whether it agrees with your account and that of other witnesses, perhaps also by whether it is plausible in the light of what is known about you and me and the circumstances yesterday, and perhaps by still other things. But when I speak of 'remembering' a dream there is nothing outside of my account of the dream (provided that I understand the words that compose it) to determine that my account is right or wrong. . . . Since nothing counts as determining that my memory of my dream is right or wrong, what sense can the word 'memory' have here?

> [Malcolm admits that] it is no misuse of language to speak of 're-membering a dream.' We are taught this expression. Only we must be mindful of its actual use *and* of how sharply this differs from the use of 'remembering' that appeared in our paradigm.[5]

Malcolm thinks that failure to notice the difference between the use of 'remembering' in the paradigm and that in 'remembering a dream' leads to a belief that dreams must be conscious experiences of which the dreamer is aware.[6] But it is not at all clear to me how the latter view is a necessary or even plausible outcome of failing to observe a difference between the use of 'remembering' in Malcolm's paradigm and its use in 'remembering a dream.'[7] And I shall argue that there is no difference

3. V. C. Chappell, "The Concept of Dreaming" [Chapter 13 below].

4. *Ibid.*, p. 308, note.   5. *Dreaming*, pp. 56–57.

6. This latter thesis he quotes from Yost and Kalish, "Miss Macdonald on Sleeping and Waking" [Chapter 3 above].

7. Certainly, there is nothing in the above-quoted passage from *Dreaming* that would indicate Malcolm's *reasons* for making this claim. Nevertheless, one might be led to speculate as to their nature, especially on the basis of remarks in the third of his recently published lectures on memory, "A Definition of Factual Memory". Factual memory (logically the most primitive of various "forms"

between these two uses of the concept (or two concepts) of remembering. 'There are differences between remembering what happened yesterday and remembering a dream, but I do not think that the differences are differences in the use of the word or concept 'remembering'. If the concept of remembering (in its ordinary sense?) fails to apply in cases where upon first awaking one reports dreams, then neither does it apply in cases of certain other phenomena reported in the past tense. But since we unhesitatingly admit that the concept of remembering has application in its ordinary sense to reports of the latter phenomena, there is no reason why it should not have application in the same sense to reports of dreams.

It can also be shown that Malcolm holds the more general thesis about "correctness". To be able to remember the colour of something one must at some time have been able to pick out the colour. Unless a man can (has learned to) identify the colour magenta he could not sensibly say that he remembers that a particular object was magenta. Upon learning to identify magenta, he might say that he remembers having seen the colour before but did not know that it was magenta. Though this is possible, it is possible only because he has already learned to identify something as having some colour. That is to say, he has learned the concept of colour. In short, being able to identify magenta is psychologically and logically prior to

---

of memory since all other "forms" imply it) is defined as follows: "A person, B, remembers that *p* from a time, *t*, if and only if B knows that *p*, *and* B knew that *p* at *t*, and if B had not known at *t* that *p* he would not know that *p*" (*Knowledge and Certainty*, [New York, 1963], p. 236). Malcolm admits that "often the knowledge that one had a dream is memory, e.g., when one knows that one had a dream last week or last month. But if a person awakened suddenly from sleep and immediately declared that he had a dream, should we call this *remembering* that he had a dream? I am not sure: but if so then this use of "He remembers that *p*" does not fall under our analysis of factual memory. . . . [For] we should not know how to determine a previous time at which he dreamt" (p. 240). Malcolm's claims about dream reports appear to commit him to the peculiar view that when I awake and tell a dream, I cannot *logically* at that moment report the fact that I dreamt, either because it is not yet a fact that I dreamt or because (in virtue of his conditions for factual memory) I am not yet in a position to report it. Even if Malcolm's *definition* of factual memory is correct, it provides no more grounds for his conclusion that we are using different senses of 'remembering' when we speak of remembering facts and remembering dreams than for the alternative conclusion that facts are different from dreams.

being able to make a correct memory claim to have seen magenta. Seeing magenta as a colour and not knowing its name could be psychologically prior to learning to identify magenta (learning the name). But seeing magenta as a colour could not be prior to being able to identify something as having some colour.

Furthermore, learning to identify the colour magenta involves having a public referent for the word 'magenta'. The public referent serves as a criterion for the correctness of an identification. The public referent is employed in correcting initial mistakes, and corroborating identifications, until the technique of identification has been mastered. With regard to dreaming it is not that these truths change, but that reporting a dream is different from remembering a colour.

One might think that it works this way: because being able to make a present-tense identification of what one is dreaming is not logically prior to being able to report a dream, this shows that reporting a dream is different from reporting what one saw yesterday. There is no criterion for correctness in reporting a dream, while there is in reporting what one saw yesterday. In the case of yesterday, the report is about something public, and in the case of a dream the report is not about something public. There is no way of corroborating one's dream reports with other people's reports of one's dreams. This shows that the concept of correctness has no application to reporting or remembering a dream. The sincere report of the dream would be the criterion of what the dream was.[8]

This sketch of an analysis seems to be mistaken. And I think that the mistake lies in recognizing the beginning but not the whole of a truth. It is true to say that neither reporting what one is presently dreaming, nor recognizing that one is presently dreaming is a logical prerequisite for reporting a dream. (Nor could it be a logical prerequisite, for logically it cannot be done.)[9] But from this it does not follow that the concept of correctness does not apply to reporting a dream, that there is no difference between thinking that one remembers a dream and remembering a dream.

One might well learn to report dreams in the way suggested

8. Cf. *Dreaming*, p. 56.   9. Cf. F. Ebersole, "De Somniis", *Mind*, 1959.

by Wittgenstein[10] and Malcolm.[11] A child awakes and tells a story about a frightful event and his parents comfort him with "It was only a dream, nothing really happened, you were only dreaming". In the future the child precedes such stories with "I dreamt". He may still be frightened by his dreams, and look under the bed for the bears of his dreams. Or, if the child has overheard adults talking about their dreams, he will use the expression 'I dreamt' similarly to report his own dreams. He need not and could not have learned to say 'I am dreaming', but he must *logically* have learned to make or understand present-tense reports of the *kind* of incidents which he reports to have dreamt. He must have learned to apply the descriptive concepts employed in dream reports. If he can be said to report correctly having dreamt that a lion was eating him, he must be able to recognize a lion or a photograph of a lion, etc. If he can correctly employ the descriptive concepts of "lion", "eating", etc., and if he has a good memory in general, then, generally, he can report correctly what he has dreamt.

But Wittgenstein suggests [12] and Malcolm argues [13] that the ordinary concept of memory is not relevant in reporting one's dreams. It is true that one does not always *speak* of remembering what one dreamt, but neither does one always speak of remembering what one knows to have happened in the past. I tell my wife that I put the car keys in the drawer, but not always that I remember that I put the car keys in the drawer. I say that I remember that I put the car keys in the drawer only under special circumstances, say, when I was unsure where they are, and I managed to reconstruct where I left them. But this does not mean that the concept of memory does not apply when I do not say "I remember".

Wittgenstein asks concerning reports of dreams: "Now must I make some assumption about whether people are deceived by their memories or not . . . ? Do we ever ask ourselves this when someone is telling us his dream? And if not—is it because we are sure his memory won't have deceived him?" [14] Ask the same question about reports of the recent past. My wife tells

10. *Philosophical Investigations* (Oxford, 1953), p. 184.
11. *Dreaming*, p. 55.   12. *Philosophical Investigations*, pp. 222–223.
13. *Dreaming*, pp. 56–57.   14. *Philosophical Investigations*, p. 184.

me that she baked a cake during the afternoon. Do I ever ask myself whether my wife is deceived by her memory? Is this because I am sure that her memory will not have deceived her? These questions sound as queer in the case of my wife's reports of what she recently did as they do in the case of my wife's dream reports. We do not ordinarily question such reports, but this might well show merely that we do not ordinarily err in such reports. One is more prone to question the reliability of memory in cases in which we say "I remember" because it is often in cases of uncertainty that this phrase is used. But this does not preclude the possibility of erring in cases in which we do not say "I remember". And the error could be an error in memory.

One might want to say that any past tense report is a memory report, on the ground that memory is a necessary condition for making such reports. There is reason for resistance to such a cavalier act of labelling. Memory in one sense is also a necessary condition for talking. If one has no memory then he cannot remember the meaning of words; he cannot learn to identify something as the same as what he has seen before.

We do speak of remembering in a way which is not so extensive. A man can be said to have a terrible memory or even to have lost his memory without forgetting how to talk or forgetting what he heard or said a moment ago. But to speak of remembering a dream is not to extend the concept of remembering beyond its ordinary scope. To say that a man remembers his dreams need only indicate that he might very well not remember his dreams but be able to talk and report other things in the past tense. One thing that might seem odd about remembering dreams is that a man who cannot fully remember his last night's dream might perfectly well remember last evening's party, and the dream he had two nights ago. But perhaps this need not strike us as being so very peculiar. One can often remember some parts of the past more easily than others. Think of the time it takes some people to remember the Roman Emperors and their dates; think of how easily others or even the same people remember the ages, names, and race-histories of horses.

Wittgenstein and Malcolm are struck with the fact that ordi-

narily when I report a past event, there is in principle the possibility of public corroboration, and that this feature is not
present in reporting a dream. This difference does not seem to
merit the conclusion that the ordinary concept of remembering
does not apply to dream reports. Nor is this public-private distinction clear.

In the first place if every one of one's own memories *must* be
checkable by those of others, then how are the memories of
others to be checked? In terms of still others? Why is checking
one's own memories against another's memory different in
principle from checking one of one's memories against another
of one's memories? And if this latter is like buying several copies of the same newspaper, then why is not the former like buying several copies of several newspapers? Several copies of the
same newspaper will not resolve a concern about the correctness of a story, but several copies of several newspapers
need not resolve concern about the correctness of a story either. All the newspaper reporters could have been taken in by
a hoax. But the problem about the past is that it is gone. And
sometimes memory is all we have.

The objection to this argument runs as folows:—For there to
be genuine remembering there must be a distinction between
remembering and merely seeming to remember. For there to
be such a distinction, however, one must be able to find out for
sure that one's "memory" (what one claims to remember) is
mistaken. But one cannot find out for sure, with certainty, that
one's own memory claim A is mistaken by appealing to another
of one's own memories B. For why would one not be just as justified in holding on to A and rejecting B, as in holding on to B
and rejecting A? No appeal to others of one's own memories
could possibly "settle the issue with certainty" that some particular case of ostensible remembering is really a case of merely
seeming to remember. Hence, for there to be a genuine case of
remembering, it must be possible that there should be evidence
independent of one's own memory (e.g. the memory of others)
which could show that the memory claim in question is mistaken.

Now this objection may be taken in two different ways. On
the one hand it may be meant to show that every particular

memory claim must be open to the test of independent evidence. On the other hand it may be meant to show that the concept of memory cannot have a private genesis. That is, if there were never any possibility of an appeal beyond one's own memory there could be no such thing as remembering. This latter way of taking the objection seems to be unchallengeable. And it seems to be one clear point that Wittgenstein was making against epistemological theories in which knowledge is built out of private images, ideas or impressions. But from this it does not follow that every particular memory claim must be open to the appeal of independent evidence. That is to say, though the genesis of the concept of memory is necessarily interpersonal or public, it is not the case that the logical status of every particular memory claim is necessarily public. Nor is it clear that Wittgenstein's argument was meant to establish that every memory claim must be open to the appeal of independent evidence.

In the second place, there are cases in which although, in principle, others could have been able to corroborate a memory report, in fact all one has is one's own memory. Say I tell you that yesterday when I saw a photograph of De Gaulle, I thought of Napoleon's personal prestige. I might have, and in principle could have, expressed this thought to somebody, but suppose I did not. I now report it in the past tense to somebody. Why should it be essential that I *could* have expressed my thought in the present tense to somebody else? Does that improve my memory? No. But it makes my report a kind of report which I could have learned to make. I could learn to report my thoughts which I kept to myself yesterday only after I have learned to express my thoughts in the present.

Now if in order to be able to remember my dreams I must be able to report dreams in the present, then I could not learn to *remember* my dreams. But I do not think that this *is* a necessary condition for being able to remember my dreams. Nor do I think that every other particular case of memory must in principle be checkable by others.

Imagine a man who is prevented by ropes and a gag from talking or writing. Later he tells me that he was lamenting

Mozart's early death. The factual impossibility of his expressing his thoughts in the present tense does not weigh against the application of the concept of truth (as opposed to truthfulness) to his memory report. Notice that the fact that he did not express himself in the present tense makes it logically impossible for us to have a public check on what he says in his memory report. But this does not weigh against the application of the concept of truth to his memory report.

Imagine that while re-reading the crime passage in *Crime and Punishment* I become so deeply engrossed that I am not aware of my wife's entrance into my study. I cannot hear her question, "What are you doing?" In such a state I could not in principle express my thoughts.[15] This, of course, eliminates the possibility of a public check on what I was thinking at that time. Someone could check my later report ('I was reading about Raskolnikov's mounting the stairs, etc . . .') against the book, but how does one publicly check that I was reading the book at that time, and not just remembering a previous reading of that passage? Furthermore, imagine a case in which there is no book. I am deep in thought and out of communication. My later report of what I was thinking is not checkable by others, but that does not seem to tell against the application of the concept of truth to what I report. Nor does it suggest that the ordinary concept of memory does not apply in such cases.

I could report (remember) correctly what I was thinking because I have learned to express my thoughts in the present tense, but it is not necessary that in this particular case I be able in principle to express *these* thoughts in the present tense. If this is so then it is only necessary that I have learned to express my thoughts in the present tense in order to be able to remember them correctly. It is not necessary that I be able in principle in every particular case to express the thoughts in the present tense. I think that the theoretical reasons for this will

15. Under the description 'I was reading X' it seems correct to say that I could in principle express my thoughts about what I am reading, but under the description I was deeply engrossed in reading X' it seems incorrect to say that in principle I could express my thoughts, since being deeply engrossed or lost in a book seems incompatible with expressing one's thoughts.

be clear from an examination of the distinction between the pedagogical genesis of memory reports and the logical status of particular memory reports.

For a child to learn to report in the past tense there must be public criteria in order that one may be able to correct mistakes. A child learns to have confidence in his memory reports, and others gain confidence in his memory reports by checking them against independent evidence. But after a child has learned the technique of reporting in the past tense, he is in a position to make memory reports in cases for which no public check is made. He says what he saw yesterday at the zoo, and if we have confidence in his *memory* we do not *in fact* check everything he says with independent evidence. We do not believe what he has said *on the ground that what he said can be publicly checked*. The fact that his report can be publicly checked puts it into a class of memory reports that can be publicly checked. But this does not exclude the existence of a class of memory reports that *cannot in principle* be publicly checked, or *cannot in practice* be publicly checked.

If a man knows how to express his thoughts in the present, and has mastered the technique of reporting what he has said and seen in the past, then he can report what he has thought under conditions where he could not express his thoughts in the present. He has acquired a technique which can be applied more widely than to situations which are necessary for teaching a person to report the past. Reporting dreams is unlike reporting a public event and more like reporting one's thoughts when in fact or in principle one was unable to express them in the present. Learning to report a dream is not learning a new technique but learning to apply a known technique to a new phenomenon.

There remains a difference between reporting dreams and reporting one's thoughts. On occasion a man might not be able in fact or in principle to express his present thoughts. Yet, if he can report these past thoughts, it is always necessarily true to say that he is able to express his thoughts in the present tense. When a man reports a dream it does not make sense to say that he is able to express or report his dreams in the present tense. This shows a difference but not an essential one between reporting dreams and reporting thoughts.[16] When a man reports his dream it is necessarily true that he understands the descriptive concepts employed in his dream report and he must know how to express his present thoughts. What is common and essential to reports both of dreams and of past thoughts is a possible error in memory. And although in learning to make memory reports the possibility and practice of a public check is necessary, once the technique is mastered it can apply to dreams as well as to unexpressed thoughts.

If a man has mastered the technique of telling what he experienced in the past, and he makes such a report, and there is no reason to suspect that he has been deceived or is lying, or has lost his powers of memory, then his report is good grounds for the truth of what he says. The reporting of dreams is similar. If a man has mastered the technique of reporting what he has experienced, and he reports that he has dreamt something, and there is no reason to doubt his sincerity, or the truth of what he says, then what he reports is good grounds for its truth. What would give reason to doubt a man's dream report aside from a doubt concerning his sincerity? If a man tells me that he dreamt something which I know to have happened, the previous day, then I might doubt that he really dreamt it. I might be led to believe that he thought that it was a dream, when it was really something that actually happened. In such a case I could tell him this. He might reply that I was right, and that he had made a mistake. And what kind of mistake would this be if not a mistake in memory? On the other hand he might tell me that he knows perfectly well what happened yesterday, and that he dreamt the thing at night also. Malcolm contends that " 'I dreamt so and so' . . . implies . . . that the so and so did not occur", [17] and this seems true, in general. But in this case the so-and-so did occur, and the man who dreamt knows it did. This possibility shows that Malcolm is mistaken in thinking that

16. This difference helps to account for our hesitation in saying that a man *knows* what it is he is dreaming *while* he is dreaming it, whereas we can quite intelligibly say that he *knows* what he is thinking *while* he is thinking it; and it suggests that the reasons for this are not to be sought in the alleged contrast between reports of thoughts and dream reports, but rather in the fact that dreams are peculiarly unlike thoughts.

17. *Dreaming,* p. 66.

"If someone were to ask you how you knew that you dreamt so and so, you could always mention something that you supposed proved or made probable that the thing in question did not occur and that therefore you dreamt it". [18] If you dream something that did already happen, you could not employ Malcolm's answer to the question of how you know it was a dream.

Furthermore, in a situation which Malcolm himself describes, questions may arise concerning the memory of a dream. Malcolm speaks of a man who "woke up in the middle of the night and *told* a dream to someone [say, of having been run over by a magenta bus], but on waking in the morning he has the impression of having had a dreamless sleep". [19] If we accept Malcolm: "The criterion of someone's having had a dream . . is that upon awaking he tells a dream", [20] then in this case the man had a dream (sincere report in the middle of the night) and he did not (sincere report in the morning). And this shows that Malcolm's criterion does not fit our concept of dreaming. In the above case we should have doubts about the man's claim to remember that he dreamt, not about his sincerity, and we should tell him about his previous testimony during the night. We might remind him of some of the details of the dream report he made, and this might remind him of the dream. His failure in this case was a failure in memory.

Malcolm says that in this case the man "believes falsely that he did not dream". [21] But how could he? Presumably because he did not *remember* the dream. Of course, we might succeed only in getting the man to remember that during the night he did awake and tell such a dream. And this, it might be alleged, is a non-problematic case quite like that of a man who remembers that he had a certain dream a month ago. Suppose, on the other hand, that the man emphatically insists that he has no memory of having given any report in the middle of the night. Nevertheless, upon reminding him of the details of his previous dream report, say, that perhaps he dreamt he was run over by a bus, he suddenly does remember the dream. Suppose

18. *Ibid.*, p. 65.   19. *Ibid.*, p. 60.   20. *Ibid.*, p. 49.
21. *Ibid.*, p. 60.

he reports having dreamt that he was run over by a lavender bus. Here we are inclined to say that he has incorrect memory concerning the colour of the bus. Indeed, if we question his memory ("Are you sure the bus was lavender?") and he says that he was mistaken about the colour, that the bus was magenta rather than lavender, then we *do* say that he had incorrect memory of what he dreamt. And this shows that the concept of correctness has application to our talk about what we have dreamt.[22]

Furthermore, a man who struggles in telling a dream is certainly not struggling to tell the truth; he is not struggling with his conscience, but trying to remember the details of his dream. Again, there are other grounds for doubting the truth of a dream report, or doubting that a man did not have a dream when he says that he did not. If a friend tells me of a dream he had last night, and I remember his telling me of a similar dream yesterday, I should doubt that he remembers when he

---

22. In certain circumstances one might have reason to doubt a dream report if it failed to accord in some important and obvious detail with something that actually happened. Still, there are important differences, with regard to the ways error may be involved, between remembering a dream and remembering a past event:

(a) The lion trainer sits up for the first time in his hospital bed, and tells us that it was the tiger that bit his arm off the previous night. But there were thousands of people at the circus who saw that it was a lion. What he tells us is mistaken, yet the error is not an error of his memory. At the time he believed that it *was* the tiger: some of the men close by heard him yell out the tiger's name as the big lion pounced on him from behind.

(b) Suppose that at least one of the many children at the circus who have nightmares that night wakes up and tells one of his parents that he dreamt he was attacked by a tiger. The parent might doubt that it was a tiger and perhaps ask the child if it was not a lion. Perhaps the child avows that he has misremembered the dream and corrects the account, saying that he dreamt he was attacked by a lion just like the one that tried to eat the man at the circus. On the other hand, he may insist that it was a tiger that he dreamt attacked him, since it most certainly was a different kind of beast from the one that bit off the man's arm at the circus. In the latter case, one admits that he had correct memory of the dream all along; in the former case that he at first remembered the dream incorrectly but now remembers it correctly. But there could not be any case where although there was no fault in his memory, what he reported turned out to be incorrect as a result of his having taken what he was dreaming (a lion) to be something else (a tiger) *while he was dreaming it.* We can attribute a lion trainer's error to his having turned his back on a lion, but not a dream reporter's error to his turning his back on his dream.

had the dream. I should remind him that he told me the same dream yesterday. He might realize that he mistakenly thought it was last night. On the other hand he might tell me that he has had the same dream now for five nights straight. These doubts are not concerning the sincerity of the dream reporter.

If a man's memory deteriorates we begin to lose confidence in his past-tense reports. If he says that the grocer phoned, and we want to find out whether he did, we can call and ask the grocer. But if he says that he was thinking about his next vacation, then we cannot find out whether what he says is true. We should have to wait until his memory improves, and if it does not, we shall not find out. We are in a similar position with regard to his dream reports.

Malcolm says, "what we take as determining beyond question that a man dreamt is that in sincerity he should tell a dream or say he had one".[23] And this does seem to be a truth about "our daily discourse". Similarly, it is true to say that in our daily discourse what we take as determining beyond question that a man smoked is that in sincerity he should say so. Normally, what a man says sincerely about what he has just done or seen is sufficient for saying that it is true. But that is not to say it is the *criterion* for truth. For on occasion one could and does err. And the error could be a memory error.

I said that the error in analysing the concept of dreaming arose from seeing part of a truth. That part is this: if there were *no* public referents for our perceptual or memory claims and we had only private ideas, impressions or images, then there would be no learning to remember, or learning to speak. The logic of learning to identify or remember requires having a public referent in order that there be criteria for correctness. *But* from this truth it does not follow that *every* memory claim *must* have a public referent. Once the technique of reporting the past is achieved, it can be applied to cases in which there is no public referent. In reporting a dream one is referring to something private to himself. And a man cannot describe his dreams in the present tense. These remain two of the many

23. *Dreaming*, p. 59.

truths about the concept of dreaming. They are enough to make the concept unique.[24]

24. Pears ["Dreaming," Chapter 9 above] recognizes that Malcolm's thesis rests "on the idea that every kind of statement must have a definite criterion whose fulfilment conclusively verifies it, and whose non-fulfilment conclusively falsifies it" (p. 219). He asks "Must every type of memory claim be verified sometimes, or at least confirmed sometimes?" (p. 213). But rather than pursue this question, and thereby question the basis of Malcolm's thesis, Pears attempts to discover some way of satisfying the requirements for a memory claim that Malcolm sets up, namely, that every memory claim must be open to public verification. He suggests correlations between dreaming *and* stimulus, behaviour or physiological phenomena, and also suggests that dreaming may "involve a special kind of awareness at the time" which affords us "two independent indications of this awareness, and therefore of dreams—subsequent memory claims and contemporary behaviour. . . . Each could be taken as sufficient ground for saying that a dream occurred" (p. 219). It may be that dreaming is a special state of awareness. But if my argument is correct, Pears did not have to "concede that reports of dreams are a type of memory claim that needs to be verified, or at least confirmed sometimes, in order to avoid being treated as self-supporting in the way that Malcolm recommends" (pp. 221–222).

13

VERE C. CHAPPELL

The Concept of Dreaming

The most interesting—and most paradoxical—thesis of Professor Malcolm's recent book on *Dreaming* is that "the concept of dreaming is derived, not from dreaming, but from descriptions of dreams", such that "the notion of a dream as an occurrence 'in its own right', logically independent of [one's] waking impression [thereof], and to which the latter may or may not 'correspond' ", is senseless (pp. 55 and 83).[1] This thesis also has a number of interesting and paradoxical consequences, many of which are noted by Malcolm himself in his book. In this paper I shall focus on one of the consequences of Malcolm's

Reprinted from the *Philosophical Quarterly,* 13 (1963), 193–213, by permission of the author and the *Philosophical Quarterly.*

1. This is a revised version of a paper originally intended as a Critical Study of Malcolm's book for the *Philosophical Quarterly.* The original version was itself the successor of an earlier study of the book that I wrote for the *Quarterly* but then asked to have withdrawn, when I realized that it contained some bad mistakes. The original version of the present paper was sent in to replace this earlier study. By accident, the earlier study was printed instead of its replacement, and appeared in the *Quarterly* for April 1962. The editor then kindly offered to publish the replacement paper as well, though it overlaps the printed study to some extent at the beginning. In preparing this new version, I have had the benefit of some searching comments by Professor Malcolm himself on the original replacement paper. With his permission I have quoted some of these comments in footnotes. They help, I believe, to make clear certain of his positions in *Dreaming* which I and others may have misinterpreted. I should note that I have nonetheless retained some points to which Malcolm objects, and that my failure to note his dissent on any given point in no way implies that he accepts or that I think he accepts what I say.

thesis and try to show that it is not established by the arguments that are adduced in its favour. I shall also try to show that the consequence in question is false. On the principle that a false consequent implies a false antecedent, I then conclude that Malcolm's thesis is false as well.

Briefly stated, Malcolm's thesis is that dreams are logically connected to dream reports, that the former are somehow logically determined by the latter. The consequence of this thesis on which I wish to focus has to do with the *remembering* of dreams. Malcolm's position is expressed in the following passage:

> We speak of 'remembering' dreams, and if we consider this expression it can appear to us to be a misuse of language. When we think philosophically about memory the following sort of paradigm comes most naturally to our minds: I spoke certain words to you yesterday. Today I am requested to give an account of what those words were. The account I give is right or wrong. This is determined by whether it agrees with your account and that of other witnesses, perhaps also by whether it is plausible in the light of what is known about you and me and the circumstances yesterday, and perhaps by still other things. But when I speak of 'remembering' a dream there is nothing outside of my account of the dream (provided that I understand the words that compose it) to determine that my account is right or wrong. I may amend it slightly on a second telling—but only slightly. If I changed it very much or many times it would no longer be said that I was 'telling a dream'. My verbal behaviour would be too unlike the behaviour on which the concept of dreaming is founded. That something is implausible or impossible does not go to show that I did not dream it. In a dream I can do the impossible in every sense of the word. I can climb Everest without oxygen and I can square the circle. Since nothing counts as determining that my memory of my dream is right or wrong, what sense can the word 'memory' have here?
>
> But of course it is no misuse of language to speak of 'remembering a dream'. We are taught this expression. Only we must be mindful of its actual *use* and of how sharply this differs from the use of 'remembering' that appeared in our paradigm. [Pp. 56–57]

What Malcolm is saying in this passage may be put in this way: although there is a sense in which dreams are remembered, there is no such thing as *mis*remembering a dream, and no such thing, therefore, as misreporting a dream, having misremembered it. In the case of a conversation I have witnessed, I can claim to remember and be mistaken; the possibil-

ity of mistake is part of the concept of remembering that applies to this sort of case. In the case of dreams, however, my
memory-claims are incorrigible; I cannot be mistaken in them.
Of course I can falsely report a dream I have had in the sense
of lying about it, or again in the sense of using the wrong
words to express what I think happened in it (this I take it is
the point of Malcolm's parenthetical provision "that I understand the words that compose" the account I give of my
dream). But it is impossible to misreport a dream in what has
been called "the most favoured sense", viz. by saying what I
think about it and being wrong in thinking this. For the notions
of being wrong about a dream, of being mistaken as to a
dream's contents, and of having a false impression that one has
dreamed at all, are all without sense, according to Malcolm.
These notions are excluded by the concept of remembering
that applies to dreams (and so of course are the contrary notions of being right and having a true impression). This is how
this concept differs from the concept of remembering that figures in the usual case, the case represented by Malcolm's paradigm.

The arguments by which Malcolm seeks to establish this position are simply extensions of the arguments on which he rests
his general thesis, that there is a logical connection between
dreaming and telling a dream. They are derived, in their essen-
tials, from certain suggestions of Wittgenstein. Two different
arguments or lines of argument can be distinguished. The first
runs roughly as follows. Dreaming is a private thing, an "inner
process"; hence no one can know what or even that a man has
dreamed in the way that he himself can know it. And yet we
must be capable of knowing, on occasion, when and what other
people dream. For if we were not so capable, then neither we
nor they could know what it is to dream; no one could have the
concept of dreaming. Unless we were able to teach a child when
to say "I had a dream" and "I dreamed that such and such",
the child could never learn the concept. And we could not
teach a child this unless we knew, at least sometimes, when he
dreamed and what it was that he dreamed. It follows that there
must be some external, public way or ways of telling when and
what other people dream. These, furthermore, must be ways of

telling, "determining beyond question", not merely bases for guessing or inferring inductively. As Wittgenstein put it, "An 'inner process' stands in need of outward criteria"; [2] and a criterion, in Malcolm's words, is "something that settles a question with certainty" (p. 60). The view, Malcolm goes on, that there is no criterion of someone's having dreamt, "but merely various 'outer' phenomena that are empirically correlated with . . . dreams . . . is self-contradictory: without criteria for the occurrence of [dreams] the correlations could not be established" (pp. 60–61). Now in the case of dreaming, Malcolm argues, "what we take as determining beyond question that a man dreamt is that in sincerity he should tell a dream or say he had one" (p. 59). In other words, "the report of a dream [is] the criterion of what the dream was" (p. 56). Furthermore, Malcolm claims, it is the "sole criterion" (pp. 70, 81); what a man says upon awakening—or more precisely, what he thinks upon awakening, since he may lie or misuse language—provides the only means by which others can tell either that or what he has dreamed. This means that one's dreams and one's waking impressions of one's dreams—if not one's accounts of them—are logically interdependent. "We may say that dreams and waking impressions are two different things: but not—two logically independent things" (p. 60). But now if what I have dreamed is determined, and logically determined, by what I *say* I have dreamed, or at least by what I say when this truthfully and properly expresses what I think I have dreamed, then the question whether what I say I have dreamed *is* what I have dreamed or not simply cannot arise. If I am to misremember a dream, what I say (or think) I have dreamed must be different from what I really have dreamed, but on Malcolm's view the very idea of such a difference is without sense. There is no sense to asking whether an account of a dream "corresponds" to the dream in question, although the account *is* not the dream. For as Malcolm puts it, it is "a matter of definition that someone who [tells] a dream [has] dreamt" (p. 81); and it is similarly "a matter of definition" that someone who says that he

2. Wittgenstein, *Philosophical Investigations*, Part I, Paragraph 580. Future references to the *Investigations* are given in parentheses, as follows: (*PI*, I, 580) for paragraphs in Part I; (*PI*, II, 184) for pages in Part II.

has dreamed that *p* (and is neither lying nor misusing language) *has* dreamed that *p*.

This argument seems to me to be inconclusive at best. For the central notion upon which it turns, that of a *criterion*, remains obscure, despite efforts by Malcolm to explain it (see pp. 59 ff. especially). The relation between a criterion and that of which it is the (or a) criterion, Malcolm says, is a logical relation. But does he mean that the relation is that of logical entailment? In his review of Wittgenstein's *Philosophical Investigations*, Malcolm maintained that Wittgenstein did not think so, and since 'criterion' is a technical concept of Wittgenstein's creation it is reasonable to suppose that this is Malcolm's view as well.[3] On the other hand, it is not clear that what Malcolm said in his review has application to the present case. He noted there that something is a criterion only *in certain circumstances*, and that the number of these circumstances is indefinite. Hence no proposition which merely describes what in the appropriate circumstances *would* be a criterion of some phenomenon *can* entail (a proposition stating) the occurrence of the phenomenon; and no proposition which *does* entail this can be formulated, since it is impossible to specify all the circumstances that might be "appropriate". But as Albritton points out in his discussion of Wittgenstein's use of 'criterion', there is reason to think that this is true only in cases in which there are a number of different criteria (or potential criteria) of the same phenomenon.[4] When something is the only (and hence "defining") criterion of X, Albritton shows, it *is* "a logically necessary and sufficient condition of X" for Wittgenstein, and he further suggests that it may be so *because* it is the only criterion. Now according to Malcolm, "waking testimony" *is* "the sole criterion of dreaming" (p. 81). Hence there is reason to conclude that waking testimony must be "a logically necessary and sufficient condition" of dreaming on his view, i.e. that someone's saying he has dreamed must entail his having dreamed, and saying he has dreamed that *p* must entail his having dreamed that *p*.

3. Malcolm, "Wittgenstein's *Philosophical Investigations*", *Philosophical Review*, 63 (1954), 544 ff.

4. R. Albritton, "On Wittgenstein's Use of the Term 'Criterion' ", *Journal of Philosophy*, 56 (1959), 851.

But if the relation here is that of entailment, then the statement 'Jones says he dreamed that p (and is neither lying nor misusing language), but in truth he didn't dream that p' would be a contradiction, in the same way that 'Jones is a bachelor, but in truth he is married' is a contradiction. And it does not seem to me that this statement is a contradiction, or that it is of a piece with 'Jones is a bachelor, although married'. It may in some sense be absurd to say that Jones reports dreaming one thing but in fact dreamed another, but I do not see that it is self-contradictory. If so, then it cannot be the case that dreams and dream reports are linked by any relation of logical entailment.

But perhaps Malcolm does not, after all, regard the relation between waking testimony and dreams as that of entailment, even though the former is the "sole criterion" of the latter. (Pp. 83 ff. lend some support to this suggestion.) In that case I am afraid I do not understand very well what the relation *is*. The relation is supposed to be logical and not empirical; dreams and dream reports are connected "as a matter of definition" and not merely contingently. And yet we could not *deduce* the occurrence and content of a dream from a dream report (which it seems to me we cannot do anyhow), since the latter would not entail the former. Hence the relation in question would not fit neatly into either of the two classes of relations with which philosophers are familiar, and which they often tend to think are both exclusive and exhaustive. The connection between dreams and dream reports would be neither "analytic" nor "synthetic". Now I do not say that there is no such relation; on the contrary, I am inclined to think that there are logical relations other than that of entailment. Hence I do not say that Malcolm's argument is fallacious on this interpretation of 'criterion'. But I do say that the nature of such relations has yet to be made clear, and that if Malcolm does understand by 'criterion' something other than 'logically necessary and sufficient condition' his argument is inconclusive without an exact account of what this is. Certainly the argument is, in this case, too weak to bear the weight that Malcolm wants to rest upon it. For even he grants that what we must say in consequence of it "seems paradoxical" (p. 55).

286 Vere C. Chappell

I turn now to Malcolm's second line of argument for his view that there is no such thing as misremembering a dream, and no such thing, therefore, as misreporting a dream having misremembered it. The argument runs as follows. Suppose that a dream and a truthful, linguistically proper account of that dream were not logically connected but were "two logically independent things". Then it would be possible to question the *correctness* of the account, to ask whether or not it corresponded to the dream and hence whether or not the person giving the account had remembered his dream, in the sense of remembered it *rightly*. But what does this question imply? Clearly it makes sense to ask a question only if it is possible to answer it. But *is* it possible to answer a question as to the correctness of a dream report? When I give an account of a conversation which I claim to remember, the correctness of my account can be determined, for it can be established that the conversation did run as I say it did—by asking witnesses and so forth. But how is the correctness of an account I give of a dream I have had, how is the correctness of my memory of the dream, to be determined? There seems to be no way of establishing either that my dream did or that it did not go as I say it did or as I claim to remember its doing. No appeal to other people's testimony is possible. Reference to "what is known about me" or to "the circumstances" of my dreaming (I was asleep) is either inconclusive or irrelevant. And if I try to appeal to other memories or impressions of my own I am in the position of the man who, in Wittgenstein's figure, buys "several copies of the morning paper to assure himself that what it said was true" (*PI*, I, 265). As Malcolm says, "there is nothing outside of my account of the dream . . . to determine that my account is right or wrong" (p. 57). It might be supposed that some intrinsic quality of dream-memories themselves, a peculiar clarity or force, is sufficient to guarantee their correctness. If so, we would be able to tell when some memories of dreams were right at least, if not when all were, although we still might have no basis for calling a dream memory wrong. But this will not do, according to Wittgenstein (and presumably to Malcolm as well). For no distinction could be drawn, for any memory with this peculiar quality, between its really *being* right and its only *seeming* to be right. Appearance and reality would coincide, "and that only means that here we can't talk about 'right'" (*PI*, I, 258). We must conclude that the concept of correctness has no application whatsoever to memories of dreams or to one's waking impressions thereof, and no application to accounts of dreams. From this it follows in general that the correctness of a dream report cannot be questioned and that a dream and an account thereof are not "two logically independent things"; and in particular that there is no such thing as misremembering a dream. The *possibility* of misremembering a dream, of remembering it wrongly, is not provided for. Neither, of course, can a dream be remembered rightly. One can remember a dream, but 'remember' here does not, as it does in the normal or in Malcolm's paradigm case, have the force of 'remember rightly'.

What is crucial in this argument can be reduced to a single contention, viz. that no memory or impression, whether of a dream or not, can be correct or incorrect unless there is something "outside" it, and indeed something outside the mind or experience of the person whose memory or impression it is, by which its correctness or incorrectness can be determined. (Hence an appeal to "the dream itself"—which one might otherwise suppose to be "outside" the memory—is ruled out.) Put otherwise, Malcolm's (and Wittgenstein's) claim is that a judgment of correctness can be made only if some *objective* means of establishing correctness, some objective *test* of correctness, is possible, or only if an appeal to some publicly available phenomenon will settle the question of correctness with certainty. Wittgenstein makes the same point in terms of justification: the concept of correctness applies to something only if the judgment that it is correct can be justified, "justification consists in appealing to something independent"—there is no such thing as a "subjective justification" (*PI*, I, 265). Given this central contention, Malcolm's conclusion about dreams follows easily. A dream is private to the person whose dream it is, it is not publicly available, and no objective means of determining whether a dream has occurred or what its content was is logically possible—apart, that is, from the dreamer's subsequent account. But then—on Malcolm's view—this account itself, or a memory or an impression of the dream, can be neither right nor wrong;

the concept of correctness does not apply to it. And from this it follows that dreams are logically dependent upon accounts of dreams or upon people's waking impressions—and also that a dream cannot be misremembered.

It seems to me, however, that the contention underlying these conclusions is mistaken, at least in its general form. I do not deny that memories and impressions of *certain sorts* can be correct (and incorrect) only if some objective means of showing their correctness is possible. But I do not think that *all* memories and impressions must, to be correct or incorrect, be subject to a public check or test. There are some memories, it seems to me, including memories of dreams, of which judgments of correctness can be justified "subjectively", memories, therefore, the applicability to which of the concept of correctness does not require the possibility of an objective test. If so, then this second argument of Malcolm's for the logical interdependence of dreams and waking impressions, and for the impossibility of misremembering dreams, fails, as did the first, and these conclusions at the least have not been established.

On what does Malcolm base his claim that there must, for any memory (or impression) to be correct or incorrect, be some objective means of determining its correctness? He does not undertake to support the claim in his book, but refers to his review of the *Investigations,* where (on pp. 533–34) a defence of it is offered. Malcolm's argument here is built around certain passages in the *Investigations,* paragraphs 56 and 265 of Part I in particular. In these passages Wittgenstein describes particular examples of memory, and tries to show that in each case the memory in question could not be shown to be correct were it not possible to appeal to something "independent", something outside not only the memory itself but the experience of the rememberer. In 56 the thing to be remembered is, first, the colour that a word stands for, and later, the colour that appears when two chemical substances are combined. Wittgenstein's point is that if one had only a memory of the colour—i.e. a memory *image* of (an instance of?) the colour, not a memory *that* the colour was, say, heliotrope—to go on, he could not claim to have remembered it correctly. But in fact there is something besides the memory—there is a sample in the one case, and the possibility of combining bits of the substances in question on occasion (together with the rule that the combination of the same two substances always produces the same colour) in the other—and both of these are "independent" or public things, things which make possible an objective check or test of the memory. The fact that one might decide against his memory upon appealing to the colour sample, or upon combining the chemical substances anew, shows, Wittgenstein says, "that we do not always resort to what memory tells us as the verdict of the highest court of appeal". But his main point is that we could not even bring a particular memory to trial, and so could not judge it as correct or incorrect, were it not possible to appeal beyond memory to something objective or public— the colour sample or particular instances of a certain chemical reaction. Without this possibility we would have no "criterion for remembering [something] right [in a given case]".

In 265 the thing to be remembered is the departure time of a train. The rememberer has one memory of what the time is and then, when questioned as to the correctness of this memory, seeks to check it by producing another memory, in this case the memory of how a page of the time-table looked. Wittgenstein's point here is that this move is successful only because "the mental image of the time-table [can] itelf be *tested* for correctness". And it can only be tested by "appealing to something independent"—the actual time-table, perhaps, or someone else's memory. For if nothing independent were available, the rememberer would have to fall back upon his own memory; he would have to appeal again to memory to test his mental image of the time-table. But such an appeal would only produce another mental image whose own correctness was in question—and this would be like buying "several copies of the morning paper". We have to have, Wittgenstein says, "a memory which is actually *correct*", and we cannot get such a memory as long as we stay within the compass of a single person's experience.

Now I think that Wittgenstein has demonstrated something by means of these two examples, and something important. But I do not think that he has demonstrated, as Malcolm and he himself suppose, that memories (and impressions) in general cannot be tested for correctness, and hence cannot be correct or incorrect, unless it is possible to check them against some public thing, unless, i.e., it is possible to determine their correctness in some objective way. To put my point shortly: Wittgenstein shows that (a) memories of *public* phenomena, and (b) memory *images*, as opposed to memory *beliefs* or memories *that* something is or was the case, can only be correct (or incorrect) if their correctness can be determined by some objective means; for such memories the applicability to them of the concept of correctness does depend upon the possibility at least of submitting them to some objective test or check. The memories cited as examples in paragraphs 56 and 265 of the *Investigations* are instances of both (a) and (b) above.[5] But the memory of a dream is an instance of neither (a) nor (b). Hence my claim is that Wittgenstein's and Malcolm's contention is true for memories of type (a) and of type (b) above, but that it is a mistake to generalize this contention so as to make it apply to all memories, since it is not true of memories of dreams (at least) in particular.

It is clear enough that the memories mentioned in 56 and 265 are memories of public phenomena. Neither the colour of 56 nor the appearance of the time-table page of 265 is, to be sure, a particular event or series of events, and in this respect these examples differ from Malcolm's paradigm, in which what is remembered is a particular conversation. But nor is either a component of anyone's private experience. The colour that goes with this word or that appears when these two substances are combined is not anyone's impression or "sense-datum", but a thing that all can see—or more strictly, since 'the colour . . .' here refers to a universal, a thing whose *instances* all can see and in seeing learn or confirm what the thing (universal) itself is. Similarly, the look of the page of the time-table that is called to mind is something that is available to numbers of people. It is not his own impression of how the page looked, of how it

5. This is not quite accurate, since in paragraph 265 *two* memories are mentioned—the original memory of the departure time of the train and the memory of how the page in the time-table looked—and though both of these are memories of public phenomena, only the latter is a memory image. But it is this latter memory that is used by Wittgenstein to make his main point; see below.

looked to *him*, that the rememberer recalls, but how it *looked*, and this is something that others can observe as well as he.[6] Now there is no doubt that memories of public phenomena— occurrences, objects, facts—are subject to objective tests, if only because what is remembered are public phonomena. And I think that Malcolm and Wittgenstein are right in holding that if no objective test of such a memory were possible, the memory could not, logically, be correct or incorrect. But it does not follow that the memory of a necessarily private phenome- non—a particular sensation or a dream, say—must meet the same condition of objective testability in order to qualify as cor- rect or incorrect. To draw this conclusion from Wittgenstein's examples seems to me to go against Malcolm's own admonition in *Dreaming*, that we "be mindful of . . . how sharply [the use of 'remembering' in 'remembering a dream'] differs from the use of 'remembering' that appeared in our paradigm" (p. 57). As Malcolm says, "there is no warrant for thinking that 're- membering a dream' carries exactly the same implications as 'remembering a physical occurrence' " (p. 58). Hence Malcolm's own precept would seem to forbid the inference that because certain conditions must be satisfied for a memory of a "physical occurrence" to be right or wrong, the same conditions must be satisfied for a memory of a dream to be right or wrong— especially when the conditions are such that they cannot, in the nature of the case, be satisfied.

But not only are the memories mentioned in paragraphs 56 and 265 of the *Investigations* memories of public phenomena; both are also memory *images*, as opposed to memories *that* something is so, or what are sometimes called memory *beliefs*. Actually, two different memories are discussed in 265, (1) the original memory of the departure time of the train, and (2) the

---

6. Of course he might also have recalled how it looked to him, and Wittgen- stein's words in 265 make it possible that this is what is meant—except that then it is hard to see how anyone could offer a memory of this as corroboration of the original memory in favour of the memory of how the page looked, which is different, *inter alia*, just in being a public thing. Wittgenstein might also have had his rememberer call to mind how the page in the time-table *looks*, which is different again, in that then the memory would be of a universal and not of a particular occasion, or of something that essentially figures in a particular oc- casion, as how the time-table *looked* would do.

memory appealed to for corroboration of this, the memory of how a page of the time-table looked. The first of these (*"that the train leaves at 3:10"*) is not a memory image, but it is also not this memory that Wittgenstein employs to make his main point in the paragraph. Regarding this original memory, Wittgenstein claims that it can be corroborated by an appeal to memory, an appeal to another memory of the same remem-berer. Such an appeal might seem to constitute a "subjective" corroboration, but in fact does not, Wittgenstein maintains, because the memory appealed to, the memory of how the page of the time-table looked, can "itself be tested for correctness". But now this second memory—and this I take to be Wittgen-stein's main point in 265—could not be tested for correctness unless it could in turn be checked against some "independent" thing, something outside the rememberer's experience or memory. Why is this? The answer is evidently meant to be con-veyed by the analogy of the morning paper. But it is not imme-diately clear just what this answer is.

What is absurd about buying "several copies of the morning paper to assure [oneself] that what is said was true"? Obviously, it is the fact that each copy bears the same relation to the events reported in the paper that all the others do, so that any mistake or inaccuracy appearing in one would also appear in every other. Each merely reproduces every other, or the original from which all derive; none is different in any way from any other. Hence an appeal to another copy of the paper would provide no basis whatsoever for checking the truth of what was said in a given copy; such an appeal would only turn up an-other instance of the thing whose truth was to be checked. Wittgenstein must then be saying that the same would hold of the memory of how the page in the time-table looked if it could not be tested against something outside the rememberer's memory or experience. His view must be that if the remem-berer tried to test his memory of how the page looked by call-ing up another memory—and no objective test were possible—this new memory would bear the same relation to how the page did look that the memory being tested does. The new memory might or might not be an exact replica of the first memory; here the morning paper analogy would seem not to hold. But in either case the new memory would have the same status as the first. It would itself be something to be tested for correctness, in the same way and for the same reason that the first memory is, and not something by which the latter could be tested.

Now I think this view is plausible. But I also think its plausibility depends on the fact that the memory in question here is a memory image, and not a memory belief or memory that something is so; and I do not see that Wittgenstein's point holds good for memories in general. To remember something by forming a memory image of it is to visualize it, to form a picture of it in one's mind. Such a memory is correct if it "corresponds" with or is a good "likeness" of what is remembered. One way to determine or test the correctness of such a memory is to "compare" it with what is remembered—in whatever way one does "compare" images with reality. But this procedure is only possible if the remembered thing is available at the time the test is to be carried out. And the remembered thing will not be available if it has stopped existing or cannot be made to exist again. It will also not be available if the question whether the same remembered thing exists at the later time cannot be answered definitely, if, that is, there are no clear criteria of identity through time for the supposedly remembered thing, or no clear way of applying such criteria. This means, I think, that the remembered thing must be a publicly observable phenomenon, an enduring or at least repeatable object or something esentially connected with such an object, for this way of testing the correctness of a memory image to be carried out. And this in turn means that an objective test of the correctness of the memory will be possible whenever this way of testing can be used; to use this way will indeed be to perform an objective test.

So far, then, Wittgenstein's point seems sound. The correctness of a memory image cannot be determined in the way described unless an objective test of its correctness is possible. But there is another way in which the correctness of a memory image can be determined or tested, viz. by forming another memory image of the same remembered thing and then comparing the two memories. If the two correspond, then the correctness of the first may be established or confirmed. But only may be, for there is another condition that must be satisfied if this procedure is to have any weight as a test of correctness. This is that the two memories be different from each other in some way other than just numerically. For if the second memory is an exact replica of the first it is no better than another copy of the morning paper; the second may indeed be a copy of the first. The second memory must derive directly from the remembered thing, or by a different route; it must present a different view, as it were, from that of the first memory, and the only evidence that it does so is that it differs in content from the first. Of course, the two memories must not be so different that they can no longer be said to correspond. But 'correspondence' must not be construed to mean 'exact similarity' or 'identity in all respects and circumstances'. The two memories might, e.g., be memories of the same thing at different times or in different lights or in relation to different things and so on. Normally, one's different memory images of the same thing do differ in such ways; one's memory of a face, e.g., usually includes an ability to call to mind several different pictures of the face, pictures different because they are pictures of the face itself under different conditions. For the most part, therefore, one is able to check the correctness of a memory image by calling up another memory image of the same thing and comparing the two.

There are cases, however, in which the correctness of a memory image cannot be determined in this way. For there are cases in which the condition that the two memories compared be different and yet memories of the same remembered thing cannot be satisfied. One such case is provided by Wittgenstein's colour example in paragraph 56 of the *Investigations*. A second memory image of the colour that a certain word stands for would necessarily be exactly like the first; if it were different in any way it would not be an image of the same colour. This is so because the remembered thing here, the colour, is a sort of logical "simple"; it has no conceptual articulation, no internal structure or concatenation of discriminable elements or aspects. Hence there is only one way in which an image of such a thing can be correct, can truly represent it; there are no different sides from which or respects in which it might be viewed or pictured. The correctness of a memory image of such a thing therefore cannot be tested by comparing it with another memory image of the same thing. To make such a comparison would be like buying several copies of the morning paper.

If now there are no other ways of determining the correctness of a memory image than the two I have mentioned, then the correctness of memories such as that discussed in *Investigations* 56 can only be tested objectively, by comparing them directly with the things remembered, or with something essentially connected to them—the sample or the chemical reaction in Wittgenstein's colour example.[7] And I think there are no other ways than these two. Certainly no appeal to another person's memory is possible, since there is no such thing as comparing two different people's images. And an appeal to a memory belief of the same rememberer would be successful only if the belief had some image associated with it or if it called up such an image, a memory image of the same remembered thing but different from the memory being tested in some significant way, in which case the test would actually consist in the comparison of the two images; this is so because beliefs and images are, strictly speaking, incommensurable. We may conclude, therefore, that for memory images of things like colours, if no objective test of their correctness were possible, then no test at all would be possible, no way of determining their correctness, and the very concept of correctness would have no application to them. Of course the colour in paragraph 56 is a public thing, or something essentially connected with public things, and so the correctness of a memory of it can be determined, even though it be a memory image. But what is true of colours as objects of memory, what I have called their logical simplicity or lack of conceptual articulation, seems also to be true of such private phenomena as sensations and feelings; they too have no internal structure, no sides or aspects to be

7. The qualification is necessary here because the thing remembered in 56, the colour, is, strictly speaking, a universal, and not a particular object. The connection of the colour first with the sample and then with the chemical reaction is *essential* because it is by means of these particulars, the one a simple enduring object and the other a series of similar discrete events, that the universal in question is *specified*.

distinguished and separately referred to and pictured. Hence if such things were not essentially connected with public phenomena, with behaviour, speech, and circumstances, memory images of them could not be tested for correctness, and so could not be said to be correct—from which in turn all sorts of unwelcome consequences ensue. (This I take to be the crux of Wittgenstein's so-called "private language argument" respecting sensations and the like, an argument which I am inclined to regard as sound.)

But what of the memory discussed in paragraph 265 of the *Investigations*, that of how the page of the time-table looked? The object of memory here certainly cannot be said to lack conceptual articulation, to be logically simple in the way that the colour of 56 is. And yet it is supposed to be impossible to test the memory for correctness if the possibility of an objective test is ruled out. The trouble here, I think, is this. The memory in question is a memory image, and hence there are only two ways in which its correctness could be determined. The first of these ways, comparison with the thing remembered, is ruled out by the stipulation that no objective test be possible, and we are then thrown back on the second way, comparison with another memory image of the same thing. But the unavoidable consequence of ruling out an objective test of the original memory is to make the thing remembered, how the page looked, a necessarily private phenomenon, something that only the rememberer even could have access to. And this means, not that a second memory of the same thing could not be *different* from the original memory—as would be the case if the object of memory were a peculiar sensation, say—but rather that no second memory, different or not, of the *same* thing could exist or at any rate be known to exist. There are no criteria of sameness (or, perhaps, no ways of applying such criteria) for necessarily private objects, so that the question whether a given memory image is a memory of the same such object that another memory is a memory of cannot be decided. And this rules out the possibility of testing the correctness of memories of such objects whether they are conceptually articulated or not.

I grant, then, that Wittgenstein has made his point concerning his examples in paragraphs 56 and 265 of the *Investigations*.

I think he has shown that the memories discussed in these paragraphs could not be correct or incorrect if an objective test of their correctness were not possible. But he is able to show this, I believe, because these memories are memory images; his case succeeds only because his examples have features peculiar to memories of this sort. Memory beliefs, or memories that something is so, are quite different from memory images. First, to have a memory belief is not to visualize anything or have a picture in one's mind, but to entertain a proposition; hence memory beliefs can be stated, whereas memory images can only be described. Second, the correctness of a memory belief consists not in its being a good likeness of or corresponding point for point with its object, but rather in its being *true*. This is so because the object of a memory of this kind is not a picturable thing but a fact or proposition. Hence, third, there is no possibility of comparing a memory belief with some thing in order to establish its correctness; at best one may examine a thing in order to determine whether a memory belief is true of it. Fourth, although two memory beliefs may be compared for the purpose of determining the correctness of one of them, correctness is not shown by their correspondence or resemblance but rather by their logical "accord", by their supporting one another evidentially or fitting together as parts of a single coherent description or story. Fifth, one person's memory beliefs may be confronted with another's, so that inter-subjective comparisons are possible. And there are doubtless other differences than these. But these are, I think, sufficient to make the application of Wittgenstein's point, which holds for memory images, to memory beliefs unwarranted at best, and I do not see that it would hold for memories in general.

Hence, although I grant Wittgenstein's success in paragraphs 56 and 265, I do not think he has established the position that Malcolm needs in order to prove his thesis about dreams, and the remembering of dreams.* For the memory of a dream is neither a memory of a public phenomenon nor a memory image (or series of memory images), and these are the only two sorts of memory for which, as far as I can see, Wittgenstein's position has been established. This means, then, that Wittgenstein's arguments in paragraphs 56 and 265 provide no basis

298 Vere C. Chappell

for concluding that the memory of a dream cannot be tested for correctness in a subjective way, and hence cannot *be* correct or incorrect.

There is no doubt that the memory of a dream is not a memory of a public phenomenon; the dream I had last night is not something that anyone else could (logically) have witnessed. But it may be questioned whether the memory of a dream does not, after all, stand to the remembered dream as the memory of the colour in *Investigations* 56 and the memory of how the page of the time-table looked in 265 stand to their respective objects. It may be thought, that is, that the memory of a dream is a memory image, or series of images, and that it does therefore merely reproduce the dream. But this is a mistake: a dream has the form of a series of events which the dreamer witnesses or takes part in. As Malcolm himself says, "a *dream* is supposed to involve a number of incidents connected in some fashion. Telling a dream is telling a kind of *story*"; the report of a dream is a "narrative of incidents" (p. 85). Dreams *come*, if I may so put it, conceptually articulated. This is shown by the very fact that I *tell* my dreams and do not *describe* them; furthermore, the words that I use in telling them are adequate to convey what I dreamed, as they would not be were I describing a series of appearances or were my waking impressions of my dreams a series of images. Malcolm's own arguments in the first part of *Dreaming* establish, I think, that a dream is not composed of images, and it seems to me to follow from this that the memory of a dream is not itself an image or anything like an image. Of course there may be a part or an aspect of a dream—a peculiar flavour or quality pervading or present in it—the memory of which *is* a memory image and which *does* merely reproduce that of which it is the memory; there may be elements in dreams which are like appearances or images or sensations. But these *are* not the dream, they do not constitute *what* I dream and are not what I *tell* when I tell my dream. And Malcolm's thesis has to do with what I dream and what I tell upon awakening, and not with any of my dream's special features.

So far I have claimed that Malcolm's (and Wittgenstein's) arguments do not establish that memories of dreams cannot be tested for correctness in a subjective way, that they cannot therefore be tested for correctness at all, and that they cannot, further, be correct or incorrect. If I am right in this, then these arguments also fail to establish Malcolm's thesis, that dreams and waking impressions are logically connected and that there is no such thing as misremembering a dream. But now I must try to say what a subjective test of the correctness of the memory of a dream would actually be like, for otherwise my claim remains negative and merely speculative. Suppose, then, I claim to remember the occurrence of a certain sequence of events, E, in a dream that I have had; I have a memory (or putative memory) of E's having happened in my dream. And suppose that I want for some reason to make sure that my memory is correct, that E did happen in my dream and that it happened in the way that I remember, or seem to remember, its doing. (There seems, by the way, to be no obvious absurdity in my wanting to do this, whereas on Malcolm's view it would be absurd.) How might I proceed? One thing I would do is try to remember the events that preceded and succeeded E in my dream, so as to see whether, and if so how, E "fitted in" with them. Suppose, e.g., that E consists of the following events (this is what I remember): (in my dream) I boarded a train, the California Zephyr, carrying a heavy suitcase; I walked forward to the Dome Car and took a seat on the right hand side of the dome, next to a woman who turned out to be the teacher I had had in second grade; as I was sitting down the woman said, "Young man, if you don't get rid of that suitcase I'll scream". Now to make sure that all of this did happen in my dream and in this way—that it was the *California* Zephyr I boarded, that I carried a *suitcase*, that I walked *forward* on the train, that it was my *second*-grade teacher that I sat next to, that she said she would *scream*—I would try to call to mind what else happened in the dream. What happened before I boarded the train? Well I remember myself hurrying down a station platform, and yes, it was Union Station, which is where the California Zephyr leaves from. And there was a porter who said *"California Zephyr"* as I passed, and who asked if he couldn't carry my *suitcase* for me. And I walked only as far as the last car of the train so I must have walked *forward* when I got on. As for what happened after that, I remember that the woman did scream, and that a great crowd of people clustered round, so she must have *said* that she would scream. So far everything *fits* with what I remember, and to that extent I consider my original memory to be confirmed. The fit of my original memory with these other memories corroborates the former and increases my confidence that it is correct. The appeal to these other memories provides a check upon my initial memory, and gives me a basis, a reason, for thinking it correct—it even serves to justify my confidence that it is correct.[8]

8. Here Malcolm comments: "Your account of how you would confirm your memory of a dream as right seems fantastic to me. You confirm, for example, that it was the California Zephyr you boarded, because in the dream you went to Union Station, since the Zephyr does leave from Union Station this supports your memory of the dream. What a hodge-podge of dream and reality! The Zephyr leaves from Union Station: but does it leave from Union Station in dreams? It might or might not. It might leave from a filling station. It depends on the dream. If the dream does not make it clear, then there is no sense in arguing *probabilities*. If you don't clearly remember whether it was the Zephyr you boarded in your dream, then it is *objectively* not clear.

"Suppose that while speaking to you about an old friend, I see him in my mind for a moment. I tell you so. Suppose you asked: 'In your image was he wearing a necktie?' Suppose that I do not recall whether he was or was not. Should I think: 'Probably he was because he usually did?' This would be another improper mixture. When I say, immediately after having the image, 'I don't recall whether he did or didn't have a necktie', that remark belongs to the description of the image, I am inclined to say. It is an *internal* description of the image. It means that the image was indefinite in this respect.

"If a child claimed that the Zephyr left from this filling station yesterday, you could tell him that this couldn't be so, because there are no railroad tracks at that station and a train has to run on tracks, and there has not been time enough for the tracks to be taken away, and no evidence that there have recently been tracks in this street, and so on. But you cannot talk to him in a similar way if he says that in his dream the train left from the filling station. In a dream a train does not have to run on tracks, and there is no 'usually' about it".

I have two things to say here in answer to Malcolm. First, my California Zephyr dream was not intended to be an instance of a dream that is "objectively not clear", but rather of a dream that was itself clear but has in part been forgotten or misremembered. I agree that "if the dream does not make it clear [where the train left from] then there is no sense in arguing probabilities". But in my case the dream *does* make it clear; I just cannot *remember* where the train left from, or am not *sure* about what I seem to remember. Of course Malcolm would deny that there is this difference here. He would deny that there is any such case as that I describe, as opposed to a case in which the dream is "objectively not clear"; he suggests indeed that one's not clearly remembering a dream is just the same as the dream's not being clear. But this is just the point that is at issue between us. Second, my resort to "probabilities" and to the usual connections between things was designed to help me remember my *own* dream,

So far I have mentioned one possible means of checking, subjectively, the correctness of one's memory of a dream. Another is this. In my memory (or putative memory) of the dream events *E*, related above, only certain details stand out or are explicit. I might try to check the correctness of my memory of these details by trying to remember other details that occurred within the same sequence *E*, to see whether the former and the latter fit with one another, or "went together", or were in accord. How about the woman I sat next to on the train? I remember (or seem to remember) that she was my old second-grade teacher and that she said something to me. But what was she like, what sort of features did she have, how was she dressed, etc.? I am able to remember that (in my dream) she was wearing glasses and had grey hair and a hook nose—yes, then, that was my second-grade and not my third-grade teacher, whom I remember (literally, not in my dream) as young and clear-eyed and decidedly pretty, whereas I always (outside of dreams) think of my second-grade teacher as old and hook-nosed and wearing glasses.[9] So the new memory, of a suppressed or overlooked detail, corroborates the original memory (or part of it), that it was my second-grade teacher whom I sat next to on the train. The one memory corroborates the other because the two do accord with one another. This accord does not, of course, *prove* the correctness of the one, but it provides some basis for preferring the view that the original memory is correct to the view that it is not. And this is all that is essential for the memory to have been checked or tested, or at any rate for the concept of correctness to apply to it.

Here, then, are two particular procedures for checking the correctness of one's memories of a dream that one has had, and procedures which are, as they must be, purely subjective. They are procedures—and there may be others as well—yield-

---

not to enable me to determine the content of someone *else's* dream or to inform another person as to what *couldn't* have been so in a dream of his. This difference is, I think, crucial.

9. Notice that the question whether someone (or something) I dream about is a certain person (or thing) is decided by determining whether he (or it) has the characteristics that I *think* (literally, *not* in my dream) of that person (or thing) as having, not whether he (or it) has the characteristics that that person (or thing) in fact *does* have.

ing a result that makes application of the concept of correctness possible, even if they do not yield conclusive proofs or sometimes, even, any result at all. But they are sufficient for the notion of correctness to gain a foothold; people do in fact regard them as checks or tests of the correctness of memories of dreams, and do in fact employ them as such. And it is legitimate for people to do so. The situation here is not like that of a man who buys several copies of the same edition of the morning paper but rather like that of a man who buys several different papers carrying accounts by different reporters of the same sequence of events. The fact that Beckett's description of a riot in the *Post* tallies with Malone's in the *Star,* both reporters having witnessed the scene, gives me some reason to believe that Malone's account, which I first read by itself, is correct; the agreement of the two accounts corroborates the one, and justifies my confidence in its correctness, to some extent at least.

There is, however, an objection that may be made to treating different memories of a single dream event as an analogue to different reporters' accounts of a single public event. The agreement of two reporters' accounts does provide a basis for believing them both to be right, it may be said, but only because the things reporters write about, public events, are governed by certain principles and rules—laws of logic and of nature, regularities of human behaviour and motivation, and the like— principles guaranteeing or making it likely that certain connections will hold between and within events. Without such principles, without such connections to rely on, there would be no basis for inferring that, if the things reported by one witness happened, then the things reported by the other witness must have happened too, or probably did; and it is on this inference that the judgment of correctness rests. But the things that happen in a dream seem not to be governed by such principles; dream events seem not to be connected in any regular, predictable way. Malcolm says: "In a dream I can do the impossible in every sense of the word. I can climb Everest without oxygen and I can square the circle" (p. 57). Surely, if contradictions can occur in dreams, no inference from any dream event or detail of any dream event to any other has the slightest warrant. Hence the fact that two memories of a dream event accord or fit with one another has no tendency whatsoever to show that one or the other of them is correct.

This objection, however, will not stand. In the first place, it is not the case, despite what Malcolm says, that in a dream I can do what is *logically* impossible. I cannot square the circle in a dream. I might do something in a dream that in the dream I *call* "squaring the circle". But this *is* not squaring the circle, even in my dream, as is shown by the fact that I would not, in telling my dream, normally *say* that I had squared the circle; I would say rather that in my dream I *thought* I was squaring or had squared the circle, or *said* to myself that that is what I was doing, or some such. If I cannot know what something would be like, as I cannot if the thing in question is a "contradiction in terms", then I cannot report the occurrence of that thing in a dream. The best I can do is report the utterance by someone of the contradictory terms, the putative name or a putative description of the thing; or else the occurrence in myself of the contradictory thought of the thing—in the dream.[10] And secondly, though it is true that anything, save what is logically impossible, is *possible* in a dream, it is not the case that the events in a dream occur in no regular order and exemplify no familiar pattern of connections among themselves. Malcolm acknowl-

---

10. Malcolm comments here as follows: "You seem to me to be wrong about contradiction. A man could tell you that he *knew*, in his dream, that he had squared the circle. He does not have to say that he *thought* he did, or *said* he did. Just as he can say that he knew that the lady on horseback in his dream was his mother. He does not have to say that he thought it was. In fact, these would be different accounts of the dream.

" 'If I cannot know what something would be like . . . then I cannot report the occurrence of that thing in a dream.' Moore, in a dream, mistook a table for a proposition. Did he 'know what that was like'? On your view he should have said: 'In my dream I thought I mistook a table for a proposition'. But how could he even *think* he did something with regard to which he did not 'know what that was like'? If your principle were a genuine principle, it ought to even keep him from reporting that in his dream he *thought* he squared the circle".

I think my position is damaged by Malcolm's counter-attack, but not totally destroyed. I am inclined to stick by my main claim while granting that my explanation and attempted justification of it are faulty. Certainly I must abandon the "principle" to which Malcolm refers—even though there is a difference between mistaking a proposition for a table and squaring the circle (the former is not logically impossible). And I do not know what to put in its place. Nonetheless, I am still convinced that one cannot, in a dream, do what is logically impossible.

edges that a dream "is supposed to involve a number of incidents connected in some fashion" (p. 85), and it is just not
true that the connections are unique and peculiar, *sui generis*,
for each different dream. The patterns in which dream events
occur, especially the more general patterns, are those of the
real world of our waking life—things happen in temporal
sequence, move by passing through intermediate points (at
least sometimes), preserve their identities (at least for a while),
exhibit their familiar accidental features as well as their necessary defining properties, behave in characteristic ways (at least
for the most part), and so on. When something bizarre or "impossible" (by waking standards) does happen in a dream it is
against the background of such and other familiar patterns.
The connections are looser in a dream, to be sure; the patterns
are more often broken or transformed. But there are connections, enough to justify inferences from one dream event to
another, and hence to support judgments of the correctness of
memories of dream events. For even in waking life the familiar
connections and patterns are broken; people do behave un-
characteristically and capriciously, and yet we do not suppose
that our predictions about what they will do or our hypotheses
about what they have done are therefore altogether baseless.

I hope now to have shown that Malcolm's claim that there is
no such thing as misremembering a dream, and with it his general thesis that dreams and dream reports are logically connected, is not established by what I have called his second line
of argument, involving the concept of correctness, any more
than it is by the first line, which turns upon the notion of a criterion. And I conclude that both claim and thesis, as presented
by Malcolm in his book, are unfounded. But it also seems to
me, in addition, that both are false, and I want now, briefly, to
try to show that they are. Since the claim about remembering
dreams is a logical consequence of the wider thesis about the
connection between dreams and waking impressions or reports,
I can show the falsity of both by showing the falsity of the
former alone.

To do this I shall rely upon two arguments, one based upon
the ordinary use of the phrase 'remember a dream' and one
consisting in an appeal to an actual case. First, then, as to the
use of 'remember a dream'. It is important to note that not

every case of someone's *telling* a dream is a case of someone's *remembering* a dream. Often, indeed usually, when I wake up and give an account of a dream I have just had I am not remembering my dream at all—I am just telling it. It is only in special circumstances that I remember my dreams. I remember a dream, e.g., if I cannot just tell it on awakening, straight off, but have to think or make an effort of some kind in order to be able to say what it was that I dreamed; I remember if the effort is successful. On the other hand, making such an effort seems not to be necessary to remembering a dream; I also remember if, having no impression that or what I dreamed on a particular occasion, it suddenly just occurs to me that I dreamed or that I dreamed that such and such. In any case, remembering a dream is an achievement, a triumph over uncertainty or ignorance, and the fact that I can remember a dream at all implies that I can be uncertain and ignorant about the existence and content of dreams; the words 'remember a dream' are *used* in this way. Further, the ignorance and uncertainty that are removed when I remember a dream constitute my *not* remembering it, so the fact that I can remember dreams implies that I can not remember them as well. Of course, not remembering may not be misremembering, since not remembering includes failing to remember as well as remembering wrongly—just as remembering includes both getting something and getting it right. And it may be that in all cases of remembering a dream the achievement represents a victory over ignorance simply, and not over error or even uncertainty. I do not think that this is true, but if it is, then (a) my present argument does not show that misremembering of dreams occurs but only at most that failing to remember them does—in which case I must rest my case against Malcolm entirely on my second argument, below; and (b) even so, my argument does show that failing to remember a dream is possible, and this may be enough to destroy Malcolm's general thesis about the connection between dreams and dream reports. For if this thesis is true, then even failing to remember (and then remembering) a dream that one has had ought not to be possible.

My second argument against Malcolm consists in showing that cases of misremembering dreams in fact do occur, or rather—since no philosophical demonstration of a matter of fact is possible—that there is no logical reason why such cases should not occur, since they can be described in logically impeccable terms. Since Malcolm's claim is the logical one that no such thing as misremembering a dream can possibly occur, it is sufficient to describe one such case. Suppose, then, that I am telling a dream and I say that the sequence of events which I called *E* above—my boarding the California Zephyr, etc.—occurred in my dream. If I am just telling my dream then, as I argued a moment ago, I am not *remembering* that *E* occurred. But now suppose that in the course of reporting *E* I falter; things seem for a moment to be a bit uncertain, and I am not altogether sure, say, that it was a woman whom I sat next to in the Dome Car and who spoke to me. I reflect for a moment, trying to get clear, and then it does seem clear to me—it was a woman, my old second-grade teacher in fact. It just *comes* clear to me; I do not first get the impression that it was a woman and then corroborate this impression by appealing to some other impression, or to some memory of some other event in my dream to see how it fits with this impression. Hence I say "I remember", not "I seem to remember" or "I think that it was a woman"; and this is a case in which I do remember (something in) my dream, or at least in which I think I remember my dream. Suppose now that I go on with the telling of my dream. I begin to recount what happened next, after I sat down next to the woman (as I now believe it to be, having remembered that it was a woman). But what I want to say is that I had an interesting conversation with the *man* sitting next to me about his work as a deep-sea diver. But this cannot be; it was a *woman* that I sat next to. So I pause again; my memory that it was a woman does not fit with my present impression that it was a man. So I think about that, and after recalling details of our conversation, conclude that it was a man; my present memory—for it now is a memory and not just my immediate impression—is correct. But then this means that my earlier memory, that it was a woman I sat next to, is incorrect. I was unsure to begin with; then I remembered, or thought I remembered, but I must have been wrong; I remembered wrongly or misremembered. And so I go back and revise my account—it was a man I sat next to on the train, and I don't know where I got the idea that it was my second-grade teacher (and then I may remember that that came from another dream—or I may not).

Here, then, it seems to me, is a case of misremembering a dream the description of which is free of any logical fault, and a case, furthermore, which could actually occur. It may be said that my conclusion, that my first memory was wrong, was un-warranted, that I had no business deciding that, since my later memory was of a man, my first memory of a woman must have been wrong. For—it may be said—both memories could have been right; people change identities in dreams, or one person fades into another or simply is replaced by another, without notice. True enough, but this does not always happen, and when it does we (often) remember that it does—else how would we know that this sort of thing does happen in dreams? Hence I do not say that the judgment of incorrectness here is final, or that it is made on very firm grounds. I am only claiming that the judgment is possible, that people do make such judgments, and that in the case that I have described the judgment is one that I myself might well have made. I do not see that I would have to be confused, unaware of the logical proprieties, in order to do so—as on Malcolm's view I would.

But there is a final qualification that I must make. It is just possible that Malcolm would allow the case that I have just de-scribed, i.e. would grant that such a case could occur, whether or not he would want to call it a case of misremembering a dream. For he says that "I may amend [an account of a dream] slightly on a second telling" (p. 57), and this seems to imply that some change of mind on the part of a dream teller is provided for in the concept of telling a dream. If so, then my case would not constitute a counter-example to Malcolm's claim, and my inclination to speak of my rejection of the one account in fa-vour of the other in terms of the incorrectness of the former could be explained away as a piece of uncritical analogising, the product of a tendency to over-emphasize similarities and over-look differences, whereas in fact the terms I use, if taken liter-ally, commit me to logical nonsense. Perhaps; but Malcolm also says that I may amend the account of a dream "only slightly" on a second telling: "if I changed it very much or many times it would no longer be said that I was 'telling a dream' " (*ibid.*). The question is, how much is "very much" and how many times are "many times"? Malcolm does not answer this question, and I do not see that he could answer it. But the resulting uncertainty threatens his claim in a new way. Malcolm may save his point by refusing to treat my case as a genuine counter-example; it then does not follow that, as I have argued, his claim is false. But if Malcolm did this very much or many times, then we could legitimately suspect that he was making his claim true by definition—in which case it would no longer command our attention as a point of any significance. This is the old Scylla and Charybdis of original philosophers, of whom Malcolm certainly is one: on the one hand, falsehood through conflict with plain facts, on the other, triviality through tautology. Perhaps, after all, Malcolm has steered clear; I am a good deal less confident that he has not than the tone of much of this paper would indicate.[11]

11. Malcolm's comment on this final paragraph is as follows: "My view was not meant to deny that a person can have a dream but fail to remember what it was, or that he can forget a dream, or that he can misremember a dream. All of these notions have a sense that is compatible with my basic doctrine that the concept of dreams is based on the telling of dreams.

"As far as misremembering is concerned, I may tell a dream and then later tell it in a way that disagrees with the original telling. If the original telling was immediately after waking, and the second telling a month later, this would surely be called misremembering: the original telling would be taken as the criterion of what the dream was. More interesting, perhaps, is the case in which a person *revises* his account in the original telling. Your conjecture . . . is right: I think we would say that when a person wavers in the first telling, then corrects himself, and finally comes down firmly on a somewhat different account, which he now stands by—I should say that we would say that at first he misremembered his dream and then remembered it correctly. Here the basis for determining what the dream was is still the telling of it. This sort of thing happens and we call it telling a dream, and with regard to what he first said and then amended we would say: 'At first he did not tell it right' or 'At first he did not remember it exactly right'. But if I had talked like this: 'I dreamt of a man on a horse riding up the steps: no, that is wrong, it was a dream of a cat and a bird talking outside my window: no, now I have it right, it was a baseball game and I was at bat: no, . . . etc.'—no one would say that I was telling a dream. This illustrates both 'too much' and 'too many'.

"You then make a remark which I find puzzling. 'Malcolm may save his point by refusing to treat my case as a genuine counter-example'. Counter-example of what? Your case was an example of misremembering, as it applies to a dream. Of course I accept such a case. 'But if Malcolm did this very much or many times, then we could legitimately suspect that he was making his claim true by definition'. I do not understand you. What claim? That one cannot misremember a dream? I do not make that claim".

14

CHARLES LANDESMAN

Dreams: Two Types of Explanations

In his monograph *Dreaming*, Norman Malcolm argues that dreams are not identical with or composed of phenomena such as thoughts, judgments, impressions, feelings, images, presentations, or any episodes,[1] processes, and states which are designated by mental nouns. He argues first that any observation of a person which would show that any such mental phenomena were occurring would be inconsistent with that person's being asleep, and second that the sleeper's testimony upon awakening could never establish these occurrences (pp. 37–43). He then claims that their presence could not be established by physiological phenomena. For suppose that when a person is awake, whenever he reports that he is making, say, a judgment, it is ascertained that a certain brain event is taking place and that the event does not take place in the absence of a judgment. Suppose also that the same type of event occurs while he is asleep. Could we say then that the person was making a judgment in his sleep? No, for "the attempt to extend the inductive reasoning to the case of sleeping persons could yield a conclusion that was logically impossible of confirmation. It would be impossible to know whether this conclusion was true or false" (p. 43).

From this passage it would seem that Malcolm accepts the

Reprinted from *Philosophical Studies*, 15 (1964), 17–23, by permission of the publisher (D. Reidel Publishing Co., Dordrecht).
1. Norman Malcolm, *Dreaming* (New York: Humanities Press, 1959). The page references in parentheses are to this work.

following principle (P): if two types of events x and y have been ascertained to occur together in a number of instances, then, if an instance of x is known to occur, we are justified in inferring that an instance of y also occurs only if it is logically possible to verify that y occurs independently of the occurrence of x. Now the scope and mode of application of P is significantly ambiguous. Consider that at some time a person says something to himself (while fully awake) but neither communicates what he said to anyone nor records it in any way. Later he remembers (or seems to remember) what he said. Can his memory judgment be justified according to P? One might argue that it cannot, because the hypothesis excludes the possibility of there being any access to the event other than his putative memory. But one might reason to the contrary that it can be justified because saying something to oneself is the sort of event such that it is logically possible that there be independent evidence for it. But again one might reason that it cannot, for saying something to oneself without leaving any record at all is the sort of event such that it is logically impossible that there be independent evidence for it. What the results of applying P turn out to be depends upon how the event is described; what is or what is not possible depends upon our choice of description. Consider now the case of making a judgment while asleep, a judgment whose presence we are trying to test by physiological evidence. If we describe it by the phrase "a judgment made while asleep," then according to P (and Malcolm's arguments) it is logically impossible to have independent evidence for it. But if we describe it simply by "a judgment" then this is the sort of thing for which we can have independent evidence. An advocate of the view that dreams may consist of judgments will argue that the inaccessibility of judgments made while asleep is a contingent matter in respect to the species 'judgment' just as the inaccessibility of an instance of talking to oneself is a contingent matter in respect to the species 'talking to oneself,' and that the validity of Malcolm's argument hinges upon the arbitrary decision to include the contingent inaccessibility within the description of the event itself so as to make its inaccessibility a logical matter. It would be begging the question to reply that the inaccessibility of judgments made while asleep is not contingent, for this reply would represent a *decision* to determine contingency or the lack of it by reference to the subspecies rather than the species of event. What is possible or impossible relative to some *x* is a function not merely of the *x*-in-itself but also of our choice of description. Describing someone as a bachelor excludes the possibility of his being married, but describing him as a man does not.

Because of the difficulty in formulating a nonarbitrary application of P, it would be better if we could find another sort of argument to support Malcolm's rejection of the view that dreams consist of mental phenomena. Now, there is an argument at which he hints in several places (e.g., pp. 51–52) but which he does not employ as his major thrust, for it entails a weaker conclusion. The premise is that dreaming is an intentional 'act' like hoping, expecting, believing, and the like; that is, these are 'acts' whose objects do not necessarily exist. From the fact that someone hopes for something, it does not follow that it will occur; from the fact that someone is expecting another to arrive, it does not follow that he will arrive; from the fact that someone believes something to be so, it does not follow that it is so; and finally from the fact that someone dreams that so-and-so happened, it does not follow that it did happen. Obviously if I dream that I have murdered my friend, it does not follow that I did murder him. By parity of reasoning, if I dream that I was judging, thinking, or imagining something, it does not follow that I was judging, thinking, or imagining at all. It is important here to note that the lack of entailment between "dreaming *x*" and "the existence of *x*" is due to the concept of dreaming and not to the nature of *x*. Hence the existence of *x* does not follow from the dreaming of *x* no matter whether *x* is a physical or mental phenomenon.

Now suppose someone claims that his dreams must consist in part of mental phenomena because he remembers making a judgment while dreaming. The argument then is that if it was a judgment that he dreamt he was making, it does not follow that he was making a judgment at all, and if it was a judgment he actually made and not merely dreamt he made, then it does not follow that the judgment was part of his dream. The conclusion is, then, that it is not part of our concept of dreaming (i.e., it is not implied or entailed by our concept) that dreams necessarily consist of mental phenomena. But this is weaker than Malcolm's conclusion which is that it is part of our concept of dreaming that dreams necessarily do not consist of mental phenomena. The weaker conclusion leaves open the possibility that dreams in fact, though not as a matter of necessity, consist of such phenomena.

II

After having mentioned what sorts of things it is *not* necessary that dreams are, can we go on to say further what they are? Among the things that Malcolm says of dreams are the following: a person's report of his dream is the criterion for others that he dreamt and of what he dreamt (p. 55) but not for himself (p. 63). The criterion is not, however, a definition of 'dream' but something that settles with certainty that a person dreamt, something that "gives the conditions that determine whether the statement 'He dreamt' is true or false" (pp. 60–61). As far as giving the nature of dreams, this is all that can be said. "Indeed I am not trying to say what dreaming *is:* I don't understand what it would mean to do that. I merely set forth the reminder that in our daily discourse about dreams what we take as beyond question that a man dreamt is that in sincerity he should tell a dream or say he had one" (p. 59).

Now when we raise the question "What is x?" we can be asking at least two different sorts of questions. In one sense, we may be asking for a criterion and/or definition of 'x' to be arrived at by examining what the concept expressed by 'x' entails or by determining what justifies us in affirming that something is an x. In another sense we may be asking for the composition of x, for a theory which will tell us what x consists of. Thus in the first sense we all know what, say, lightning is, that is, we have criteria which enable us to identify something as a flash of lightning. In the other sense we have to go to physical theory to learn that lightning consists of moving electric charges. Similarly we all know what dreams are; they are something that occur during sleep, that leave us with an impression when we awake, and that can be narrated to ourselves and others. But when we ask further, "What is this something that occurs during sleep?" we are, I think, asking for a theory to explain what dreams are in the same sense that physics provides us with a theory explaining what lightning is. From the standpoint of common sense, there is no more reason for us to know what dreams are in this sense than for us to know what lightning is. The question "What is dreaming?" can, I think, be given a sense.

Now I want to suggest a situation which, if it holds, would give meaning to the hypothesis that dreams are, that is, consist of, brain processes and then to counter an argument that Malcolm would raise against the hypothesis. When we wake up in the morning with a dream-impression, the impression is something we find ourselves with, something in respect to which we are passive; it is not the product of any deliberate effort of ours. It is the sort of thing for which it is natural to say that it was caused by something that was happening to us while we were sleeping and that this something was the dream. Suppose it is possible to discover some interesting correlations between the brain processes of a sleeping person and his reports of his dream-impression such that to each type of dream report there corresponded a particular type of brain event. Suppose also that the sort of correlation established suggested that the brain event caused the dream-impression. Since it is not necessary that dreams be mental phenomena, it would then be natural to identify the dream with the brain event.[2] This identification would be contingent and hence liable to empirical refutation; it does not follow logically from the concept of dreaming.

Now this hypothesis has several virtues. In the first place, it would eliminate the apparent strangeness of dreams; dream phenomena would turn out to be similar to the neurological events that go on in us when we see, think, imagine, and so on.

2. Malcolm discusses (in Chapter 13) correlations between eye movements and dream reports. Suppose there were such a correlation. Yet it would not be natural to identify eye movements with dreams. Then isn't it just as absurd to identify brain events with dreams? The reply is that because dreams reflect our previous learning and our past experiences and because it is probable that the brain 'stores' in some way what we have learned and experienced, the identification of dreams with brain processes is more natural than with eye-movements. The identification is natural only relative to certain theories about the functions of the brain. It would not have been natural for, say, Aristotle.

In the second place, it would enable us to render plausible facts about dreams discovered by psychoanalysis without accepting Freud's metaphysic of unconscious mental processes. In essence what Freud tells us is that our dream-impressions provide us with information about ourselves which, during our waking life, we resist admitting to ourselves. If the brain can be conceived as a mechanism for storing information, and if, during sleep, some of this information is transformed into brain processes by a lowering of resistances, then it is not at all surprising that our dream-impressions are informative.

I doubt whether anyone is in a position to confirm this hypothesis. My interest is in the prior question as to whether it is intelligible, whether it has sense. Malcolm would, I think, deny its intelligibility. He says: "Physiological phenomena, such as rapid eye movements or muscular action currents, may be found to stand in interesting empirical correlations with dreaming, but the possibility of these discoveries presupposes that these phenomena are *not* used as the criterion of dreaming. The desire to know more about dreaming should not lead scientists into transforming the concept in such a way that their subsequent discoveries do not pertain to *dreaming*" (pp. 81–82). What concerns Malcolm is that if x is the criterion of y then y cannot be logically independent of x. But if a dream is a brain process, then it would seem that dreams are events which are logically independent of our dream-impressions and dream-reports. Then it would be logically possible that "mankind might have told dreams without ever having dreams, or might have had dreams without ever having told dreams" (p. 60), and this is absurd. But this absurdity, if it is one, is not entailed by the hypothesis. For if dreams are in fact brain processes and if telling the dream is the criterion of the dream's occurrence, then telling the dream is the criterion of what is in fact a brain process. Analogously, if a flash of lightning is a motion of electrical charges and if certain perceptible characteristics constitute a criterion for the occurrence of the flash of lightning, then these perceptible characteristics constitute a criterion for the occurrence of what is in fact a motion of electrical charges. More generally, if x is a criterion of y and if y is as a matter of fact z, then x is the criterion for what is as a matter of fact z. Of course from the fact that we use x as a criterion for y and that y is z, it does not follow that we must thereby know that y is z.

If x and y are any events, it makes sense to say that x is or is not logically independent of y only relative to a choice of description. If I refer to some x as the fire which caused my burn then x is not logically independent of my burn, but if I refer to it as the fire on Main Street, then it is logically independent of my burn. Similarly, if a dream is a brain process, then relatively to any purely neurological description of it it is logically independent of the dream impression and the dream narration. But if we say that dreams are only those brain processes which cause dream-impressions, then if a person awakes without a dream-impression, he can be sure he did not dream. And if a dream is any brain process which causes a dream-impression, then if a person awakes with a dream-impression he can be sure that he did dream. Thus the physiological hypothesis need not be inconsistent with the dream reports being a criterion of dreams any more than a physical explanation of the composition of lightning need be inconsistent with certain perceptible characteristics being the criterion of lightning.

In a review of Malcolm's book Donald Kalish suggested "that 'dream' should be construed as a theoretical rather than an observation term."[3] Now if an observation term is a term that refers to something whose presence or absence can be determined by perception, then it is not clear whether 'dream' is an observation term. For though I do not learn about my own dreams by perception, I learn about the dreams of others by *hearing* what they tell me. But if an observation term is one that designates something whose presence or absence can be determined without investigation, without the use of special instruments or theories, then 'dream' is an observation term as much as is 'lightning.' Thus the physiological hypothesis is not to be construed as implying that 'dream' is a theoretical term. Rather it is a suggestion of a special theoretical explanation of the composition of something whose existence can be determined without the help of theory.

It does seem that we can sensibly talk of remembering

3. *Journal of Philosophy*, 58 (1961), 439.

dreams. But isn't it absurd to talk of remembering a brain process? Now, there is a short way with this objection. If I remember seeing a flash of lightning and if lightning is in fact a motion of electric charges, then I remember seeing something which is in fact a motion of electric charges even though I may not know this at the time. But though we do talk of remembering dreams there is some reason to believe that this use of 'remember' is only analogous to and is not literally the same as uses in other contexts.[4] For the past events we say we remember are those we have witnessed or have been conscious of. And if we should ask someone whether he remembers an event, he could reply: "No I was sleeping at the time," a reply which suggests that being asleep is a good reason for not remembering something in that sense.

The similarity between remembering what we dreamt and remembering something we have experienced is that in the first case we awoke with an impression that an event occurred which, if it had occurred, we could say we remembered as in the second case. Since we know it did not occur we do not say merely "I remember . . ." but "I remember dreaming . . ." But instead of saying the latter, why instead do we not simply say "I think I remember . . ."? For if we said this there would be no difference between the two uses of "remember." The reason is that when we say that we think we remember an event we are expressing our uncertainty whether that event occurred whereas in the case of dreams we know it did not occur. Thus remembering what we have dreamt is not a straightforward case of remembering a past event, for it is not a case of our exercising our knowledge that a certain event occurred.

4. Malcolm too argues that its use is different here (pp. 56–57) but for different reasons. However, even if the case of dreams is neglected the term 'remember' has several uses which are not identical. There is the use of 'remember' to refer to *past* events which we have witnessed or experienced and the use which expresses the fact that we have learned something and not forgotten it and which has no essential reference to the past. Thus there should be no surprise at a third use.

15

E. M. CURLEY

Dreaming and Conceptual Revision

An ancient argument, already a commonplace when Plato wrote the *Theaetetus,* finds in dreams a ground for scepticism. The argument may take many forms, of varying cogency, but one interesting variation goes like this:

Sometimes, when we are asleep, we have very vivid experiences, so like our most vivid waking experiences that, when we are having such an experience, we are taken in it by and believe something to be true which is false; but since this is so, the fact that I am now having certain very vivid experiences cannot guarantee that the beliefs I form as a result of those experiences are true; nothing about my present experience can make it certain that I am not now asleep and dreaming.

The conclusion we are meant to draw from these considerations is that no belief based on present experience can be fully certain.

There are many ways in which we might try to avoid this conclusion. But one of the most radical challenges to the dream argument is that offered by Norman Malcolm, first in an article entitled 'Dreaming and Skepticism',[1] and again three years later, in his book *Dreaming.*[2] Malcolm's attack is an exception-

Reprinted with emendations from the *Australasian Journal of Philosophy,* 53 (1975), 119–141, by permission of the author and the *Australasian Journal of Philosophy.*

1. *The Philosophical Review,* 64 (1956), pp. 14–37. Reprinted in Doney, W., ed., *Descartes, a collection of critical essays* (1968). Hereafter cited as 'DS' [with page references to Chapter 4, this volume—ED.]

2. *Dreaming* (1959). Hereafter cited as 'D'.

ally bold one. Not only does he deny that we can have beliefs (and *a fortiori*, false beliefs) while asleep; he also denies that we can have experiences (and *a fortiori*, vivid experiences) while asleep. Malcolm, indeed, claims to have a 'schema of proof' capable of showing the unintelligibility of supposing that any psychological state—any mental activity, like thinking, reasoning, or imagining, or any mental 'passivity', like having an emotion, or an illusion, or imagery—might occur in sleep. (D, p. 45)

In this paper I propose to expound and criticise Malcolm's arguments for this thesis. Those arguments have frequently been rejected as depending on an unjustifiably strong version of the verifiability theory of meaning. In the end, I think this rejection is valid. But criticism of Malcolm is often based on inaccurate or contentious exposition, permitting the Straw Man Defence (examples will be cited later). And certainly Malcolm's statement of his case raises problems which have not been adequately explored. So influential writers still presume that it is possible, and even necessary, to go at least part of the way with Malcolm. Kenny, for example, while allowing that imagery might occur in sleep, agrees with Malcolm that we cannot make judgements or entertain beliefs in sleep.[3]

There are, moreover, grounds for re-opening the case against Malcolm which go beyond any narrow concern with the cogency of his arguments or the truth of his conclusions. Dreams pose problems not only for epistemology but also for the philosophy of mind. And we might hope that an examination of Malcolm's work would, indirectly, throw light on the thought of that most enigmatic of modern philosophers, Ludwig Wittgenstein. The *Philosophical Investigations* is clearly one of this century's most important contributions to the philosophy of mind. But its literary style makes it peculiarly difficult to understand, and even sympathetic interpreters have sometimes thought that in it Wittgenstein commits himself to *some* form of behaviourism. Malcolm's essay is an extended attempt to apply one of the key themes of the *Investigations*, the contention that ' "inner processes" stand in need of outward criteria', (*Investigations*, I, §580) to one especially puzzling inner process. Written

3. See his *Descartes* (1968), pp. 30–1. Cf. also A. R. Manser's article on 'Dreams' in the *Encyclopedia of Philosophy*, v. 2, pp. 414–7.

by someone who knew well both Wittgenstein's work and the man himself, it has the advantage of presenting a comparatively clear and straightforward argument. Perhaps Malcolm misapplies the insights and techniques of the master, and in so doing arrives at untenable conclusions. But if so, then it would be a challenging task for someone to work out what a truly Wittgensteinian position on dreaming would be.

There is a further reason for paying close attention to this landmark work on dreaming. We are often invited, in philosophical discussions of mental concepts, to consider what we should say if experimental research discovered a close correlation between some mental process and some physiological process. In the case of dreaming, empirical research has, on the face of it, replaced philosophical science-fiction with fact, and the search for a physiological correlate has been spectacularly successful. Hence the question of what we should say is quite pressing. Malcolm's approach has led him to challenge a great deal of recent experimental work on dreaming. Not only does this raise issues about conceptual change, and the relation of scientific concepts to ordinary ones, it also provides an opportunity for considering whether the work of experimental psychologists has any implications for philosophical problems about dreaming. I shall argue that it does, and that its main effect is to strengthen the sceptical argument based on dreaming.

I

Malcolm's argument: Before outlining Malcolm's argument, I want to call attention to the strength of its conclusion. Malcolm is arguing against the intelligibility of supposing that *any* psychological state occurs in sleep. This needs to be stressed, because some have wanted to agree with Malcolm that *beliefs* cannot occur in sleep, while disagreeing with him by holding that experiences, imagery, and the like *can* occur in sleep. This compromise position would apparently be sufficient to evade the dream argument for scepticism. If we cannot have beliefs while asleep, then it cannot be true that we are sometimes deceived, while asleep, by our dreams. But Malcolm's argument provides no basis for such a compromise. It is a quite general argument against supposing that *any* psychological state occurs in sleep. If his argument fails, supporters of any compromise position need to show how it could be modified to provide good grounds for accepting a weaker claim.

Malcolm's argument is complex, but the following seems a fair summary: In the case of adults and older children we have two criteria for saying whether someone is (sound) asleep: behaviour and testimony. If a person is lying down, with his eyes closed, breathing regularly, is relatively inert and relaxed, does not react in the characteristic waking manner to stimuli in his immediate vicinity, acts dazed or groggy when (ostensibly) waking up, then he satisfies the criterion of behaviour. If he is unable subsequently to report on things going on now in his immediate vicinity, he satisfies the criterion of testimony. On the other hand, in the case of animals and human infants, there is only the criterion of behaviour. Hence, according to Malcolm, 'The concept of sleep is not exactly the same in the two cases.' (D, pp. 22–34)

Similarly, we have behavioural and testimonial criteria for saying that someone is in a particular psychological state. If a person says in standard circumstances, 'It's going to rain', and shows by his present behaviour that he is aware of what he is saying, and has shown by his past behaviour that he understands the use of that sentence, or if he acts in some other, non-verbal, manner characteristic of someone who believes it is going to rain, then he satisfies the behavioural criterion for believing that it is going to rain. If he subsequently reports seriously that he had believed it was going to rain and shows by his present behaviour that he is aware of what he is saying, then he satisfies the testimonial criterion for having believed that. (D, chapters 3 and 4)

Now, it is self-contradictory to suppose that the criteria for being (sound) asleep and for being in a psychological state might both be satisfied for the same person at the same time. If he satisfies the behavioural criterion for being in a psychological state, then he cannot satisfy the behavioural criterion for being (sound) asleep. For any behaviour which showed that he was in a particular psychological state would demonstrate a degree of bodily activity and awareness of his surroundings which would be incompatible with the inertness and obliviousness required for (sound) sleep. And if he subsequently reports having been in a particular psychological state at a time when he satisfied the criteria for (sound) sleep, we must ask how he could know now that he had been in that state then. Malcolm argues that there can be no satisfactory answer to this question. (D, chapters 9 and 10)

Since the criteria for (sound) sleep and psychological states cannot both be satisfied, it is impossible to *verify* that someone is both (sound) asleep and in some psychological state. It is not impossible that someone should *be* both (sound) asleep and thinking, or having an experience. But the supposition is unintelligible, or senseless, because logically incapable of verification.[4]

What are we to make of this? A natural first reaction is to regard Malcolm as maintaining that dreams do not occur. After all, it is common for dictionaries to give, as the primary sense of 'dream', some such paraphrase as: 'a train of thoughts, images, or fancies passing through the mind during sleep; a vision during sleep; the state in which this occurs . . .'. This account comes from the *OED*, but other dictionaries use much the same language. Malcolm typically ascribes to 'philosophers and psychologists' the view that when we dream, we have thoughts, images, etc., while asleep. But clearly that view is not just a philosophical psychologist's fairy tale. If it is nonsense to suppose that any psychological states occur in sleep, is it not nonsense to suppose that dreams occur? [5]

Malcolm, as we might expect from a philosopher once best known for his defence of (Moore's defence of) common sense, denies that any such conclusion follows. The criterion for dreaming, unlike the criteria for the psychological states so far

4. *Pace*, John Passmore: *A Hundred Years of Philosophy* (1968), p. 512. Cf. D, pp. 36–7. Here Malcolm shifts from the position of DS, cf. DS, n. 13.

5. I omit here, as Malcolm frequently does, the qualifying adjective 'sound.' Malcolm's arguments do not seem to touch the supposition that we have thoughts, etc., in sleep which is not sound, and he says curiously little about 'half sleep'. In DS he had allowed that 'A person who is partly awake can have thoughts (however groggy and confused) and so can be deceived. But he does not *have* to be deceived. He is not "trapped in a dream." If it seems to him that he is sailing in the air high over green meadows, he can decide to investigate— for example, to open his eyes and see where he is.' (p. 123). This line is dropped in D, and not replaced by anything more plausible.

described, is compatible with the criteria for sleep. The sole criterion for dreaming is that the dreamer is able to 'tell a dream', i.e. that after awakening he has the impression that certain incidents occurred, which he is able to relate, but which did not in fact occur. The satisfaction of this criterion is compatible with his having satisfied the criteria for being asleep at the time at which he was supposed to be dreaming. Since it is undeniable that the criterion for dreaming is sometimes satisfied, it is undeniable that dreams occur. (D, pp. 49–53)

The conclusion we are supposed to draw from Malcolm's argument is that dreams are not what philosophers and psychologists (and lexicographers) have thought they are, i.e. a series of thoughts, images, etc., occurring in sleep. Not that Malcolm offers an alternative account of what dreams are. In particular, he does not maintain that a dream *is* the waking impression of having dreamt. He evidently regards any attempt to define dreaming as misguided. The task of philosophical psychology here is to elucidate our criteria for saying that someone has dreamt.[6]

II

Malcolm on criteria: Is Malcolm's conceptual analysis right? Is it true that the language game we play with 'dream', 'sleep', 'think' and their cognates is governed by criteria of the sort Malcolm describes? What is a criterion, anyway?

On this central point, Malcolm is not a paradigm of clarity. A criterion is 'something that settles a question with certainty'. (D, pp. 60–1) A criterion for X is not merely a probable indication of X, a phenomenon empirically correlated with X; though it does not say what X is, or define X, its relation to X is a logical one. This suggests that the satisfaction of a criterion for X is a logically sufficient condition for the existence or occurrence of X. Moreover, 'the application of a criterion must be able to yield either an affirmative or negative result'. (D, p. 24) This suggests that the satisfaction of a criterion for X is also a logically necessary condition of the existence or occurrence of X.

---

6. *Pace,* D. M. Armstrong: *A Materialist Theory of the Mind* (1968), p. 71. Cf. D, p. 59.

For only if it is, could the application of the criterion yield a negative result with certainty.

If Malcolm were to explain his own use of the term 'criterion' as he explains Wittgenstein's, no doubt he would not accept this interpretation as it stands. For Malcolm's Wittgenstein,[7] the propositions describing the criterion of someone's being in pain do not logically imply that he is in pain, because a criterion is satisfied *only in certain circumstances.* We cannot state a logically sufficient condition for someone's being in pain by conjoining a description of his pain-behaviour with the negation of every proposition describing a circumstance which would count against saying that he is in pain, e.g. 'he is rehearsing for a play', because there are indefinitely many such circumstances. But we might attempt to formulate Malcolm's conception of a criterion in the following terms: a criterion is something which, in certain normal, though otherwise unspecifiable circumstances, is a necessary and sufficient condition.

Now the interpretation so far advanced is similar to suggestions which have sometimes been made about Wittgenstein's use of the term 'criterion'.[8] And students of Wittgenstein have sometimes attempted to rebut this line of exegesis by pointing out that he allowed for the possibility of there being a plurality of independent criteria for a given state of affairs. On the face of it, this seems incompatible with a criterion's being a necessary and sufficient condition. For if the criteria are independent, it is conceivable that they might point in opposite directions. And this would mean that the question was settled, with certainty, both in the affirmative and in the negative.[9]

The same problem arises in the exegesis of Malcolm. For he too allows that there can be a plurality of criteria for something, and that the different criteria may conflict. So, e.g. there are two criteria for being asleep, behaviour and testimony, and

7. Cf. his review of the *Philosophical Investigations,* reprinted in *Wittgenstein, The Philosophical Investigations,* a collection of critical essays, ed. George Pitcher (1966), pp. 83–9.

8. Cf. Rogers Albritton: 'On Wittgenstein's Use of the Term "Criterion" ', or C. Chihara and J. Fodor: 'Operationalism and Ordinary Language' [Chapter 8 above], both reprinted in Pitcher, *op. cit.*

9. Cf. Kenny's article on 'Criteria' in the *Encyclopedia of Philosophy,* v. 2, pp. 258–61.

these could conflict. (D, pp. 23–6) A man's behaviour might show that he was asleep, though his subsequent ability to give an account of what went on around him indicated that he was awake. Conversely, a man might satisfy the behavioural criterion for being awake, but subsequently be unable to say what was happening around him. In discussing these cases Malcolm says that one criterion has greater weight, or greater probative weight, than the other. Here a criterion sounds like something that settles a question with greater or lesser degrees of probability.

But Malcolm makes it plain that this is *not* what he intends. He discusses two rather different types of case without, however, distinguishing them clearly. In one kind of case, the greater weight of one criterion lies in its priority of application: 'The criterion of testimony is merely supplementary to the criteron of behaviour, being employed only when the casual observation of a person has left some doubt as to whether he is asleep.' (D, p. 25) That is, if we have insufficient evidence to determine whether or not the behavioural criterion is satisfied, we may appeal to the testimonial criterion to resolve our doubts. But if we know whether the behavioural criterion is satisfied, it is superfluous to apply the testimonial criterion. Given the impossibility of specifying exhaustively the circumstances which would count for or against our saying that a criterion has been satisfied, we might often feel uncertain that the behavioural criterion was satisfied. So this kind of case might be a common one. But it is not, strictly speaking, a case of conflict. *Ex hypothesi,* it is a case in which it is unclear whether or not one of the criteria is satisfied.

More interesting is the case where we *would* ordinarily be inclined to say that it is clear from behaviour whether or not the man is asleep, but where the testimonial evidence points to a contrary conclusion. Behaviour may indicate a waking subject, and yet the subsequent inability to testify to what happened indicate, one who was asleep. Or behaviour may indicate a sleeping subject, while the subsequent ability to testify indicates one who was awake. Malcolm discusses one hypothetical case of each kind, and in each case assigns 'greater weight' does not mean that the answer it indicates is more probable than the answer the testimonial criterion indicates. In each case Malcolm asks us to imagine that the man's behaviour makes it *quite certain* whether he is asleep or not. The subsequent testimonial 'evidence' is treated, not as evidence lending *some* probability to a particular conclusion, but as a phenomenon to be explained.

This is, when you think about it, rather a surprising line for Malcolm to take. For if, in the presence of contrary behavioural evidence, the testimonial evidence does not weaken the force of the behavioural evidence, then it is not easy to see why, in the absence of contrary behavioural evidence, we should regard the testimonial evidence as conclusive.

And in any case, it may seem that there is an alternative line available to Malcolm. He might, consistently with his general position, I think, invoke the fact that criteria are satisfied 'only in certain circumstances', and argue that any situation in which the behavioural and testimonial criteria conflict is *ipso facto* an abnormal one. Our use of the term 'sleep', he might contend, presupposes certain regularities, among which is the fact that, in the vast majority of cases, the behavioural and testimonial criteria agree. Where this agreement is lacking, we simply will not know what to say. (Cf. the *Investigations*, §142) and in one place Malcolm comes quite close to taking this line: 'It is possible that there should be cases in which there is no correct answer to the question "Was he sound asleep?"' (DS, p. 106) Indeed it seems likely that this *is* what we should say in some cases of conflict, though of course this is quite different from treating *one* kind of evidence as conclusive and the other as having no weight at all.

So in spite of the fact that Malcolm admits the existence of a plurality of independent criteria for some things, he consistently avoids a resolution of cases of conflict which would involve saying that each criterion makes the conclusion it favours more or less probable. Criteria are either conclusive evidence, or they are not evidence at all.[10]

10. So, *pace* Kenny's *Encyclopedia* article on 'Criteria', I do not think Putnam can fairly be accused of having attacked a Straw Man in his 'Dreaming and "Depth Grammar"'. (In R. Butler's *Analytical Philosophy*, first series, 1962.) But I make no attempt here to decide what implications this line of argument might have for the interpretation of Wittgenstein.

In any case, the complications which ensue from the existence of a plurality of potentially conflicting criteria do not affect Malcolm's account of dreaming. For he holds that the ability to tell a dream on awakening is the *sole* criterion of having dreamt. (D, pp. 49, 55, 81) So a person's ability, on waking, to tell a dream must, in normal circumstances, be a necessary and sufficient condition of his having dreamt.

III

Dream-reporting as necessary for dreaming: Is this a true account of the way we use the verb 'to dream' in ordinary life? Well, do we take a person's inability to tell a dream to establish with certainty that he has not dreamt? Or are we not prepared to allow that if he cannot tell a dream he may have dreamt and forgotten his dream? Freud writes that 'Most dreams are forgotten soon after waking; or they persist throughout the day, the recollection becoming fainter and more imperfect as the day goes on. . .'.[11] And surely this is a familiar fact about dreams. If we can forget a dream soon after waking, why cannot we forget it as we wake, or before we wake? We may not, at first, know what to make of the suggestion that some dreams are forgotten before we wake. We may be inclined to dismiss it as impossible to verify. But reflection may suggest methods of verification that are not obvious at first.

The hypothesis that many dreams are forgotten before we wake guided some of the earliest systematic studies of dreams. Equipping themselves with paper and pencil, candle and matches, researchers undertook to record as many dreams as possible, in as much detail as possible, sometimes relying on spontaneous awakenings, sometimes on an alarm clock set to go off at random times during the night.[12] One result of this was a reversal of the then widespread belief that the deep sleep of the middle hours of the night is dreamless. There was no time during the night when dreams were not recalled. Clearly this kind of experiment would never have been undertaken if it had been thought that a person's inability to recall a dream on

11. *A General Introduction to Psychoanalysis*, trans. Joan Riviere (1964), p. 95.
12. See F. Snyder: 'In Quest of Dreaming', in *Experimental Studies of Dreaming*, ed. by H. Witkin and H. Lewis (1967). Cited hereafter as WL.

awakening established conclusively that he had not been dreaming.

Further confirmation that many dreams are forgotten before we wake may be found in the fact that dreams are often recalled, not on awakening, but only some time later, when a chance external stimulus or internal association 'triggers' the memory of a dream.[13] It is reasonable to infer that many dreams are lost forever, due to the lack of such a stimulus.

These methods of confirmation require no very elaborate equipment, and raise no particular conceptual problems. More esoteric procedures produce more spectacular, though more contentious, results. Recent experimental work, first reported in 1953, has shown that, when we sleep, a state now known as the REM state recurs periodically, at intervals of about 90 minutes, and lasting, on the average, for about twenty minutes. 'REM' abbreviates 'rapid eye movements', the first feature of the state to be discovered. But there are a number of other features associated with this state: a distinctive brain wave pattern, more like that of drowsing than those of non-REM sleep or waking, increased irregularity of pulse, respiration and blood pressure, sporadic muscular twitches, reduced neck and chin muscle tone, and penile erections, all of which 'suggest a more highly aroused level of nervous activity' (WL, p. 12) than is present in non-REM sleep. It is not clear, however, that the REM state is a period of 'light' sleep. Psychologists find 'deep sleep' a difficult notion to define operationally, but by some indices, e.g. awakening threshold, REM sleep is often as deep as non-REM sleep.[14] We might note that sleep researchers now take the characteristic brain wave pattern, and not the rapid eye movements themselves, as definitive of the REM state.

The REM state is considered by psychologists working in this area to be a highly reliable indicator of dreaming. When people are wakened from REM sleep, they usually report that they have been dreaming and are able to give a very vivid and detailed account of their dream, the length of the narrative being

13. See Domhoff: 'Home Dreams Versus Laboratory Dreams', in M. Kramer: *Dream Psychology and the New Biology of Dreaming* (1969).
14. WL, pp. 40–1. Cf. also Goodenough: 'Some Recent Studies of Dream Recall', in WL, pp. 131–2.

roughly proportional to the length of the REM period.[15] Awakenings in non-REM sleep produce reports of dreams much less often, and when they do, those reports are much less detailed than those that come from REM sleep. The frequency and detail of dream reports on being wakened from non-REM sleep decrease sharply as the length of time since the last REM period increases. One plausible interpretation of these phenomena is that dreams occur in conjunction with REM periods, and that reports of dreams from non-REM periods reflect memories of a dream in a previous REM period.

If this interpretation is accepted, then we spend a great deal more of our sleeping life in dreams than one would have expected—about one-fifth of total sleep time. But only 'an insignificant fraction' of these dreams are normally recalled. (O, p. 68) Hence the 'hypothesis' that many dreams are forgotten before we wake seems to be not merely verifiable, but quite probably true, and true to a surprising extent.

Consider, now, two objections which have been made to the above argument. First, it may be contended that the question 'Why can't dreams be forgotten *before* we wake?" is improper, like the question 'Why can't I make my bet after the race?' The analogy may be an unfortunate one, since there is nothing conceptually impossible about placing a bet after the race. Usually they will not let you; but sometimes they will, as the confidence tricks (like that in *The Sting*) illustrate. Nevertheless, there is a serious point to the charge of impropriety. Forgetting, the objector may continue, is ceasing to know something that one once knew. But on Malcolm's view there is no *knowing* that I am dreaming, or have dreamt, while I am asleep. So to suggest that dreams may be forgotten before we wake is the beg the question against Malcolm.

Reply: This objection proves too much, if it proves anything. For the account of forgetting which it presupposes makes it just as problematic to say that *any* dreams can be forgotten. So when Malcolm, in his lectures on memory,[16] defines factual

15. Cf. Ian Oswald: *Sleep* (1966). Cited hereafter as O.
16. 'Three Lectures on Memory', in *Knowledge and Certainty* (1963). See pp. 239–40.

memory as 'knowing that p because one knew that p', he considers the following objection: we can remember dreams, but we cannot know that we are dreaming while we are dreaming; so remembering that we had a dream cannot be analysed into knowing that we had a dream because we previously knew it. Malcolm finds the objection sound and concludes that his analysis of factual memory does not capture the sense of 'remember' in which we can claim to remember dreams.

Second objection: You say that normally many of our dreams are completely forgotten because experiments suggest that, though people are not usually awakened and questioned during REM sleep, if they were awakened, they would usually report a dream. Why, then, not say that people see the moon during sleep whenever it comes through their window at night? Of course, they do not report seeing the moon. But that is because they forget. If they had been awakened, they would have said they saw it!

Reply: What they would report is *seeing* the moon, not *having seen* it. And this would lend no support at all to the theory that they saw the moon while asleep. If they did report *having* seen the moon, and if they had just previously satisfied the criteria for being asleep, this might be evidence that they had dreamt they saw the moon, but not that they saw it. Seeing requires a waking subject whose eyes are open.

IV

Conceptual revision: When Malcolm first wrote on dreaming in 1956, the only experimental work he referred to was that summarised in *Recent Experiments in Psychology,* by Crafts, *et al.,* published in 1938. The discovery of an impressive correlation between the occurrence of a physiological process during sleep and subsequent dream reports was something we were asked to imagine, though Malcolm knew what he would say about it if the discovery were made. (DS, pp. 119–120)

When he published *Dreaming,* Malcolm was in a position to discuss one of the earliest of the REM studies, Dement and Kleitman's 'The Relation of Eye Movements During Sleep to Dream Activity: An Objective Method for the Study of Dreaming'.[17] This article showed good correlations between the duration of REM periods and subjects' estimates of the length of their dreams, and between specific eye movement patterns and the visual imagery subsequently described in dream reports. For example, one dreamer reported a dream in which he was throwing basketballs at a net, first shooting and looking up at the net, then looking down to pick another ball off the floor. The eye movements in the associated REM period were wholly in the vertical plane. Writing in 1965, Dement characterised this latter type of correlation as 'the most conclusive evidence that dreaming takes place during the REM period'.[18]

In *Dreaming* (ch. 13) Malcolm is highly critical of the Dement and Kleitman study, and develops in some detail the line which had been anticipated in 'Dreaming and Skepticism'. Dement and Kleitman, he argues, have implicitly adopted rapid eye movements as their *criterion* of dreaming. In doing so, they are not 'consciously and deliberately', but 'without an adequate realization of what they are doing', proposing a new concept of dreaming, involving radical conceptual changes, and only remotely resembling our present concept of dreaming. If their 'stipulation' were accepted, the concept of dreaming would be so transformed that subsequent discoveries would not pertain to dreaming. (D, pp. 75, 80–2)

On what sort of evidence does Malcolm claim that Dement and Kleitman are using REMs as a *criterion* of dreaming? He notes their contention that an increase in the length of REM periods was 'almost invariably associated with a proportional increase in the length of the dream', and asks:

But what is their criterion of the *length* of a dream? It should not be the duration of the associated REM period, for that would make non-

17. Originally published in the *Journal of Experimental Psychology* (1957), this classic study is now most conveniently available in W. B. Webb's *Sleep: An Experimental Approach* (1968). Cited hereafter as Webb. For discussions of this, and similar studies, see WL, pp. 19 ff, and W. Dement's 'An Essay on Dreams', in *New Directions in Psychology*, II, ed. W. Edwards, et al. (1965). Cited hereafter as Dement.

18. Dement, p. 173. The 'scanning hypothesis' has been fairly controversial. For a more recent evaluation of the evidence, see Dement's 'Brain and Mind: Are They Related During REM Sleep?' in *Proceedings of the XXth International Congress of Psychology*, 1972, p. 239.

sense of their assertion of a *proportional relation* between the two. Yet their article contains an indication that this is their criterion. In giving an account of their experiment . . . (where [subjects] were awakened after either 5 or 15 minutes of rapid eye movements and 'required on the basis of their recall of the dream to decide which was the correct duration') they report that all subjects save one 'were able to choose the correct dream duration with high accuracy'. . . . How is it decided what the correct dream duration was? Nothing explicit is said on this point in the article. The most plausible conjecture is that their criterion of the duration of a dream is the duration of the associated REM period. (D, p. 78)

Now this seems an incredible caricature of a perfectly sensible piece of scientific reasoning. To begin with, why should we suppose that Dement and Kleitman had *any* criterion, in Malcolm's very strong sense of that term, for the duration of dreams? After all, one stated purpose of the experiment was to *find* a reliable method of determining the duration and temporal location of dreams. What they were operating with was, not a criterion, but a theory, which says that dreaming occurs in conjunction with a particular physiological process. This theory had already been made more or less probable by previous experiments. If the theory is correct, then the duration of the physiological process should be a reliable indicator of the duration of the dream. One way of testing the theory is to check the results of using that way of measuring the duration of the dream against those we get by asking the dreamer. If there is a good agreement between these two supposed indices of dream duration, then we infer that they are indeed both measures of the same thing. As it happens, the results did agree in about 83% of the cases.

This procedure assumes, of course, that a person's own impression of how long his dream was is likely to be at least roughly accurate, i.e. that if he is asked to make gross discriminations, he will be right most of the time. The assumption seems a plausible one. But it also helps to explain why, even if the theory we are testing is correct, we should not expect a 100% agreement between the two indices. Suppose we were doing an experiment with waking subjects, who were watching a play or listening to a lecture. Suppose we asked them to estimate whether they had been watching, or listening, for 5 or 15 minutes. Would we expect to get correct answers in every case? Of course not.

Part of Malcolm's evidence for claiming that Dement and Kleitman employed REMs as their *criterion* of dreaming lies in their treatment of 'one exceptional "inaccurate" subject'. (Malcolm's description, D, p. 71) Noting that this subject had made most of his 'inaccurate' estimates after being awakened from 15 minute 'dreams', Dement and Kleitman suggest that: 'This is consistent with the interpretation that the dream was longer, but he was only able to recall the latter fraction and thus thought it was shorter than it actually was.' (Webb, p. 85) To Malcolm this is evidence of the adoption of a convention, a decision to regard REMs as a criterion of dreaming. But surely Dement and Kleitman's 'interpretation' is no more than a plausible auxiliary hypothesis. Consider the evidence. Assuming that REMs *are* a reliable indicator of dream-duration, the 'exceptional "inaccurate" subject' estimated correctly in 80% of his 5 minute dreams, but in only 50% of his 15 minute dreams. Surely this discrepancy calls for some explanation. Here we should note that there was a similar, though less marked, variation in the figures for the other subjects (who estimated correctly in 90% of their 5 minute dreams, as opposed to 84% of their 15 minute dreams). Of course the interpretation suggested by Dement and Kleitman is not forced on us by the phenomena. Other interpretations are possible. But if that is all Malcolm means by calling it a convention, we shall find precious little in science which is not convention.

Suppose, however, we grant that Dement and Kleitman *are* adopting a new criterion of dreaming. Does it follow that they are engaging in conceptual revision so radical that their subsequent discoveries do not pertain to dreaming?

Malcolm claims that a wide range of consequences follow from using REMs as a criterion of dreaming: e.g. that (a) people would have to be informed on waking that they had dreamt, that (b) the new concept would have to be taught differently, and that (c) 'it could turn out that there was a tribe of people among whom the phenomenon of telling a dream was quite unknown—and yet physiological experiments proved that all of them dreamt every night.' (D, p. 80) But neither (a) nor (b) follows. People would not *have* to be informed on waking that they had dreamt. And we should not need to explain the workings of an EEG to teach someone what a dream is.

These conclusions might be validly drawn if the only alternative to the use of waking testimony as the *sole* criterion of dreaming were to use the REM-state as the *sole* criterion of dreaming. But why should we not operate with a plurality of criteria? No doubt Malcolm might say that by adopting a second criterion we alter the concept—just as he says that the concept of sleep we employ in the case of adults and older children (where we have two criteria: behaviour and testimony) is 'not exactly the same' as the concept of sleep we employ in the case of animals and human infants, where we have only the criterion of behaviour. But this would hardly support charges of radical conceptual revision.

On the other hand, (c) does follow, even if the REM state is not treated as the sole criterion of dreaming. And in fact, recent work on dream recall presents us with something fairly close to the situation Malcolm hypothesises. Studies of non-reporters—people who claim that they rarely or never dream at home—show that they undergo as regular a cycle of REM periods as reporters do. When awakened in the laboratory during an REM-period, they do report dreams, but with much less frequency than reporters do: about 50% of awakenings, as opposed to 80–90% in those who claim that they often dream at home. There has been no one who has not reported some dreams in laboratory experiments, even among those who claim that they never dream at home.[19]

There is, nonetheless, a fairly high incidence of non-reporting in the laboratory among people who are non-reporters at home. Psychologists take this, not as disconfirming the correlation between REM-states and dreaming, but as setting a problem of explanation: why do these subjects 'fail to report' dreams? Shall we say, then, that these psychologists have so radically revised the concept of dreaming that their discoveries do not pertain to dreaming?

19. See Goodenough: 'Some Recent Studies of Dream Recall', in WL.

Clearly that would be premature. That psychologists treat 'failure to report' a dream as a phenomenon requiring explanation is certainly good evidence that they are not taking the REM-state as their *sole* criterion of dreaming. And the hypothesis that many dreams are completely forgotten had occurred to people before anyone had ever heard of the REM-state. Indeed there is, as we noted above, evidence to support it which is independent of the correlation between dreams and REM states.

In any case, before we dismiss as *ad hoc* the claim that non-reporters do dream even when they fail to report a dream, it seems prudent to consider whether experimental psychologists are able to offer plausible explanations of 'failures to report' a dream. Goodenough, in his survey of recent work on dream recall, distinguishes three types of failure to report a dream, and suggests that the different types may require different explanations:

(1) Sometimes subjects say that nothing was going through their minds before they were awakened, that they were in a dreamless sleep. Typically a dreamless sleep report is given when the subject is considerably more difficult to awaken than he is on those occasions when he produces dream reports. Goodenough thinks that the explanation for this type of failure may be that consolidation of memory traces is essential for long-range memory, that consolidation is impaired by sleep, and more seriously impaired by deeper sleep. The theory of memory invoked in this explanation is a controversial one, but there is evidence to support it.

(2) Sometimes subjects say that they were dreaming, but cannot recall any content. This is counted as a failure to report a dream, and there is substantial evidence to suggest that this type of experience may be accounted for by a tendency to repress anxiety dreams. One way of testing this hypothesis is to expose subjects, in the pre-sleep period, to films thought likely to induce anxiety dreams and see whether no-content dream reports are more frequent. Of course some no-content dream reports may result from nothing more exotic than a deliberate withholding of embarrassing dreams.

(3) Sometimes subjects claim to have been awake and think-

ing rather than asleep and dreaming. Goodenough's description of the experimenters' initial reaction to these cases is worth quoting for what it illustrates about the attitude of practicing experimental psychologists to conceptual revision. The concept at issue here is that of sleep:

> At first we were inclined to take the subject's claim at face value and discount the EEG indications of sleep. . . . As more and more data accumulate, we are becoming increasingly confident that in most of these cases the subjects are asleep. In some awakenings the sound of the bell has reached an intensity of 80–100 decibels above the ordinary perceptual threshold before these subjects respond to it. . . . That is a sound of almost painful intensity, and certainly a lot of sound for a waking person to ignore. In some cases we have heard people claim that they never even fell asleep, when, in fact, by any criterion, they had been deeply asleep for hours. (WL, pp. 140–1)

Some awake-and-thinking reports may be accounted for as reports of dreams which are classed as thinking because insufficient vivid or bizarre detail is recalled to make it seem like a dream: when subjects are asked to describe *what* they were thinking, they sometimes are able to recollect features of the experience which lead them to revise their classification of it. Other reports may be 'arousal artifacts', reports of mental content occurring, not during the REM-period but during a gradual period of arousal; and some awake-and-thinking reports turn out to involve mental content which may be better classed as dream-like rather than thought-like.

We might note at this point that many psychologists use 'dream' more strictly than the *OED* definition would suggest. For example, Snyder (WL, p. 28) defines dreaming as an hallucinatory state occurring in sleep, marked by complex perceptual imagery and dramatic development over time. Some psychologists' subjects are even stricter, refusing to class mental contents as dream-like unless they contain quite bizarre elements (cf. O, p. 67). The question 'What counts as a dream report?' is now recognised by psychologists as constituting a serious methodological problem (cf. Dement, pp. 185–92). Malcolm, by contrast, is quite hostile to the possibility that there might be a significant degree of irregularity in people's application of the term 'dreaming'. (D, p. 54)

It would be too much to say that every case of 'failure to report' a dream when wakened from an REM-state can now be convincingly explained. But unless we have unreasonable expectations, we should be able to understand why experimental psychologists treat 'failure to report' as setting a research problem, rather than as disconfirmation of the correlation between REM-states and dreaming. To dismiss their discoveries as not pertaining to dreaming would be a reckless exercise in conceptual legislation.

V

Dream-reporting as sufficient for dreaming: So far I have been arguing that we do not, and should not, even in normal circumstances, treat someone's inability to tell a dream as establishing conclusively that he did not dream. The ability to tell a dream is not a necessary condition of having dreamt. Is it a sufficient condition?

Here we need to distinguish two questions: (i) Does the fact that a person (sincerely) reports having dreamt establish conclusively that he has dreamt? and (ii) Does the fact that a person (sincerely) reports having dreamt a particular sequence of events establish conclusively that he had *that* dream?

As regards (i), perhaps there are *some* cases in which we would treat a person's waking impression that he has just had a dream as establishing conclusively that he *has* just awakened from a dream. But there are certainly a good many cases in which we would not, or at least would not on reflection. One kind of case which Malcolm allows is that in which a person wakes with the impression that certain events occurred, is persuaded by others conspiring to deceive him that those events did not occur, and concludes erroneously that he dreamt the events in question. (D, pp. 64–5)

In discussing this case Malcolm reports an inclination to believe that statements of the form 'I dreamt so and so' are always inferential in nature. (D, p. 65) It is easy to see why he would want to say this. Often, presumably, a dreamer wakes with the impression of having experienced something, and then decides that he must have been dreaming, either because of the extraordinary content of the experience or because of its lack of connection with present experience. But, then, not all dreams are extraordinary or disconnected with waking experience. So the dreamer himself might often be uncertain whether his impression that he has been dreaming is correct. Sometimes we might be in a position to resolve his doubts. ('Yes, there was a knock at the door just then.') But sometimes we might not. And even where we are, it seems that our judgement that he has been dreaming will be just as inferential as his—an inference from his report of what it seems to him has happened *and* our knowledge of the situation. And if that is right, then it does not seem that we are treating his waking impression as being conclusive by itself.

As regards (ii), the answer is pretty clearly 'no'. If dreams can be forgotten, they can also be mis-remembered. So we cannot take the dreamer's sincere telling of the dream as establishing with certainty *what* he dreamt. Malcolm cites with approval Freud's statement that 'Any disadvantage resulting from the uncertain recollection of dreams may be remedied by deciding that exactly what the dreamer tells is to count as the dream, and by ignoring all that he may have forgotten or altered in the process of recollection.' (*op. cit.*, p. 89) But what is methodological policy in Freud is elevated to the status of a conceptual necessity in Malcolm. 'Dreaming is not to be conceived of as something logically independent of dream reports.' (D, p. 122)

If Malcolm meant by this only that it is senseless to suggest that *all* dreams are completely mis-remembered, then there would be no reason to quarrel with it. But Malcolm's account of the logic of dreaming makes it self-contradictory to suggest that any dreams are at all mis-remembered. And surely this is false.

The claim that this part of Malcolm's account is certainly wrong must be made with some care, for here Malcolm is plainly able to invoke the authority of the master. There are not many passages in the *Investigations* in which Wittgenstein discusses dreams directly. But in one of them he does say that 'The question whether the dreamer's memory deceives him when he reports the dream after waking cannot arise, unless we introduce a completely new criterion for the report's "agreeing" with the dream, a criterion which gives us a concept of "truth" as distinct from "truthfulness" here.' (*Investigations*, pp. 222–3; cf. D, pp. 54–7) Now I think it must be admitted that as a rule we do not, in fact, question whether a particular person really had a particular dream, or whether it merely seems to him that he did. But is it really true that the question *cannot* arise? Certainly the *general* question arises. For example, psychologists do sometimes wonder whether perhaps some of their subjects are 'unwittingly embellishing' their dream reports. (Cf. O, p. 67) And I think it would be very surprising if psychoanalysts were not frequently sceptical about the details of some particular dreams that are reported to them (cf. Masserman, quoted in Dement, p. 140).

'What meaning has this question?—And what interest?' (*Investigations*, p. 184) Dreams being what they are, the question probably has very little interest for most people. And *if* it is required, for the meaningfulness of a question, that there should be a way of settling it, and *if* 'settling' here means 'settling with certainty', then very likely the question is meaningless.

On the other hand, we do now have *some* correlations between certain physiological phenomena and dream content, e.g. between the direction and degree of rapid eye movement and the type and degree of activity witnessed in the dream, and between the degree of penile erection and the affective content of the dream (cf. WL, pp. 19, 109–14). And there is no reason not to expect other correlations to be discovered. It is easy enough now to imagine a situation in which we had good, though of course inconclusive, reasons to think that someone's sincere report of a dream was in error. For example, he might, prior to sleep, have been shown a film calculated to produce an anxiety dream, and he might, during an REM period, show some of the physiological symptoms of anxiety (e.g. irregular breathing, irregular penile erection), and yet he might, on being awakened from that REM period, report a dream free of features suggesting anxiety. If he appeared, in giving his report, to be having difficulty in 'recapturing' the dream, we might reasonably suspect that certain features of the dream were being repressed, and that probably some of the features which gave the dream its coherence were 'unwitting embellishments'. I do not see how we could ever think we had *conclusive* evidence for such an interpretation, since the establishment of the correlations we would be employing has proceeded on the assumption that, for the most part, dream reports are fairly reliable. But we might easily have good, though inconclusive, evidence.

No doubt it will be said that in treating these physiological symptoms as evidence of dream content we are introducing 'a completely new criterion' of dream content, and radically revising the concept of a dream. But the argument of section IV has shown the inadequacy of that line of defence.

I conclude that Malcolm's positive account of the concept of dreaming is seriously in error. But what of his negative thesis, that dreams are not a series of thoughts, images, etc., occurring in sleep?

VI

Mental activity and sleep: Malcolm maintains that dreams *could* not be a series of thoughts, images, etc., occurring in sleep, because it is self-contradictory to suppose that we might verify that someone who is asleep is also in some particular psychological state. Here again, the results which Malcolm's philosophical psychology produces clash with those which experimental psychologists produce. Consider the following experiment, related by Oswald (O, pp. 32–4, 69).

Subjects were told to respond by clenching their fist if they heard their own name or certain other names called out during their sleep. They then went to sleep, while a tape recorder played a long series of names, including their own and the other designated names, over and over, in different orders. It was found that subjects were often able to respond as instructed to their own and the other designated names, even when their sleep was quite sound as measured by the EEG pattern. The frequency of fist-clenching was much greater than could be ascribed to chance. If fist-clenching did not occur, the EEG of sound sleep was usually at least disturbed by the speaker's own name and the other designated names. Oswald infers that the sleeping brain was maintaining an unconscious scrutiny of outside noises, discriminating between the names, and selectively arousing the subject when certain names were recognized. Discrimination between meaningful and meaningless noises is clearly a fairly complex piece of mental activity, and one conclusion drawn from the experiment was that some mental activity is sometimes present in sound, non-REM sleep.

Clearly Malcolm could not accept this reading of the experiment. But where would his attack fall? There seem to be no good grounds for denying that these subjects were mentally active. Perhaps Malcolm would deny that they were really sound asleep. By taking the EEG pattern as his criterion of sound sleep, Malcolm might say, Oswald is proposing a new concept of sound sleep, involving radical conceptual change, and only remotely resembling our present concept of sound sleep. If his 'stipulation' were accepted, the concept would be so transformed that subsequent discoveries would not pertain to sound sleep.

But this line is no more satisfactory in the case of sound sleep than it is in the case of dreaming. Sleep researchers do not in fact use the EEG pattern of sound sleep as their sole criterion of sound sleep. They also use other, more familiar, criteria, such as degree of movement and auditory-arousal threshold. The EEG pattern would not be used as a criterion of sleep depth at all if there were not a good agreement between its answers and those of the more familiar criteria. If it is sometimes given priority, that is partly because it lends itself to greater precision and can be used without disturbing the subject's sleep, but partly also because it seems to be more reliable than some more familiar criteria. So, for example, Oswald notes that in a comparison of normal volunteers with patients complaining of insomnia 'the difference [sc. in EEG patterns] was much more consistent among the different individuals than the difference in number-of-times moved.' (O, p. 22) In any case, the links with ordinary criteria are such that talk of radical conceptual revision would be absurd.

If experimental psychologists like Oswald are right, or even if they are saying something intelligible about sleep and mental activity, then something must be amiss with Malcolm's schema of proof. But what?

Well, Malcolm's schema presumes that if it is logically impossible for the criteria for p and q to be jointly satisfied, then it is logically impossible for p and q to be jointly verified, so that the conjunction of p and q is senseless. Clearly some form of the verifiability theory of meaning is at work here. Perhaps that is all right. It may be that in some form the verifiability theory of meaning is defensible. What does seem clearly objectionable is this: Malcolm assumes that if it is impossible for a criterion for p to be satisfied, that is sufficient to show the impossibility of verifying p. But since a criterion for p is supposed to establish *with certainty* whether or not p is true, this amounts to taking *conclusive* verifiability as a necessary condition of meaningfulness.

This may seem an unlikely mistake for a philosopher of Malcolm's intelligence to make. The objections to taking conclusive verifiability as a criterion of meaningfulness are strong, and have long been well-known.[20] And in his article on Wittgenstein in the *Encyclopedia of Philosophy* (v. 8, p. 334) Malcolm rejects verificationist interpretations of both the *Tractatus* and the *Investigations*. Since he takes himself, in his work on dreaming, to be applying Wittgensteinian insights, there is no doubt that he would reject any attempt to represent his argument as verificationist. But it is difficult to see how the argument would go if we dropped the moves from 'impossible to satisfy criteria for p' to 'impossible to verify p' to 'p is meaningless'.

At this point some may wish to concede that Malcolm's own argument is unsatisfactory because his concept of a criterion is too strong. But, it may be contended, by adopting a different account of criteria we might be able to formulate a roughly similar argument in favour of a roughly similar conclusion. Well, suppose we were to adopt the (increasingly popular) account of criteria proposed by Sydney Shoemaker,[21] according to which a criterion for some state of affairs is something which is necessarily evidence for that state of affairs, though not necessarily decisive evidence for it. Would we be able, using this

20. See, e.g. C. G. Hempel: 'Problems and Changes in the Empiricist Criterion of Meaning' in *Revue Internationale de Philosophie*, 4 (1950), 41–63, and widely reprinted.

21. In his *Self-Knowledge and Self-Identity* (1963). Discussed in Kenny's encyclopedia article on criteria and in W. G. Lycan: 'Noninductive Evidence: Recent Work on Wittgenstein's "Criteria" ', *American Philosophical Quarterly*, 8 (1971), 109–25.

concept of a criterion, to derive any paradoxical conclusions about dreaming? I cannot see how to do it. If we accept Oswald's interpretation of his experiment we shall want to say that there is evidence that mental activity sometimes continues during sound sleep. This does not commit us to saying that *any* of the things which are ordinarily taken to be evidence of sound sleep have ceased to be evidence for that state.

VII

Conclusions: That Malcolm's argument for his conclusions should turn out to be quite inadequate to support them, and that those conclusions should be in conflict with empirical evidence, will scarcely surprise anyone who has felt fully the paradoxical nature of Malcolm's conclusions. Any interest the argument of this paper has must stem from the light it may shed on larger problems in epistemology and the philosophy of mind. I would claim the following results:

(1) Whatever someone means who says that inner processes stand in need of outward criteria, he had better not mean 'We cannot talk intelligibly about inner processes unless we have some means of establishing with certainty whether or not a particular inner process is occurring.' Interpreting Wittgenstein's dictum in that way would really be just what it looks like it is, viz. adopting an untenable form of behaviourism. Dreams are a paradigm inner process. We can talk intelligibly about them, but we lack anything like an outward criterion for their occurrence, in Malcolm's sense of the term 'criterion'.

(2) We may, nonetheless, concede that dream reports are the basic criterion for dreaming, in the following sense. They do constitute a peculiarly privileged, though inconclusive, type of evidence for dreaming. Their peculiar privilege lies in the fact that the development of alternative criteria for dreaming has proceeded (and, I think, *must* proceed) on the assumption that dream reports are, for the most part, fairly reliable evidence of dreaming. But this does not entail that we may not, without radical conceptual change, use other criteria as well, or that we may not, without radical conceptual change, come to regard those other criteria as more reliable than the basic criterion.

(3) At the beginning of this paper I suggested that recent ex-

perimental work on dreaming strengthened the argument, based on dreaming, for scepticism about the 'external world'. How? Some philosophers who have used the dream argument—most notably, Descartes—have supposed that some dreams are so like our paradigms of waking experience that they cannot be distinguished from waking experiences with certainty. Other philosophers—most notably, Austin—have denied this.

If we leave aside bad *a priori* arguments like Malcolm's, the question 'What are dreams like, as experiences?' is an empirical one, which each of us who dreams should, it seems, be able to speak about with equal authority. This makes the conflict of testimony between Descartes and Austin puzzling, and may lead to the view that some people just have dreams which are much more vivid than those other people have. And perhaps this is true.

But recent experimental work on dreaming has at least two consequences which are relevant here: (a) there are very great individual differences in the ability that people have to recall their dreams; and (b) the conditions under which we ordinarily try to recall our dreams are not optimal; most people who have been awakened from an REM-period in a sleep laboratory find that they can recall much more detail than they ordinarily can. The experience seems to them to have been much more vivid. So what look like individual differences in dream vividness may be individual differences in dream recall. It may well be that each of us, every night, has dreams as vivid as those Descartes reports, without recalling them in the morning, or at least without recalling how vivid they were. And so Descartes may well be right about what many dreams are like as experiences.

Suggestions advanced recently by one leading experimental psychologist would make Descartes' thesis more than just a possibility. In his 'Essay on Dreams', Dement argues for what amounts to a theoretical redefinition of the concept of dreaming. There are two main motives for this. First, whereas REM studies have, with remarkable uniformity, shown high incidences of dream reports when subjects were awakened from REM periods (80–90%), the results are not so consistent for awakenings from non-REM periods. They vary as the criteria for a dream report vary. If we adopt fairly exclusive criteria, requiring high degrees of detail and temporal development, then the figures go as low as about 7%. If we count as a dream report any report of mental content occurring during sleep, and any report of a 'no-content dream', then the figures go over 50%.

Partly as a result of this kind of evidence, but partly also because of studies like the one by Oswald, described above, Dement thinks that some form of mental activity, sometimes involving imagery and sometimes not, occurs throughout sleep. If we were to adopt an inclusive definition of dreaming (along the lines of the *OED* definition), we should be inclined to say that dreaming occurs throughout sleep, and not only in conjunction with REM periods. We should still be free, of course, to distinguish two different kinds of dreams—those which occur in conjunction with REM periods and which are strikingly more vivid, and those which occur in non-REM sleep and which may involve no perceptual imagery at all.

But as we have seen above, there is significant irregularity in the ordinary use of the verb *to dream,* so that a stricter definition would be consistent with much ordinary usage. And scientific considerations—so Dement argues—give us reason to adopt a stricter definition. Physiologically REM sleep is quite distinct from non-REM sleep. 'The physiological data describe a central nervous system that is, in fact, behaving as if it were receiving a high level of sensory input from the environment . . . its neurophysiological properties resemble those of the active waking state.' (Dement, p. 107) Dement hypothesises that in the REM state the central nervous system is somehow generating 'sensory input' by itself, independently of the environment, and that, from the psychological point of view, REM mental activity is 'not only more complex, but presents an essentially complete perceptual field . . . just as in the waking state, all sensory modalities are ordinarily present in the dream . . . with many details in each mode.' (Dement, p. 205) So Dement proposes that we define dreams as a kind of experience occurring during REM periods of sleep, in which the brain is generating, on its own, the sort of perceptual experience which otherwise occurs normally only in waking subjects as a result of interaction with the environment.

It would be impossible to reconstruct here the whole of Dement's complex argument for this (quite conscious and deliberate) exercise in conceptual revision. But in view of our previous discussion it should be stressed that Dement has grounds which go beyond empirical considerations of the sort so far described. Partly there is the desire to work with a concept of dreaming 'verifiable by physiological experimentation'. But partly there is also the conviction that, because the vivid REM experiences are more likely to be subsequently recalled than are non-REM experiences, "it is quite likely that REM experience has contributed most of the material that has been labelled "dreaming" in the past, and will constitute the major share of the "dreams" that will be collected by daytime interview and questionnaire techniques in the future.' (Dement, pp. 210–1) So he does not see himself as radically revising the extension of the concept, and argues that the REM definition is 'consonant with generally accepted meanings'.

However that may be, it does seem probable that Descartes's thesis is true, and that many dreams, at least, *are* very like waking experiences. I close with one picturesque illustration of this. Many philosophers have held that dreams are to be distinguished from waking experience by their lack of connection with waking experience. Even Malcolm allows that this lack of connection may be used to help us answer the question '*Was* I dreaming?' If we awake with a certain impression and wonder whether it belongs to a dream or to reality, we can consider whether it 'fits in' with what we remember, or are presently perceiving. (D, p. 113) Of course we cannot, on Malcolm's view, engage in any such reflection while asleep.

There is one interesting pathological condition in which the usual discontinuities are not preserved. Sufferers from narcolepsy are abnormally liable to fall asleep (O, pp. 98–9, Dement, p. 221). They undergo brief 'sleep attacks', lasting from 10 to 20 minutes, at odd and inconvenient times during the day, e.g. when walking down the street, or eating dinner. It has been discovered that narcoleptic patients, unlike other adult subjects who have been studied, often go into REM sleep as soon as they fall asleep and that the sleep attacks they suffer

during the day usually consist only of REM sleep. It frequently happens that the immediate environmental setting is maintained as the background in the dreams that are experienced during these attacks. Under these circumstances, when the patients awaken, they are never quite sure whether or not the dream really took place. . . . One patient fell asleep during the day in the laboratory and apparently dreamed that he was in the exact same situation but that the experimenter entered the recording room and had him take a pill. When he awakened a few minutes later he asked, 'What was in that pill you had me take?' When the experimenter assured him that no such event had taken place, he said with surprise, 'Oh, I must have been asleep.' (Dement, p. 221)

So the confusion of dream appearance with waking reality which the dream argument postulates is evidently a fact. Whether sceptical conclusions really do follow from this fact is a question best left for another day.[22]

22. This was originally (though no longer) part of a chapter on dreaming in what may now be described as a forthcoming book, to be titled *Descartes Against the Skeptics*. In the book I defend the soundness of Descartes' version of the dream argument.

Bibliography of Philosophical Writings on Dreaming

Essays included in this anthology are not listed below. Entries preceded by an asterisk (*) do not concern themselves directly with Malcolm's writings.

Armstrong, D. M. *A Materialist Theory of the Mind.* London, 1968. See pp. 70–71.

Ayer, A. J. "Rejoinder to Malcolm." *Journal of Philosophy,* 58 (1961), 297–299.

*Baker, M. J. "Sleeping and Waking." *Mind,* 63 (1954), 539–543.

Bennett, Philip W. "The Sleeper's Dream and the Stoic's Pain: a Reply to Simpson." *Analysis,* 34 (1973), 57–59.

*Botkin, Robert. "Descartes' First Meditation: A Point of Contact for Contemporary Philosophical Methods." *Southern Journal of Philosophy,* 10 (1972), 353–358.

——. "What Can We Do When Dreaming: A Reply to Professor Davis." *Southern Journal of Philosophy,* 10 (1972), 367–372.

*Broad, C. D. "Dreaming and Some of Its Implications." *Proceedings of the Society for Psychical Research,* 52 (1959), 53–78.

Brown, Robert. "Sound Sleep and Sound Scepticism." *Australasian Journal of Philosophy,* 35 (1957), 47–53.

Cerf, Walter. "Studies in Philosophical Psychology." *Philosophy and Phenomenological Research,* 22 (1962), 537–558. (Malcolm is discussed on pp. 551–556).

Chappell, Vere C. "Critical Study." *Philosophical Quarterly,* 12 (1962), 178–185. (This article was published by mistake; Chappell had requested that it be withdrawn.)

Davis, Ralph. "I Have on Rare Occasions While Half Asleep Been Deceived." *Southern Journal of Philosophy,* 10 (1972), 359–365.

Dilman, Ilham. "Dreams." *Review of Metaphysics*, 15 (1961), 108–117.

——. "Professor Malcolm on Dreams." *Analysis*, 26 (1966), 129–134.

Dunlop, Charles E. M. "Performatives and Dream Skepticism." *Philosophical Studies*, 25 (1974), 295–297.

——. "Dreams, Skepticism, and Scientific Research." *Philosphia: Philosophical Quarterly of Israel* (forthcoming).

*Ebersole, F. "De Somniis." *Mind*, 67 (1959), 336–349. Reprinted, with changes, as "The Objects of Perceptions and Dreams," in F. Ebersole, *Things We Know* (Eugene, 1967), pp. 89–112.

Hacking, Ian. "Norman Malcolm's Dreams." In Ian Hacking, *Why Does Language Matter to Philosophy?* Cambridge, 1975. Pp. 103–112.

Hasker, William. "Theories, Analogies, and Criteria." *American Philosophical Quarterly*, 8 (1971), 242–256.

*Hodges, Michael, and W. R. Carter. "Nelson on Dreaming a Pain." *Philosophical Studies*, 20 (1969), 43–46.

*Hunter, John. "Some Questions about Dreaming." *Mind*, 80 (1971), 70–92.

*——. "A Puzzle about Dreaming." *Analysis*, 36 (1976), 126–131.

Kalish, Donald. Book review of *Dreaming*. *Journal of Philosophy*, 57 (1960), 308–311.

Kantor, Jay. "Pinching and Dreaming." *Philosophical Studies*, 21 (1970), 28–32. (This is a reply to the paper by Nelson [1966].)

Kenny, Anthony. "Criterion." *The Encyclopedia of Philosophy* (New York, 1967), Vol. II, pp. 258–261.

Kneale, Martha. "Dreaming." In *Knowledge and Necessity*. Royal Institute of Philosophy Lectures, Vol. 3 (1968–9), pp. 236–248. London, 1970. See also the editor's remarks in the "Foreword", pp. xix–xx.

*Lacey, A. R. "Is Life a Dream?" *Review of Metaphysics*, 14 (1961), 433–451.

Lewis, H. D. *Dreaming and Experience*. L. T. Hobhouse Memorial Trust Lecture No. 37. London, 1968.

*von Leyden, W. "Sleeping and Waking." *Mind*, 65 (1954), 241–245.

*Linsky, Leonard. "Deception." *Inquiry*, 6 (1963), 157–169.

——. "Illusions and Dreams." *Mind*, 71 (1962), 364–371.

——. "Malcolm and the Use of Words." *Analysis*, 21 (1961), 121–123.

*——. "On Misremembering Dreams." *Philosophical Studies*, 7 (1956), 89–91.

Locke, Don. *Myself and Others*. Oxford, 1968. Pp. 124–131.

Malcolm, Norman. *Dreaming*. London, 1959, 1962.

——. "Dreaming and Scepticism: A Rejoinder." *Australasian Journal of Philosophy*, 35 (1957), 207–211.

——. "Professor Ayer on Dreaming." *Journal of Philosophy*, 58 (1961), 294–297.

Mannison, D. S. "Dreaming an Impossible Dream." *Canadian Journal of Philosophy*, 4 (1975), 663–675.

*Manser, A. R. "Dreams." In *Proceedings of the Aristotelian Society*, Supp. Vol. 30 (1956), pp. 208–228.

——. "Dreams." In *The Encyclopedia of Philosophy* (New York, 1967), Vol. II, pp. 414–417.
Nagel, Thomas. "Dreaming." *Analysis,* 19 (1959), 112–116.
*Neisser, Hans. "The Phenomenological Basis of Descartes' Doubt." *Philosophy and Phenomenological Research,* 25 (1965), 572–574.
* Nelson, John O. "Can One Tell That He Is Awake by Pinching Himself?" *Philosophical Studies,* 17 (1966), 81–84.
——. "An Inconsistency in 'Dreaming.' " *Philosophical Studies,* 15 (1964), 33–35.
Palmieri, L. E. "To Sleep, Perchance to Dream." *Philosophy and Phenomenological Research,* 22 (1962), 583–586.
*Pearl, Leon. "Is Theaetetus Dreaming?" *Philosophy and Phenomenological Research,* 31 (1970–71), 108–113.
Price, J. T. "Dream Recollection and Wittgenstein's Language." *Dialogue,* 13 (1974), 35–41.
Putnam, Hilary. "Dreaming and 'Depth Grammar.' " In R. J. Butler, ed. *Analytical Philosophy,* First Series (Oxford, 1966), pp. 211–235. Reprinted in Hilary Putnam, *Mind, Language and Reality* (Cambridge, 1975), pp. 304–324.
Sibajiban. "Descartes' Doubt." *Philosophy and Phenomenological Research,* 24 (1963), 106–116.
*Siegler, F. A. "Descartes' Doubt." *Mind,* 72 (1963), 245–253.
Simpson, R. L. "Stoics, Sleepers and Stones." *Analysis,* 32 (1972), 164–167.
*Smith, Brian. "Dreaming." *Australasian Journal of Philosophy,* 43 (1965), 48–57.
Squires, Roger. "The Problem of Dreams." *Philosophy,* 48 (1973), 245–259.
Suter, Ronald. "The Dream Argument." *American Philosophical Quarterly,* 13 (1976), 185–194.
*Thomas, L. E. "Waking and Dreaming." *Analysis,* 13 (1953), 123–124.
*——. "Dreams." *Proceedings of the Aristotelian Society,* Supp. Vol. 30 (1956), pp. 197–207.
Thompson, Janna L. "About Criteria." *Ratio* 13 (1971), 30–43.
Wolfe, Julian. "The Criteria of Sleep." *Theoria,* 34 (1968), 62–65.
*——. "Dreaming and Scepticism." *Mind,* 80 (1971), 605–606.
*——. "On Knowing One Is Awake." *Philosophy and Phenomenological Research,* 33 (1972–3), p. 268. (This is a reply to the article by Pearl.)
Yost, R. M., Jr. "Professor Malcolm on Dreaming and Scepticism—I." *Philosophical Quarterly,* 9 (1959), 142–151.
——. "Professor Malcolm on Dreaming and Scepticism—II." *Philosophical Quarterly,* 9 (1959), 231–243.

Index

Library of Congress Cataloging in Publication Data
(For library cataloging purposes only)

Main entry under title:
Philosophical essays on dreaming.

    Bibliography: p. 347
    Includes index.
    CONTENTS: Bouwsma, O.K. Descartes' skepticism of the senses.
—Macdonald, M. Sleeping and waking—Yost, R.M., Jr., and Kalish, D. Miss
Macdonald on sleeping and waking. [etc.]
    1. Dreams—Addresses, essays, lectures. 2. Sleep—Addresses, essays,
lectures. I. Dunlop, Charles, E.M., 1943–
BF1078.P53   154.6'3   77-4582
ISBN 0-8014-1015-0
ISBN 0-8014-9862-7 pbk.